Arteriovenous Hemofiltration

A Kidney Replacement Therapy for the Intensive Care Unit

Edited by P. Kramer

With 125 Figures

Springer-Verlag Berlin Heidelberg New York Tokyo

Prof. Dr. med. Peter Kramer
Georg-August Universität Göttingen
Medizinische Klinik und Poliklinik
Robert-Koch-Straße 40
D-3400 Göttingen, FRG

ISBN-13:978-3-540-15317-7 e-ISBN-13:978-3-642-70370-6
DOI: 10.1007/978-3-642-70370-6

Library of Congress Cataloging in Publication Data. Arterio-venous hemofiltration. English. Arteriovenous hemofiltration. Translation of: Arterio-venöse Hämofiltration. 1. Artificial kidney. 2. Hemodialysis. 3. Blood–Filtration. I. Kramer, Peter, 1938–1984. II. Title. [DNLM: 1. Blood. 2. Kidney, Artificial. 3. Ultrafiltration. WJ 378 A7865a] RC901.7.A7A6913 1985 617'.461 85-12657
ISBN-13:978-3-540-15317-7 (U.S.)

Typesetting: Brühlsche Universitätsdruckerei, Giessen

Peter Kramer

April 8., 1938 October 7., 1984

Just in the middle of preparing and organizing the English edition of this book Peter Kramer died unexpectedly on October 7., 1984.

Peter Kramer was born on April 8., 1938 in Mödling near Vienna. He studied medicine in Innsbruck, Freiburg, and Göttingen where he took his doctor's degree in 1964 with experimental investigations on early hypertension. After a one and a half years Rotating Internship at the Middlesex General Hospital, New Brunswick, N.J., USA, he passed a theoretical scientific education at the Division of Physiology of the Max-Planck-Institute for Experimental Medicine in Göttingen, and in 1968 he joined the Division of Nephrology in the Department of Internal Medicine of the University of Göttingen. 1978 he was nominated professor of medicine.

Peter Kramer's far-reaching scientific interests included all the manifold problems of clinical and theoretical nephrology, he was enthusiastic about the technical aspects of dialysis as well as about intricate questions of clinical pharmacology. The results of his comprehensive studies on the pharmacokinetics of cardiac glycosides in chronic renal failure have proved to be essential for the treatment of the uremic patient. From the very start in the Division of Nephrology in Göttingen he had a decisive share in the development of hemofiltration, and owing to his power of observation finally the almost wide-spread method of continous arteriovenous hemofiltration became available for intensive care medicine. His investigations were supported by the Artificial Kidney Program of the NIH, Bethesda, USA, and 1979 he was elected as a member of the Registration Committee of the EDTA.

Peter Kramer was a passionate physician and nephrologist, a delighted and inspiring academic teacher, and an inventive scientist. Enthusiasm for his ideas and future plans, an indefatigable activity, and catching optimism were his main qualities. The fate did not allow him to accomplish his promising scientific career. So I hope confidently that this book as Peter Kramer's legacy and according to his ideas will successfully contribute to our attentions in helping our patients.

Göttingen, November 1985 Fritz Scheler

Table of Contents

Arteriovenous Hemofiltration: Principle

The process of arteriovenous hemofiltration imitates glomerular filtration, a function of the natural kidney.

The pumping force of the heart is utilized: blood is conducted through a bundle of capillaries, which we call "hemofilter," via a tubing system, from a large artery (usually the femoral artery) and returned to the patient through a large vein (usually the femoral vein). The driving force for blood flow and filtration is the difference between arterial and venous pressure: That is why this filtration method is called arteriovenous. A pressure difference of 70 mmHg is sufficient to maintain the "filtration of blood," the "hemofiltration."

To inhibit coagulation, heparin must be added continuously to the blood as soon as it enters the artificial circulation.

The walls of the capillaries through which the blood flows are permeable to water and all substances not bound to plasma proteins up to a molecular weight of approximately 10000 daltons. Blood cells and protein are retained.

During arteriovenous hemofiltration approximately 8 ml/min (11.5 l/day) are filtered through the capillaries. In the natural kidney, the filtrate of the glomeruli is further processed by the tubuli of the nephrons; therefore, a healthy person eliminates only 1–2 l of urine enriched with uremic toxins per day. With arteriovenous hemofiltration, however, it is necessary to discard the filtrate with a relatively low concentration of uremic toxins, and to replace it with a simple salt solution (potassium-free Ringer's lactate solution).

Since the great advantage of this procedure lies in its continuous use, it is increasingly referred to as continuous arteriovenous hemofiltration (CAVH) in international publications.

Introduction

Discovery and Relative Importance of Continuous Arteriovenous Hemofiltration

Lee W. Henderson

Continuous arteriovenous hemofiltration (CAVH) has seen a brisk upswing in popularity in Europe since its introduction by Dr. Kramer and colleagues from Göttingen, West Germany in 1977 [1]. In the United States, the technique received approval as a clinical tool from the Food and Drug Administration in April 1982. This approval flowed, in no small measure, from the extensive experience reported from Europe and in particular West Germany [e.g., 2, 3]. Reports of its clinical utility now have begun to appear in the United States [4].

Removal of excess total body water using synthetic membranes in an extracorporeal circuit dates back to the work of Alwall and the artificial kidney that he designed which permitted utilization of a hydrostatic pressure gradient to motivate water flow across the membrane [5]. Kolff's original rotating drum with its unencased membrane required an osmotic driving force [6]. Hemofiltration, the use of the filtration process to remove uremic solutes with the artificial kidney, in analogy with the glomerulus, was reported in 1967 [7]. This was made possible by the availability of synthetic membranes with far higher hydraulic permeability (approximately 10 times higher) than conventionally used cellulosic hemodialysis membrane. Specific applications of these "high flux" membranes to the removal primarily of excess total body water followed shortly thereafter [8]. One may now obtain these high flux membranes in a variety of formulations (polysulfone, polycarbonate, polyamide, cellulosic) and formats (hollow fiber, sheet) as well as complex and sophisticated fluid balancing systems to conduct hemofiltration.

In my view, the critically important contribution of the Göttingen group in 1977 was the casting away of the complexity of the hemofiltration system with its arteriovenous shunts, pumps, and monitors in favor of the far simpler filtration system driven by arterial blood flow and systemic blood pressure, utilizing percutaneous vascular access for the removal of excess body water and its attendant solutes. Longer treatment time was substituted for performance efficiency to arrive at a more physiologic way of sustaining the patient with acute renal failure (ARF), i.e., devoid of "peak and valley" blood chemistry perturbations. Technical innovations and improvement in CAVH methodology have occurred since 1977 in the form of better catheters and tubing sets for vascular access, the design of replacement solutions that address the unique nutritional needs of the patient with ARF, and fluid balance systems that make treatment monitoring easier, but so far nothing has compromised the basic simplicity of the system.

At present, there is no clear demonstration that patients with ARF treated with CAVH have either a lower mortality or incidence of morbid events. This is not surprising given the difficulty in conducting controlled experiments in such a critically ill population. I remain confident, however, that time will provide experimental confirmation of the clinical perception that both morbidity and mortality are lower when CAVH is employed in the treatment of ARF secondary to acute tubular necrosis.

Finally, it is apparent that much of the methodology being worked out currently for continuous application of artificial kidney treatment in patients with ARF will be brought to bear on patients with chronic renal failure in a manner historically analogous to acute intermitent hemodialysis. The exciting prospect of a simple, continuously functioning artificial kidney that is easily "wearable" is brought nearer by the pioneering clinical experimentation reported in this book edited by Dr. Kramer.

References

1. Kramer P, Wigger W, Matthaei D, Scheler F (1977) Arterio-venous haemofiltration: a new simple method for treatment of overhydrated patients resistant to diuretics. Klin Wochenschr 55:1121
2. Kramer P, Böhler J, Kehr A, Grone HH, Schrader J, Matthaei D, Scheler F (1982) Intensive care potential of continuous arteriovenous hemofiltration. Trans Am Soc Artif Intern Organs 28:28
3. Olbricht C, Mueller C, Schurek HJ, Stolte H (1982) Treatment of acute renal failure in patients with multiple organ failure by continuous spontaneous hemofiltration. Trans Am Soc Artif Intern Organs 28:33
4. Lauer A, Saccaggi A, Ronco C, Belledonne M, Glabman S, Bosch JP (1983) Continuous arteriovenous hemofiltration in the critically ill patient. Ann Intern Med 99:455
5. Alwall N (1947) On the artificial kidney. I. Apparatus for dialysis of the blood in vivo. Acta Med Scand 128(4):317
6. Kolff WJ, Berk HJJ (1943) Artificial kidney: dialyzer with great area. Ned Tijdschr Geneskd 87:46/47
7. Henderson LW, Besarab A, Michaels A, Bluemle LW Jr (1967) Blood purification by ultrafiltration and fluid replacement (diafiltration). Trans Am Soc Artif Intern Organs 12:216
8. Silverstein ME, Ford CA, Lysaght MJ, Henderson LW (1974) Treatment of severe fluid overload by ultrafiltration. N Engl J Med 291:747

Physical Determinants of Continuous Arteriovenous Hemofiltration

Mass Transfer in Arteriovenous Hemofiltration

M. J. Lysaght, B. Schmidt, and H. J. Gurland

Background

Both the glomerular basement membrane of the human kidney and the synthetic hemofilters used in arteriovenous (AV) hemofiltration are ultrafilters. Both employ fine hollow capillaries arranged in parallel configuration. Both have membranes which produce an albumin-free filtrate containing electrolytes and metabolic waste products.

Figure 1 illustrates the construction of a capillary hemofilter: Proximal to the patient is a fluid inlet region, followed by a "tube sheet" where the inner lumina of the fibers are presented to the blood, then a filtration region, and finally an outlet region. Fiber inside diameter is typically 200 μm; the fiber walls are carefully engineered for high fluid throughput. On the filtrate side of the membrane is both a chamber in which the ultrafiltrate is collected and a port from which it exits. The filtrate side and blood path are separated from each other by an epoxy or urethane potting compound.

The design of the entry region broadly resembles that of a shell and tube heat exchanger. It differs substantially from – and in many ways is less satisfactory than – the bifurcating network found in anatomy and in the real kidney. However, reasonably satisfactory results can be obtained with sufficiently large fiber diameters (about 200 times that of the natural kidney), adequate heparinization, and attention to design details. Alwall [1] and Kolff [8] had evaluated ultrafiltration for treatment of acute renal failure (ARF) but early membranes lacked sufficient water permeability to render the process feasible. Early interest by Henderson [6] and Quellhorst [24] in convective solute removal for treatment of chronic renal failure prompted the development of efficient biocompatible devices for the high rate, in vivo ultrafiltration of blood. Henderson, working with anisotropic

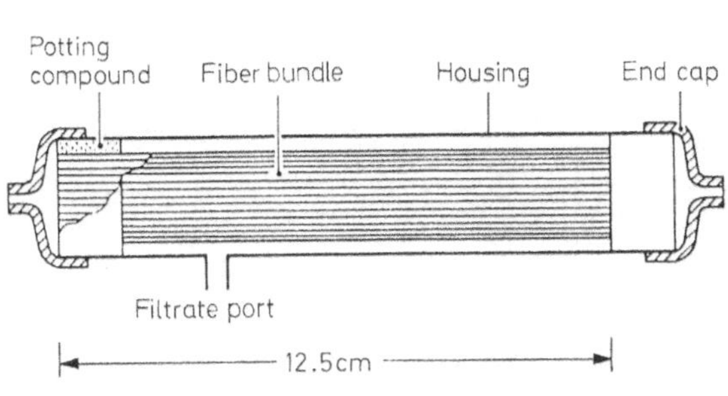

Fig. 1. Schematic illustration of the hollow fiber ultrafilter used in AV filtration. Commercial devices range in length from 12 to 22 cm and contain 4000 to 6000 capillaries

hollow fiber membranes, rapidly appreciated the pertinence of such technology to the management of intractable fluid overload. In 1974 [27], he and his colleagues reported on the construction and clinical use of a small (less than 10% of the size then used for chronic hemofiltration) ultrafilter for the treatment of edema and hypervolemia. Other reports followed [13, 17, 19, 21–23], including the use of ultrafiltration to concentrate blood during or immediately following cardiac surgery [25]. However, the clinical modality of isolated ultrafiltration remained relatively obscure until the development in 1977 by Kramer of the remarkably simple protocol termed "AV hemofiltration" [9, 10]. Since that time, the process has entered into the main stream of ARF therapy [4, 7, 11, 12, 20]. Kramer's circuit comprised arterial and venous catheters, short lengths of tubing, the ultrafilter, originally the Diafilter-20 (Amicon), and one peripheral access line for heparin. All the remaining bricolage of hemodialysis (blood and dialysate pumps, fluid cyclers, monitors, alarms, etc.) was eliminated. The AV process has proven sufficiently simple and nontraumatic to allow patients to be treated continuously, and has thus avoided the saw tooth patterns of parameter excursions and the associated stresses found in intermittent therapy. Significantly, in Kramer's AV method, the pumping action of the human heart provides the full driving force for blood flow through the filter and also for filtrate flow through the membrane. This highly cybernetic approach represents the first clinically realized artificial organ system in which mass transfer is achieved without an external power source.

Membranes and Devices

Figure 2 is a schematic drawing of a hollow fiber ultrafiltration membrane. The inner diameter is ~200 μm. The overall wall thickness is 75–150 μm, but the wall is divided into two distinct regions: First, a "skin" or "active layer" which is ~1 μm or less in thickness and second, a substrate which comprises the remaining 75–150 μm. The skin region contains pores which may be thought of as cylindrically shaped holes whose inner diameters are larger than water, salts, and other low molecular weight catabolites but smaller than the hydrated radius of albumin. Such a diameter is on the order of 100 Å. The substrate contains much larger, micron-sized pores.

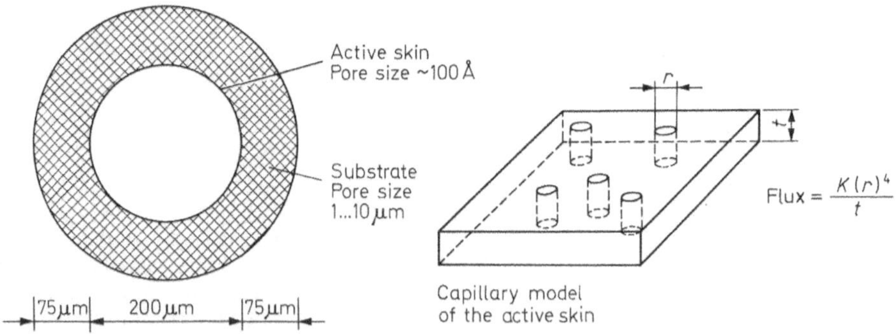

Fig. 2. Schematic illustration of pore-flow model for anisotropic membranes

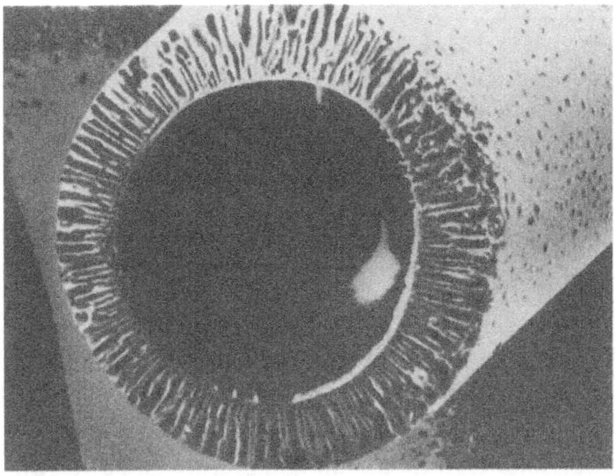

Fig. 3. Scanning electron photomicrograph of a single hollow fiber in cross section ("XP" grade polysulfone capillary from Amicon). Note the consolidated structure forming the inner skin to the fiber

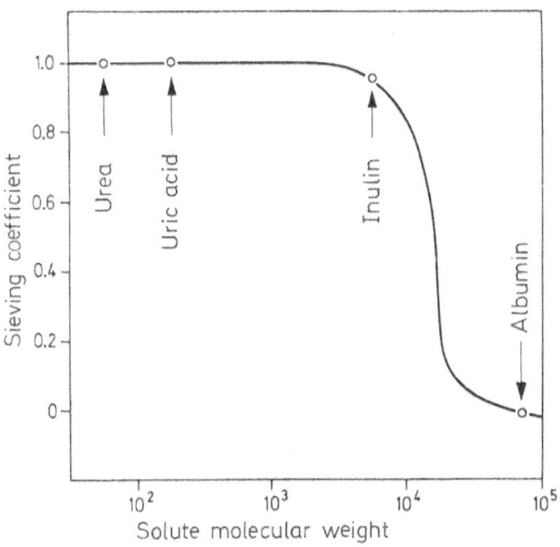

Fig. 4. In vivo sieving coefficient to typical hemofiltration membrane [2, 5]

All transport-related activity is controlled by the skin; the substrate is present only for mechanical support. The success of the structure rests upon the fact that the geometry-dependent discriminatory ability of ultrafiltration membranes is principally a function of pore diameter and is independent of thickness, while the throughput decreases linearly with thickness. Thus, if the hollow fibers illustrated in Fig. 2 were homogeneous and the skin extended from the inside diameter to the outer diameter, then the selectivity and solute rejection characteristics would be the same as for the anisotropic analogue, but the water permeability would be 100–200 times lower.

Figure 3 shows a scanning electron micrograph of a cross section of a hollow fiber membrane made of polysulfone (Amicon). Similar fibers have recently become available from other manufacturers. Note again the very compact active skin resting atop the open substrate. The hollow fiber in Fig. 3 is prepared from

Table 1. Properties of three filter devices

Designation	Manufacturer	Fiber material	Fiber internal diameter	No. of fibers	Length (cm)		Area (cm^2)
					Full	Active	
Diafilter-20	Amicon	Polysulfone	200	4000	12.5	8.5	2100
Diafilter-30	Amicon	Polysulfone	200	6000	20	16	6000
HF-101	Gambro	Polycarbonate	215	5200	22	8	6300

polysulfone thermoplastic resin. It adsorbs no water and is opaque because the pore diameters in the substrate are of the same magnitude as the wave length of visible light.

Figure 4 is a plot of the sieving coefficient of the asymetric membrane as a function of increasing molecular weight of the permeated substances. Small molecules and inulin pass the membrane completely while albumin is quantitatively held back. These data are taken from an early in vivo study [3, 5]; the overall curve should probably be shifted slightly to the left as membrane formulations have tightened somewhat over the years.

In addition to the original Diafilter-20, two more hollow fiber devices (Diafilter-30; Amicon; HF-101, Gambro) are now offered for AV filtration. Their properties, based upon manufacturer's specification, are shown in Table 1.

These devices generally deliver between 500 and 1000 cm^3/h in clinical service. There has been at least one report [2] of the use of a high-flux, flat sheet hemodialyzer (Biospal 1200S) for AV filtration and no doubt other such devices might also function in this mode.

Transport Relations

Under normal conditions of AV filtration, the blood flow rate ranges from 50–150 cm^3/min. Note that blood flow is a dependent variable determined by available pressure drop and device geometry. This runs counter to the normal experience in extracorporeal circulation where blood flow rate is set by a pump and device pressure drop is the dependent variable. This distinction has important consequences for device performance. The magnitude of the dependent flow rate may be very well estimated by the Hagen Poiseuille relationship for incompressible Newtonian laminar flow, as expressed in Eq. (1).

$$Q_B = \frac{\Delta P N \pi r^4}{\mu L_d} 10^{-10} . \tag{1}$$

Q_B is the blood flow, ΔP is the end-to-end pressure drop, i.e., arteriovenous pressure difference less circuit resistance, N is the number of fibers, μ is the average blood viscosity, r is the internal fiber radius, and L_d is the device length. (Units for all equations are given in the table of nomenclature following the text.)

Equation 1 implicitly assumes that blood flow rate is limited by the hydraulic resistance of the extracorporeal circuit and not by the capacity of the access; this is generally true for the types of access employed in AV filtration.

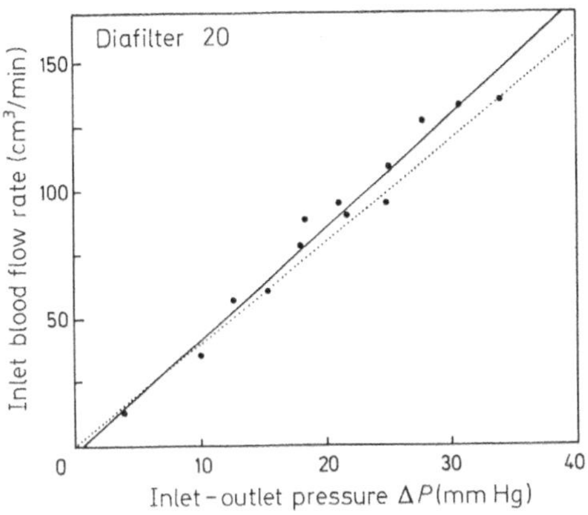

Fig. 5. Blood-flow rate in the Diafilter vs end-to-end pressure drop. Hematocrit=25%; methods in [18]. *Dotted line* is linear regression; *solid line* is from Eq. (1) with μ=2.5 cps

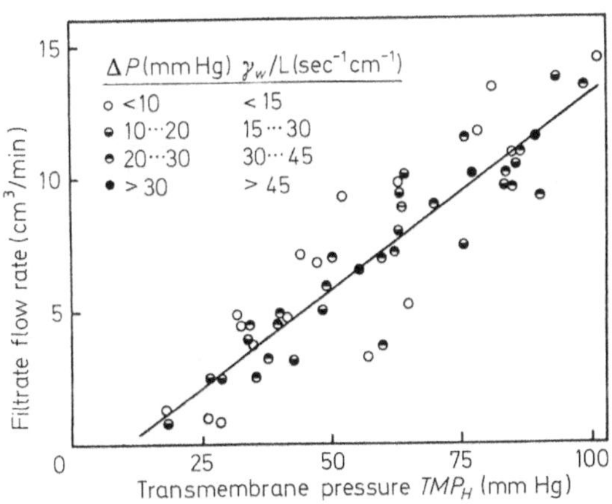

Fig. 6. Filtration rate vs TMP_H over normal operating range of AV filtration for the Diafilter-20. In vitro, hematocrit=25%, methods in [18]. P and γ_w/L (see [3]) do not appear to directly influence filtration rate

Although more rigorous methods are available, Eq. (1) is generally evaluated with inlet values of blood flow and viscosity: the decrease of Q_B along the length of the filtering fibers more or less cancels the concomitant increase of μ. Figure 5 is a representative in vitro plot of Q_B vs end-to-end pressure drop, ΔP, for the Diafilter-20; there is excellent agreement between the linear regression line and the behavior predicted by Eq. (1). The pressures and flows given in Fig. 5 cover the ranges of those encountered in vivo under normal operating conditions. At a given ΔP, blood flow will scale linearly with Nr^4/L_d (0.94 and 0.99 for the Diafilter-30 and HF-101, respectively, relative to 1.0 for the Diafilter-20).

Filtration rate Q_F in AV circuits ranges from 5–20 ml/min. In normal circumstances, Q_F for a particular filter is linear with transmembrane pressure, TMP_H, and independent of blood-flow rate. More complex circumstances can arise, however, and these will also be discussed below. Transmembrane pressure is the average of inlet and outlet (gauge) pressures upstream of the membrane less filtrate pressure.

Typical behavior during AV filtration is illustrated in Figs. 6 and 7. Filtration rate is clearly seen to increase linearly with TMP_H and to intersect the TMP_H axis

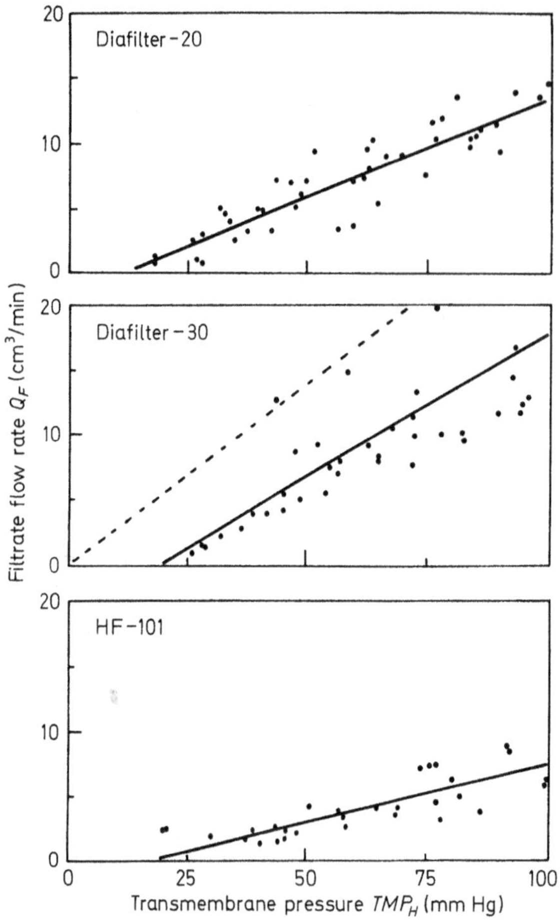

Fig. 7. Filtration rate vs TMP_H over normal operating range of AV filtration for the Diafilter-20, Diafilter-30, and HF 101. In vitro, hematrocrit = 25%, methods in [18]. Data are intended to illustrate Q_F vs TMP_H relationships and, since only a limited number of each device was tested, should not be used for general comparison of device performance

at roughly the value for plasma oncotic pressure. In Fig. 6, the data points are segmented according to end-to-end pressure drop and the wall shear rate divided by length and these factors do not appear to directly influence filtration rate. In Fig. 7, the water permeability, taken postexposure to blood because of possible protein adsorption, is parallel to the plasma filtration line but intersects the TMP_H at 0; water has no colloid-osmotic pressure. Such behavior is described mathematically as:

$$Q_F = AK_p(TMP_H - \Pi), \tag{2}$$

Q_F is filtration rate, A is area, K_P is membrane hydraulic permeability, TMP_H is hydraulic transmembrane pressure, π is mean plasma oncotic pressure.

In transport theory, Eq. (2) represents the classic description for filtration rate limited by a noncompressible membrane; the same behavior is seen in hemodialysis, though at much higher pressures. Equation (2) predicts that filtration rate will increase with area but otherwise be independent of length and fiber radius, in fact, as seen in Fig. 7, Diafilter-30 does have a greater filtration rate than Diafilter-20 but the increment is not as large as would be expected from Eq. (2); this could be due to device-to-device variation in membrane properties.

In general, then, filtration behavior is straightforward. Two special cases arise:

Oncotic Pressure Effects

As first suggested by Bosch and Lauer [14, 15], at high filtration fractions the oncotic pressure towards the outlet end of the filter may exceed the hydraulic pressure. In this case, no further filtration will occur and the distal end of the filter would be wasted. Such a condition can be created in vitro; in fact, if TMP_H is reduced below ~15 mmHg, "reverse filtration" from the filtrate chamber into the fibers is observed. In clinical practice, however,it is highly unlikely that colloid-osmotic pressure would exceed the outlet hydraulic pressure. The collection reservoir is usually at least 50 cm below the filter, creating a siphon pressure of −30 mmHg. The venous pressure is at least 10 mmHg, even neglecting the pressure drop across the venous return line and catheter. Thus, the minimum TMP_H at the outlet is 45 mmHg which will only be reached at the unrealistically high outlet protein concentration of 35 g/100 cm³ [25] corresponding, at an inlet hematocrit of 25%, to a filtration fraction of 0.25. Higher filtration fractions could be reached by imposing higher values of *TMP* but this would have the effect of preserving the TMP_H-Π differential.

Boundary Layer Limitations

As illustrated in Fig. 8, the linear dependence of filtration rate upon TMP_H does not extend indefinitely but eventually reaches a new fluid dynamic regime where further increases in pressure do not lead to further increases in filtration rate. Physically, a "secondary membrane" has been formed by the proteins which, at the higher filtration rates, are being brought to the surface more rapidly than they can diffuse away. The secondary membrane has a greater hydraulic resistance

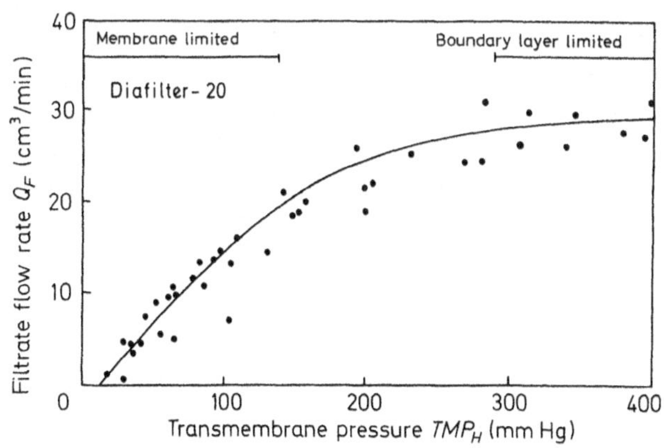

Fig. 8. Filtration rate vs TMP_H for the Diafilter-20. Data in vitro, hematocrit = 25%, methods in [18]. The high values of TMP_H were obtained by placing a tubing pump on the filtrate line. ΔP ranged from 10 to 30 mmHg

than the underlying polymeric membrane and thus it controls or limits filtration rate. This so-called "boundary-layer controlled" regime is well understood [3, 5]. In the spontaneous circuit, filtration rate limited by a secondary membrane is described by Eq. (3) [16, 18] and is seen to be independent of both TMP_H and of the permeability properties of the primary synthetic membrane.

$$Q_F = \left(\frac{\Delta Pr}{2\mu L_f L_d}\right) 8.3 \times 10^{-3}. \tag{3}$$

L_f is the effective fiber length and other terms are as described previously. The constant inlet plasma protein concentration was assumed to be 7 g/100 cm^3.

The value of TMP_H at which the flux plateau begins can be estimated by combining Eqs. (2) and (3).

$$\overrightarrow{TMP}_H = \left(\frac{\Delta Pr}{2\mu L_f L_d}\right)^{0.5} \times \frac{8.3 \times 10^{-3}}{K_p} + \Pi. \tag{4}$$

$\overrightarrow{TMP}_H$ is the value of transmembrane pressure at which the maximum filtration rate is first reached and other terms are as defined previously.

Solution of Eq. (4) demonstrates that as long as ΔP exceeds 20 mmHg, the transition $\overrightarrow{TMP}_H$ will be well above 100 mmHg for all present devices. TMP_H in AV filtration rarely exceeds 100 mmHg and thus the boundary layer regime is unlikely to be encountered. This situation could change, however, if devices with higher membrane permeabilities become available.

To summarize with an example, consider an AV circuit employing the Diafilter-20. Inlet hematocrit is 25%, protein concentration 7 g/100 cm^3, viscosity 4 cps. Mean pressure at the device inlet is assumed to be 50 mmHg and at device outlet 20 mmHg; these are typical values from in vivo measurements, the inlet value being lower and the outlet value being higher than the physiologic and arterial and venous pressures, owing to the pressure drop across the arterial and venous catheters. Pressure in the filtrate side is -35 mmHg which would be obtained by placing the collection reservoir 50 cm below the AV filter. ΔP is 30 mmHg and TMP_H is then 70 mmHg. From Fig. 5, blood-flow rate through the filter is 125 cm^3/min and from Fig. 6, filtration rate is 8 cm^3/min. Filtration fraction, Q_F/Q_B, is 0.064. Membrane permeability, K_p, is 4×10^{-5} cm/min mmHg. The outlet protein concentration is 7.8 g/100 cm^3 corresponding to a colloid-osmotic pressure of 17 mmHg (using the correlation of Reusser [26]) which is less than the TMP_H of 55 mgHg at the distal end of the filter. From Eq. (3), the boundary layer limited flux would be 28 cm^3/min but according to Eq. (4), this level would not be reached below a TMP_H of 350 mmHg. Additional calculations show that the mean luminal blood velocity is 1.6 cm/s and filtration velocity only 0.6 μm/s. Wall shear rate is 670 s^{-1} and Reynolds number is 1.

Implications

Several implications attend this understanding of the relationship between filtration rate and available pressure driving force. First, for a given device, blood-flow rate is normally determined by ΔP (Eq. 1, Fig. 5), while filtration rate is determined by TMP (Eq. (2), Figs. 6 and 7). At high values of TMP_H and low values of ΔP, and providing that the constraints of Eq. (4) are not violated, filtrate could become a dangerously high fraction of incoming blood flow rate. In our experience, this situation is unlikely in normal AV filtration but can be encountered at low ΔP's or Q_B's if a pump or suction greater than 100–200 mmHg is applied on the filtrate side. The result is excessive dewatering of the blood and the formation of a red cell puree which could easily be mistaken for a clot. Accordingly, considerable caution should be applied by those using the suction-assist method of CAVH described by Kaplan [7]. Second, since filtration rate is a consequence of membrane water permeability postexposure to plasma, manufacturers should emphasize this property in device quality control. Moreover, device filtration rate can most easily be improved simply by increasing membrane permeability to the level where the boundary layer becomes controlling. Attention should also be paid to the uniformity of fiber diameter in a given cartridge: as can be seen from Eq. (1), blood will preferentially flow through larger bore fibers (the flow through a fiber with a radius of 105 μ will be 50% greater than through a parallel fiber with a radius of 95 μ). The flow in the small fibers may in fact be so low as to lead to excessively high local filtration fractions and fiber plugging. Much of the "clotting" seen in existing filters may reflect this phenomenon. Finally, there appears to be little reason for maintaining fiber diameter at 200 μ ID. Increase to 300 μ would give substantially higher blood-flow rates, with no loss of filtration rate, thereby minimizing the likelihood of clotting and of excessive filtration fractions.

The general understanding of transport in spontaneous AV filtration has advanced considerably in the past few years and can provide assistance in selection of optimal process conditions and improved device design. Future research is likely to concern the role (if any) of pulsatility, the effects of membrane material, time-dependent phenomena such as compaction of the adsorbed or polarized proteins, and methods to minimize flux-decay and to extend filter service life.

Nomenclature

Equations 1–4 will be numerically correct using the following units

A	Membrane surface area, cm^2
K_P	Membrane permeability coefficient, cm/min mmHg
L_f	Length of fiber uncovered by epoxy and available for filtration, cm
L_d	Full length of ultrafilter, cm
N	Number of capillaries in filter
ΔP	Difference in pressure at device inlet and outlet, mmHg
Q_B	Blood flow rate, cm^3/s
Q_F	Filtrate flow rate, cm^3/s
r	Fiber radius, μm
TMP_H	Transmembrane pressure (hydraulic); average of inlet and outlet pressure minus filtrate pressure, mmHg

$\overrightarrow{TMP}_H$ Value of transmembrane pressure at which maximum filtration rate for given inlet conditions is first reached

γ_w Wall shear rate, s^{-1}

μ Blood viscosity, cps

π 3.1416

Π Plasma oncotic pressure, mmHg

References

1. Alwall N (1963) Therapeutic and diagnostic problems in severe renal failure. Svenska Bokfoerlaget, Stockholm, Chapter 1
2. Castro LA, Banthien FCA, Gurland HJ (1983) Successful clinical experience in the use of a small flat-sheet dialyzer for continuous AV-hemofiltration. In: Bonomini V, Stefoni S, Black MM (eds) Life support systems. The journal of the European society for artificial organs. Proceedings of the X annual meeting ESAO. Bologna, September 1983
3. Colton CK, Henderson LW, Ford CA, Lysaght MJ (1975) Kinetics of hemodiafiltration, I. In vitro transport characteristics of a hollow-fiber blood ultrafilter. J Lab Clin Med 85:355
4. Dodd NJ, Turnez JH, Parsons V, Weston MJ (1982) Continuous haemofiltration maintains fluid balance and reduces hemodialysis requirement acute renal failure. Proc Eur Dial Transplant Assoc 19:329
5. Henderson LW, Colton CK, Ford CA (1975) Kinetics of hemodiafiltration, II. Clinical characterization of a new blood cleansing modality. J Lab Med 85:355
6. Henderson LW, Colton CK, Bluemle LW, Bixler HJ (1970) Uremic blood cleansing by diafiltration using a hollow fiber ultrafilter. Trans Am Soc Artif Intern Organs 16:107
7. Kaplan AA, Longnecker RE, Flokert VW (1983) Suction assisted continuous arteriovenous hemofiltration. Trans Am Soc Artif Intern Organs 29:408
8. Kolff WJ, Leonards JR (1959) Reduction of otherwise intractable edema by dialysis or filtration. Cleve Clin Q 20:61
9. Kramer P, Langscheid C, Matthaei D, Rieger J (1977) Behandlung der diuretikaresistenten Überwässerung mit arterio-venöser Hämofiltration. In: Scheler F, Henning HV (Hrsg) Hämofiltration. Dustri, München
10. Kramer P, Wigger W, Rieger J, Matthaei D, Scheler F (1977) A new and simple method for treatment of overhydrated patients resistant to diuretics. Klin Wochenschr 55:1121
11. Kramer P, Schrader J, Bohnsack W, Grieben G, Groene HJ (1981) Continuous arteriovenous hemofiltration: a new kidney replacement therapy. Proc Eur Dial Transplant Assoc 18:743
12. Kramer P, Boehler J, Kehr A, Groene HJ, Schrader J, Matthaei D, Scheler F (1982) Intensive care potential of continuous arteriovenous hemofiltration. Trans Am Soc Artif Intern Organs 28:33
13. Lamar J, Briggs W, McDonald S (1978) Effective fluid removal with the amicon diafilter. Proc Ann Dial Transplant Forum 25
14. Lauer A, Saccaggi R, Belledonne M, Glabman S, Bosch JP (1982) Continuous ultrafiltration in chronic hemodialysis patients via pre-existing access. Am J Kid Disease [Suppl] 20:(abstract)
15. Lauer A, Saccaggi M, Ronco C, Belledonne M, Glabman S, Bosch JP (1983) Continuous arterio-venous hemofiltration in the critically ill patient. Annals Int Med 99:455–460
16. Lysaght MJ (1982) Die Kinetik der arterio-venösen Haemofiltration. In: Kramer P (Hrsg) Arterio-venöse Hämofiltration. Nieren-(Ersatz)-Therapie im Intensivpflegebereich. Vandenhoek and Ruprecht, Zürich

17. Lysaght MJ, Ford CA, Henderson LW (1977) A simplified approach to high rate in vivo ultrafiltration of blood. Abstracts XII. Congress Eur Dial Transplant Assoc 11
18. Lysaght MJ, Schmidt B, Gurland HJ (1983) Transport relations in AV filtration. J Blood Purification 1:178–183
19. Neff MS, Sadjadi S, Slifkin R (1979) A wearable artificial glomerulus. Proc Ann Dial Transplant Forum 26
20. Olbricht C, Mueller C, Schurek HJ, Stolte H (1982) Treatment of acute renal failure in patients with multiple organ failure by continuous spontaneous hemofiltration. Trans Am Soc Artif Intern Organs 28:33
21. O'Keefe J (1977) Diafiltration in acute renal failure. Abstracts XIV Congress Eur Dial Transplant Assoc 11
22. Paganini EP, Nakamoto S (1980) Continuous slow ultrafiltration in oliguric acute renal failure. Trans Am Soc Artif Intern Organs 26:203
23. Pogglitsch H, Waller J, Giessauf W, Holzer H, Katschnigg H (1976) Die Hämofiltration zur Behandlung generalisierter Ödeme. Acta Med Aust 3:73
24. Quellhorst E, Fernandez E, Scheler F (1972) Treatment of uremia using an ultrafiltration-filtration system. Proc Eur Dial Transplant Assoc 9:584
25. Romagnali A, Hacker J, Keats AS, Milan J (1976) External hemoconcentration after deliberate hemodilution. Abstracts of scientific papers. Ann Meet Am Soc Anesthesiol
26. Reusser P, Oberholzer M, Wolfe G (1980) Messung und Berechnung des kolloidosmotischen Drucks in ungestörtem postoperativen Verlauf. Schweiz Med Wochenschr 110:1163
27. Silverstein ME, Ford CA, Lysaght MJ, Henderson LW (1974) The treatment of intractable fluid overload. N Engl J Med 291:747

Effect of Hydrostatic Pressure and Hematocrit on Blood Flow and Filtration Rate

P. Kramer, F. Rösick, G. Biege, G. Hellige, and F. Scheler

Arterial pressure and hematocrit are the practically important determinants of blood flow through capillaries [2, 3, 6, 7]. The following figures (except Fig. 5) demonstrate results of studies on the blood flow and filtration rate studied under in vivo conditions (37 °C) [9]; oxygen and glucose substituted blood [10]; pulsatile blood flow with Harvard-pump driven membrane heart [8] in relation to blood pressure, negative filtration pressure, hematocrit, use of three-way valves in the extracorporeal tubing system and in relation to postdilution [5]. The Amicon continuous arteriovenous hemofiltration (CAVH) set (1983) including diafilter-20 (0.2 m^2) and the eight Charr-Vygon vascular catheters were used for the artificial circulation. Systolic, diastolic, and venous back flow pressure as well as the flow and pressure profiles were comparable to in vivo conditions.

Figure 1 demonstrates a linear relationship between blood pressure and blood flow. It is also obvious from the figure that the slope of the pressure-flow relationship is lowered and flattened by an increase of the hematocrit: Low hematocrit results in high blood flow rate and in a higher effect of pressure on the blood flow rate.

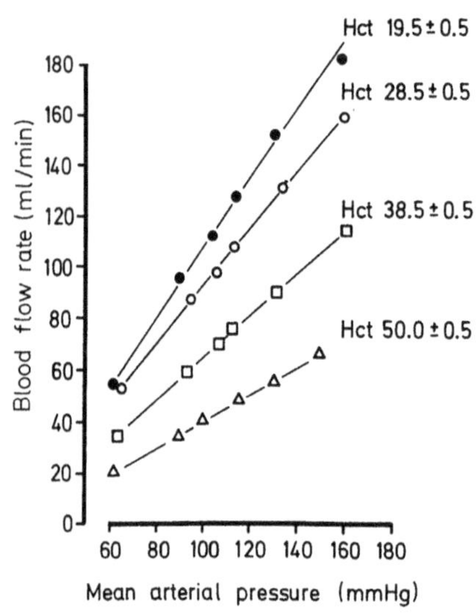

Fig. 1. Relationship between blood-flow rate, mean arterial pressure, and hematocrit

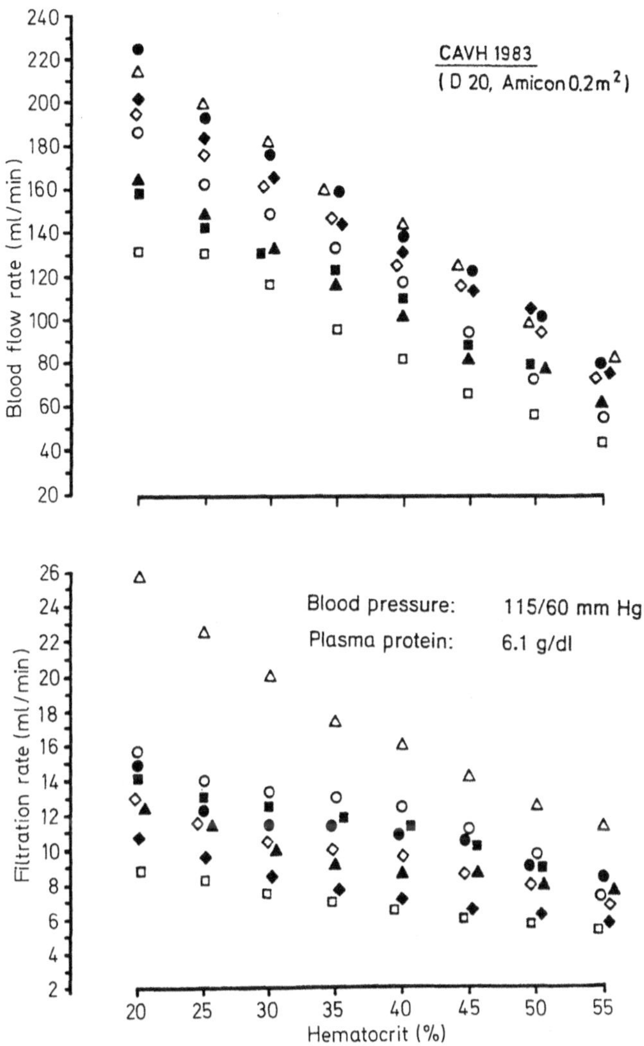

Fig. 2. Effect of increasing hematocrit on blood-flow rate and filtration rate

According to Fig. 2 (systemic pressure 120/60 mmHg, venous back flow pressure 10 mmHg) an increase of the hematocrit from 20% to 55% caused the blood flow rate to decrease from 130–230 to 40–80 ml/min, whereas the filtration rate fell only by 15% as a result of the exponential increase of the filtration fraction from 0.1 to 0.2, (Fig. 3). The hydraulic permeability, however, was slightly reduced with increasing hematocrit (Fig. 4). This can only be explained by a direct effect of the erythrocytes on membrane permeability [1, 11]. It may be speculated that the erythrocytes hinder the off-diffusion of plasma proteins from the membrane surface.

The importance of either blood viscosity or the hematocrit for the blood flow rate is demonstrated by the effect of fluid withdrawal and dilution during CAVH.

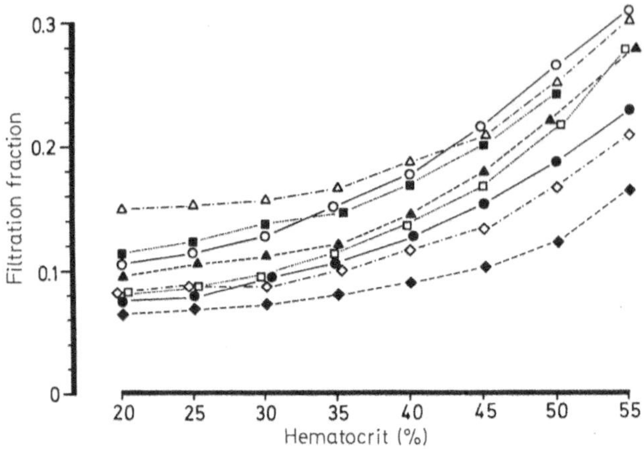

Fig. 3. Effect of increasing hematocrit on the filtration fraction

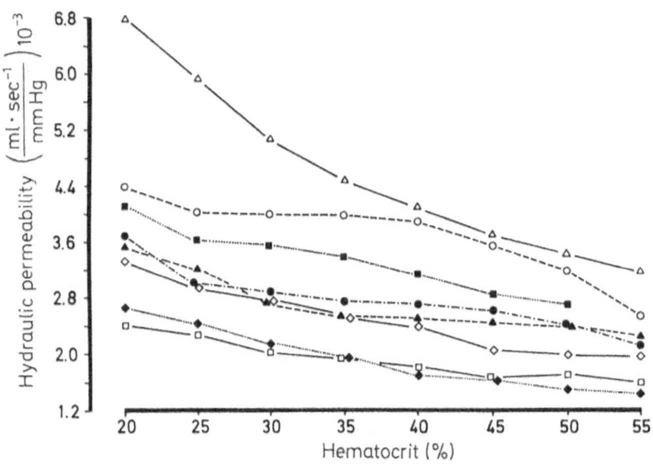

Fig. 4. Effect of increasing hematocrit on the hydraulic permeability

According to Fig. 5 an increase of negative filtration pressure caused enhanced fluid withdrawal from the blood passing the capillaries. This resulted in a fall of blood flow rate in all four patients; in one patient also filtration rate was reduced, when the negative pressure exceeded -100 cm H_2O. The only explanation is an increased viscosity due to elevated hematocrit in the capillaries.

Figure 6 shows the effect of postdilutional fluid substitution on the blood flow rate. The higher the initial hematocrit the more pronounced was the increase of blood flow by postdilution. With a hematocrit of 50 vol% postdilution resulted in an increase of blood flow by 15% due to reduced pressure drop along the venous three-way valve. In contrast to blood flow rate the filtration rate was even reduced by 3%.

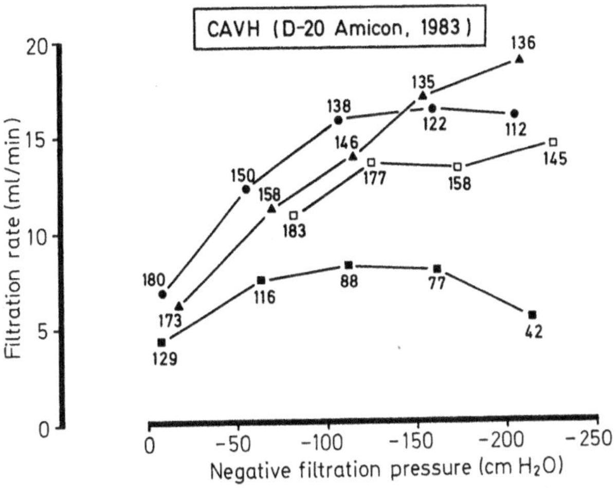

Fig. 5. Effect of increasing negative filtration pressure on filtration rate and blood-flow rate. The figures beside the symbols are the blood-flow rates determined by means of an electromagnetic flow meter during CAVH in patients

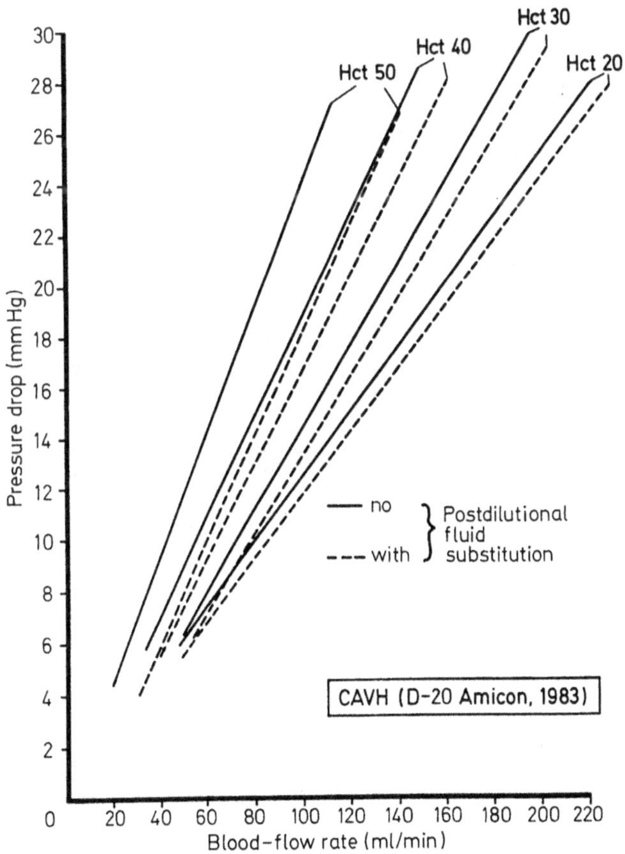

Fig. 6. The effect of postdilution and hematocrit on the pressure drop along the venous three-way valve, the blood flow rate, and the hematocrit

Conclusions for Clinical Practice

1. An elevation of the hematocrit causes, independent of the increase of viscosity, a reduction in membrane permeability.
2. The administration of packed red cells causes only slight reduction of filtration rate as long as the hematocrit is below 40 vol%.
3. Suction-assisted ultrafiltration causes reduction of blood flow due to increased viscosity and may block the hemofilter in some patients with low blood flow rate and high hematocrit if the negative pressure exceeds -100 cm H_2O. The application of slight negative pressure may be helpful in selected cases with high blood flow rate and low hematocrit [4].
4. The infusion of substitution fluid into the venous three-way valve causes, particularly in patients with high hematocrit, an increase of the blood flow rate with slight reduction of filtration rate.

References

1. Chien S, Usami S, Dellenback RJ, Gregersen BM (1970) Shear-dependent deformation of erythrocytes in rheology of human blood. Am J Physiol 219:136–142
2. Hershko C, Carmeli D (1970) The effect of packed cell volume, hemoglobin content and red cell count on whole blood viscosity. Acta Haematol 44:142–154
3. Hochmuth RM, Davis DO (1969) Changes in hematocrit for blood flow in narrow tubes. Bibl Anat 11:59–65
4. Kaplan AA, Longnecker RE, Folkert VW (1983) Suction-assisted continuous arteriovenous hemofiltration. Trans Am Soc Artif Intern Organs 29:408–412
5. Kramer P, Rösick F, Rosekranz W, Hellige G, Scheler F (1984) Determinanten der Filtrationsfraktion bei arterio-venöser Hämofiltration. Verh Dtsch Ges Inn Med 90:983–986
6. Litwin MS, Chapman K (1970) Physical factors affecting human blood viscosity. J Surg Res 10:433–436
7. Okazaki M, Yoshida F (1976) Ultrafiltration of blood: effect of hematocrit on ultrafiltration rate. Ann Biomed Eng 4:138–150
8. Olthoff G, Bleiber R, Menninger H, Olthoff D (1977) Veränderungen der Erythrocytenform durch Anwendung des extrakorporalen Kreislaufs. Z Exp Chir 10:226–232
9. Snyder GK (1971) Influence of temperature and hematocrit on blood viscosity. Am J Physiol 220:1667–1672
10. Tannert C, Schmidt G, Steinhof A, Staack R (1979) Untersuchungen zur Verformbarkeit roter Blutzellen bei Lagerung mit einem einfachen Filtrationsverfahren. Acta Biol Med Ger 38:1595–1600
11. Teitel P, Szasz I (1971) A haemorheological view on molecular interactions between red blood cell constituents. Haematologica 5:37–44

Influence of Colloid-Osmotic Pressure on the Filtration Rate During Continuous Arteriovenous Hemofiltration

F. Rösick, J. Böhler, and P. Kramer

In contrast to pump-actuated hemofiltration, where a transmembrane pressure gradient of several 100 mmHg maintains the process of filtration [1], arteriovenous hemofiltration is a low-pressure process in which the colloid-osmotic pressure has a significant effect on the filtration rate, as it does in the capillary loops of the glomeruli.

Figure 1 shows the situation in the capillary loops of the glomeruli: the blood pressure of +70 mmHg is opposed by an average (integrated) colloid-osmotic pressure of 30 mmHg and pressure in the Bowman's capsule space of 15 mmHg, so that the effective transmembrane filtration pressure is only +25 mmHg.

In contrast to the glomeruli, in arteriovenous hemofiltration we have a negative pressure of 30–50 mmHg in the extracapillary space caused by lowering of the fil-

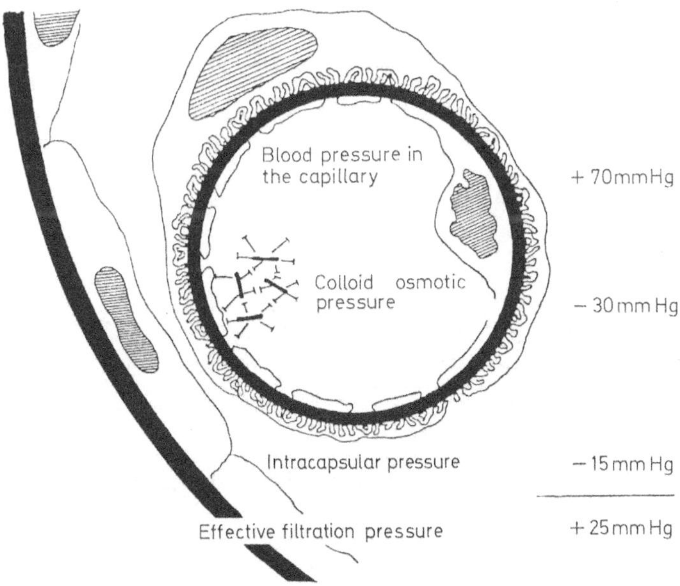

Fig. 1. Diagram of pressure conditions in the capillary loops of the glomeruli. The blood pressure of +70 mmHg is opposed by an average colloid-osmotic pressure of 30 mmHg and pressure in the capsule of 15 mmHg, resulting in 25 mmHg effective transmembrane filtration pressure. For details see text

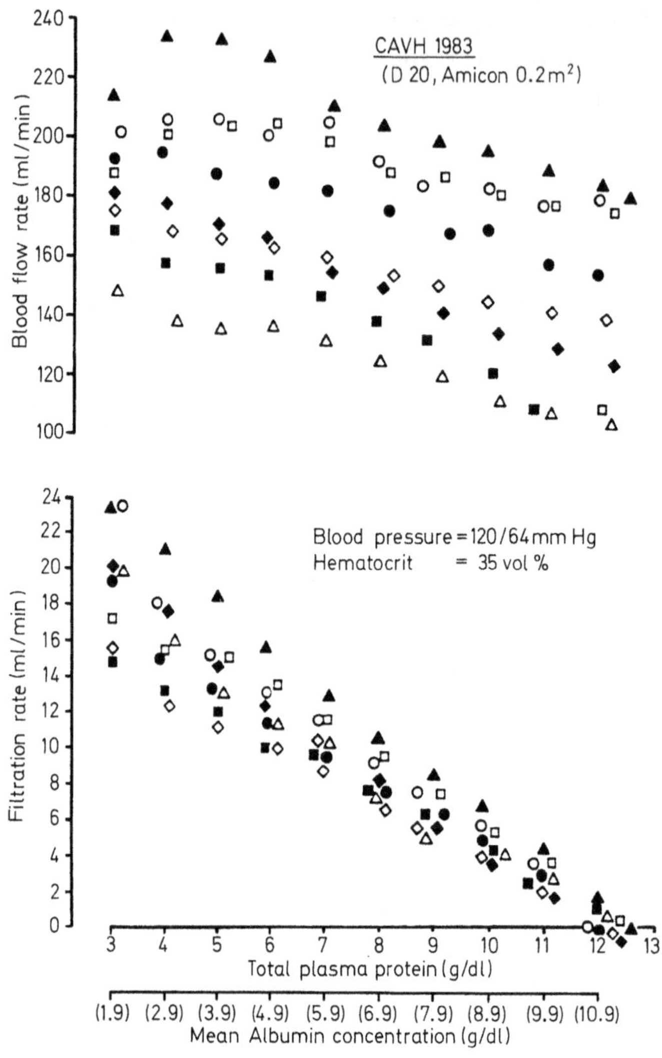

Fig. 2. Effect of total plasma protein and albumin concentration on the blood flow rate and the filtration rate

trate-collecting container on the bed of the patient. In the capillaries, the colloid-osmotic pressure acts against the filtration pressure.

This relationship is demonstrated in Fig. 2, which shows the effect of increasing plasma albumin concentration on blood flow and filtration rate. These results were obtained under in vivo conditions with oxygenated and glucose substituted blood at 37 °C temperature using a Harvard-pump-driven membrane heart for a pulsatile blood flow. The filtration rate ceased with a total plasma protein concentration of 12 g/l (90% albumin), whereas blood flow rate had fallen only from 120–220 to 110–190 ml/min. With a mean systemic pressure of 120/60 mmHg and a venous back flow pressure of 10 mmHg, the filtration fraction according to

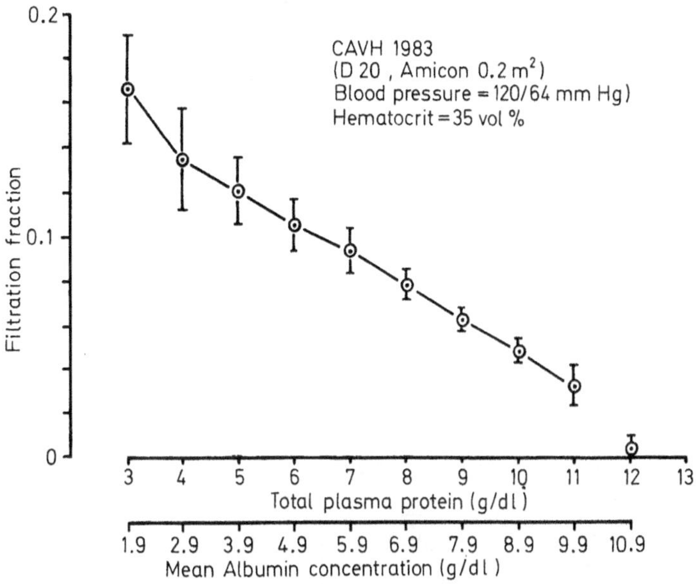

Fig. 3. Effect of total plasma protein and albumin concentration on the filtration fraction

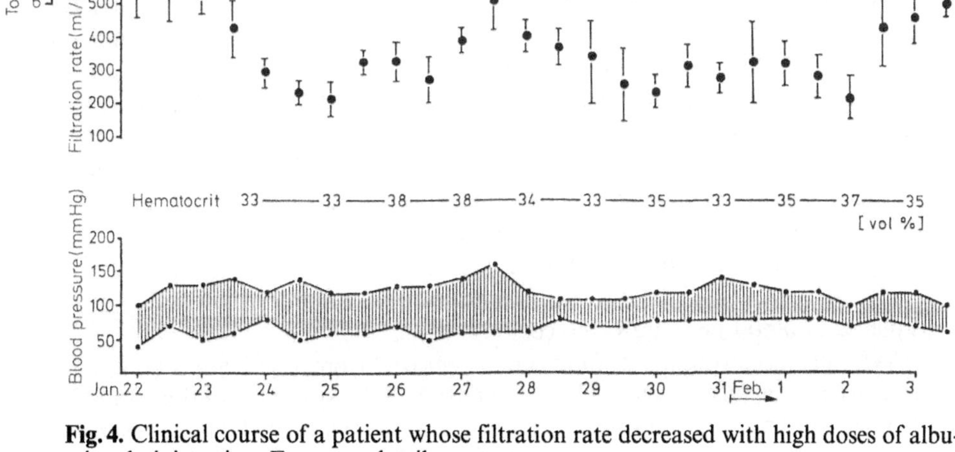

Fig. 4. Clinical course of a patient whose filtration rate decreased with high doses of albumin administration. For more details see text

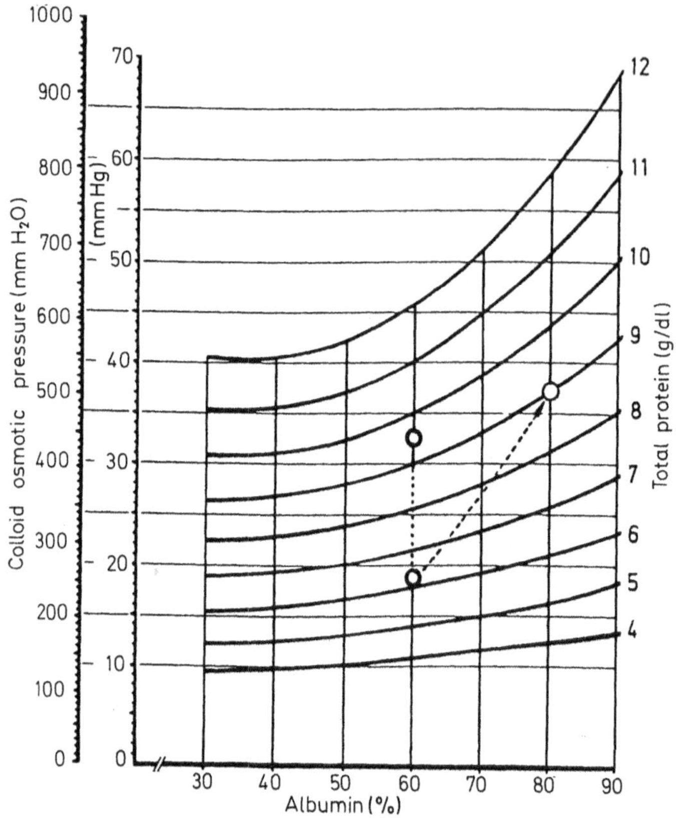

Fig. 5. Nomogram for the determination of colloid-osmotic pressure based on total plasma protein concentration and albumin portion according to the formula of Landis and Pappenheimer [3]. For details see text

Fig. 3 decreased linearly from 0.16 to 0, when albumin concentration was elevated from 2 to 11 g/l.

These results clearly demonstrate the importance of colloid-osmotic pressure. Although in clinical practice the extreme values are never observed, moderate overtreatment with albumin in surgical patients has however been observed.

In Fig. 4 a clinical course is described where large amounts of albumin where administered inadvertently, resulting in an increase of total protein up to 10 g/l. At this total protein level, filtration rates decreased to 200 ml/h without change in blood pressure. With decreasing total protein, the filtration rose again and fell down with renewed albumin administration.

Figure 4 also illustrates the influence of blood pressure: the high filtration rate in the night of Jan. 27/28 and the low filtration on Feb. 2/3 are surely a consequence of blood pressure variance.

As a rule, large volumes of fluid can be removed from a patient via continuous arteriovenous hemofiltration (CAVH) even when the systolic blood pressure has dropped to 70 mmHg and when the natural kidney no longer eliminates even with large doses of diuretics. At these low pressures, the colloid-osmotic pressure plays a significant role. This has led in practice to great reluctance in administering albumin to uremic intensive care patients. Usually the filtration process ceases at a systolic pressure of 60 mmHg since flow through the capillaries is no longer assured at this pressure.

For the estimation of the colloid-osmotic pressure, the nomogram in Fig. 5 can be used if total plasma protein and plasma albumin concentrations are known [7].

The nomogram was established by using the formula of Landis and Pappenheimer [3]. With reference to the literature, in our opinion, direct measurement of colloid-osmotic pressure can be disregarded, due to the disadvantages of this method. More accurate values can be obtained by determining total protein and albumin concentrations indirectly [2, 5–7].

The degree to which the colloid-osmotic pressure rises along the capillaries can only roughly be estimated:

If the volume of blood flowing through the hemofilter is reduced from 100 ml/min to 70 ml/min, an increase in total protein (e.g., from 6.2 g/l to 9.5 g/l) will result in a proportional increase in the colloid-osmotic pressure of approximately 14 mmHg, as shown in Fig. 5.

Since the albumin portion is responsible for 60%–80% of the colloid-osmotic pressure in the plasma, high doses of albumin administered for therapeutic purposes can raise the colloid-osmotic pressure significantly. In the example in Fig. 5, total protein rises from 6.2 to 9.0 g/l and the albumin portion increases by 20%, causing an elevation of the colloid-osmotic pressure of 19 mmHg.

Contrary to other anticoagulants, heparin does not affect colloid-osmotic pressure, even at high extracorporeal concentrations [4].

References

1. Colton CK, Henderson LW, Ford CA, Lysaght MJ (1975) Kinetics of hemodiafiltration. I. In vitro transport characteristics of a hollow-fiber blood ultrafilter. J Lab Clin Med 85:355
2. Ladegaard-Pedersen HJ (1979) Measurement of the colloid osmotic pressure in patients. Scand J Clin Lab Invest 20:79
3. Landis EM, Pappenheimer JR (1963) Exchange of substances through capillary walls. In: Down P, Hamilton WF (eds) Handbook of physiology, Vol II. Circulation. American Physiological Society, Washington DC, pp 961–1034
4. Marty AT, Intaglietta M (1970) Effect on anticoagulants on human plasma colloid-osmotic pressure measurements. J Appl Physiol 29:740
5. Morton AP, Holling J (1978) Colloid osmotic pressure in surgical patients and its relationship to serum protein and albumin estimations. Aust N Z J Surg 48:418
6. Prather JW, Gaar KA Jr, Guyton AC (1968) Direct continuous recording of plasma colloid osmotic pressure of whole blood. J Appl Physiol 24:602
7. Rowe MI, Lankau C, Newmark S (1974) Clinical evaluation of methods to monitor colloid oncotic pressure in the surgical treatment of children. Surg Gynecol Obstet 139:889
8. Weil MH, Henning RJ, Puri VK (1979) Colloid osmotic pressure: clinical significance. Crit Care Med 7:113

Leukocyte Counts and Complement Activation During Arteriovenous and Pump-Driven Hemofiltration

J. Böhler, P. Kramer, G. Schlag, H. Redel, O. Götze, and P. Schwartz

Significant leukopenia accompanied by complement activation and impairment of pulmonary function [1, 16] after starting a dialysis treatment were first observed by Kaplow and Goffinet in 1968 [13]. These changes are most striking when cuprophane membranes are used for dialysis [12]. Craddock et al. have studied these side effects of hemodialysis thoroughly and postulate the following pathogenesis: The complement system is activated during contact of the plasma with the dialyzer membrane [3, 4]. C5a fragment of the complement component C5 induces aggregation of granulocytes in the patient's venous blood [5, 10, 17]. These aggregates are trapped in the pulmonary microvessels resulting in a transient, profound leukopenia of the peripheral blood [19].

It is a matter of discussion whether aggregated granulocytes, which are shown to damage endothelial cells in vitro [17], are responsible for the transient impairment of pulmonary function [7, 8] that follows the leukopenia.

Besides the common dialysis procedure, two different methods of hemofiltration, conventional mechanical pump-driven hemofiltration (HF) and continuous arteriovenous hemofiltration (CAVH) are used in the treatment of renal failure. Figures 1 and 2 show electron microscopic pictures of polysulfone capillaries (Fig. 1) and of a cellulose triacetate flat membrane (Fig. 2) used for HF.

The surface of both membranes appear smooth, overlaid with only a few small humps.

Fig. 1 a–f. Electron micrographs of polysulfone capillaries (Amicon D-20, after rinsing with normal saline). **a** *Lower part:* capillary seen from the outside shows the support membrane with its large pores; *Upper part:* lengthwise split of capillary showing the lamellar support structure surrounding the tubular blood compartment. **b** Section of a lengthwise-cut capillary. The lamellar support structure provides stability for the 0.01–1 μ thin filtration membrane. Only this inner layer comes in contact with the blood and determines the sieving characteristics of the filter. The support structure does not increase the resistance for the filtrate flow. **c** and **e** Border between support structure and filtration membrane. View of the lamellar system (*top*) and of the inner membrane at the depth of the lumen (blood compartment). Dark spots are visible on the inner membrane. **d** and **f** Section of the inner membrane shows deposits of 1–4 μ in size. These deposits can be seen both before and after the rinsing of the filter. The chemical composition of the stratifications and the effect on biocompatibility are not known

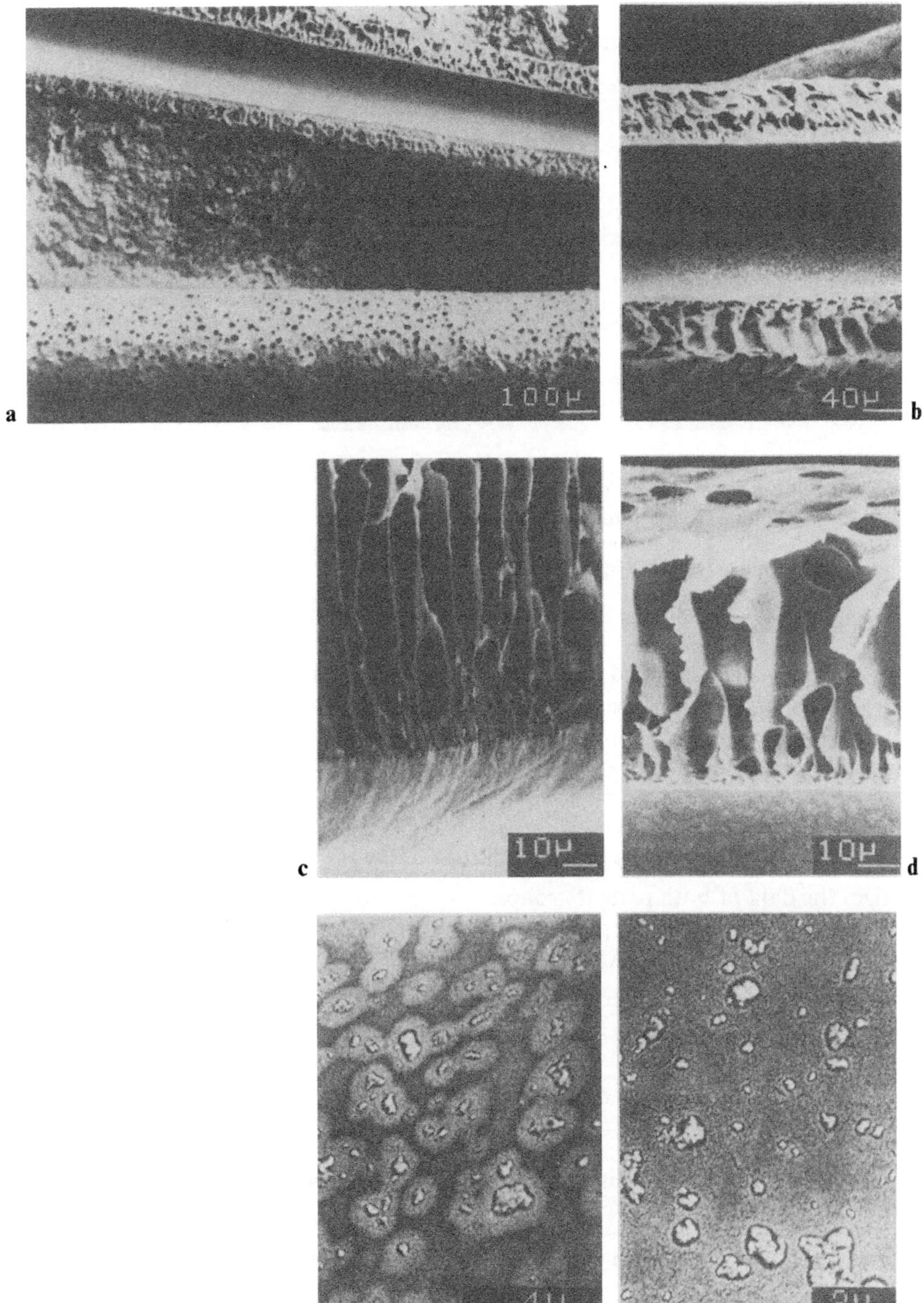
100μ
a
40μ
b
10μ
c
10μ
d
4μ
e
2μ
f

a 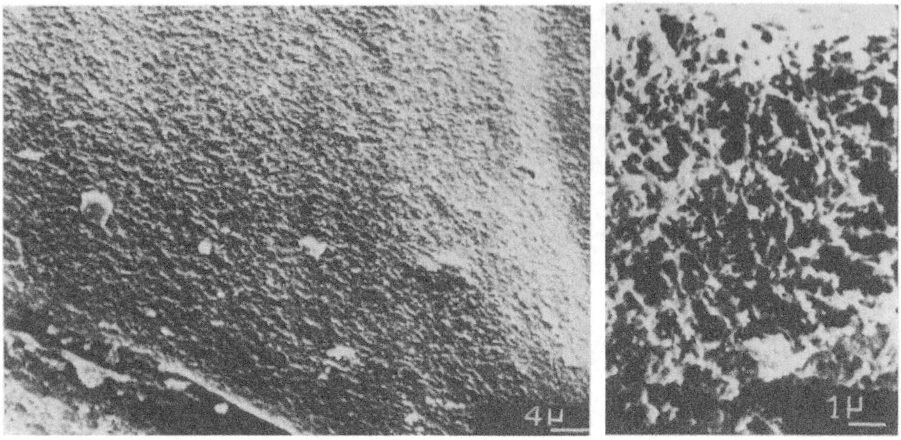 b

Fig. 2 a, b. Electron micrographs of cellulose triacetate membrane (Sartorius SM 400-04, after rinsing with normal saline). **a** *Lower left:* Net-like support structure. *Upper part:* Top view of the inner filtration membrane. There are also deposits of 1–4 µ in size that were found before and after rinsing with normal saline. **b** Higher magnification of the support fabric of cellulose triacetate membrane

Since CAVH is applied mainly in intensive care patients with pulmonary and acute renal failure, it appeared particularly important to investigate the biocompatibility of membranes used.

Patients and Methods

The hemofiltration methods have been described elsewhere [14]. Table 1 summarizes the data of both patient groups.

Prefiltration blood samples were taken from the artery after the initial dose of heparin (600–5000 IU). After onset of hemofiltration samples were taken from the arterial blood line at 5, 15, 30, 60, and 150 min. In HF the last sample was

Table 1. Patient groups and method of hemofiltration

	Group 1: Continuous arteriovenous hemofiltration (CAVH)	Group 2: Pumpdriven hemofiltration
Patients studied	Ten intensive care patients	Six chronic intermittant hemofiltration patients
Hemofilter material	Polysulfone capillary (Amicon D20, D30)	Cellulose triacetate membrane (Sartorius SM 40004)
Surface area	0.2 or 0.5 m^2	0.6 m^2
Blood access	Femoral artery and vein	Cimino a-v-fistula
Driving force	Arteriovenous pressure difference	Blood pump

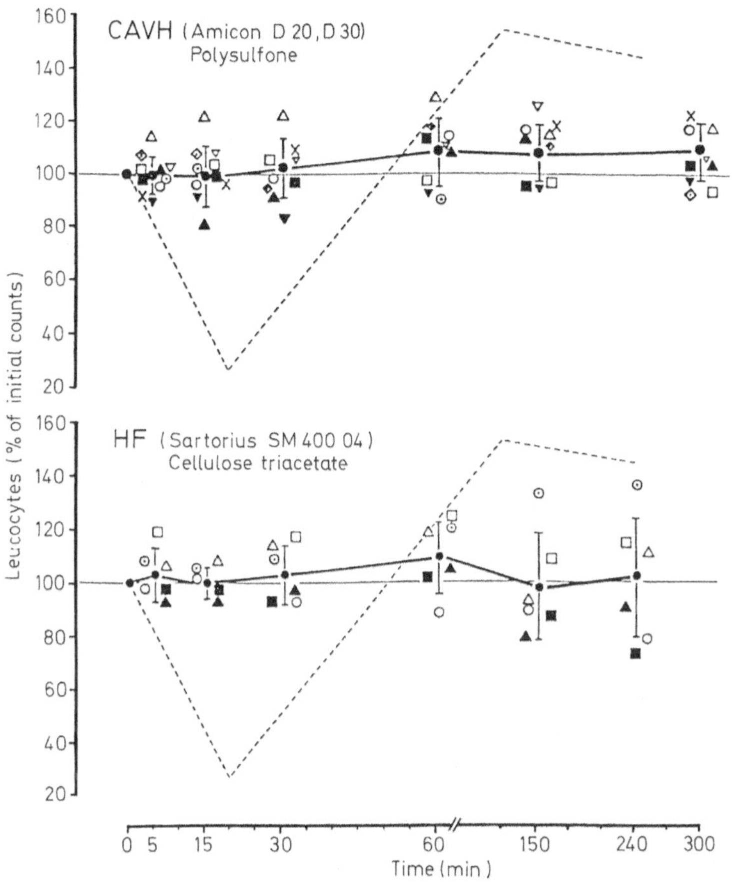

Fig. 3. Leukocyte counts during hemofiltration (CAVH, polysulfone; HF, triacetate). Results are given as percent changes of prefiltration values during treatment. *Dotted line*, cuprophane dialysis (from [12], shown for comparison)

taken after 240 min, in CAVH after 300 min (Fig. 3). In both groups some additional samples were taken from the outlet of the filter.

All samples were analyzed using the following methods (Table 2):

Table 2. Methods of measurement

Leukocyte counts, hematocrit	Coulter counter S (Coulter Electronics)
Complement	
Total hemolytic complement	Hemolytic-CH_{50}-method
C3-component	C3-laser-nephelometry
C4-component	C4-laser-nephelometry
C5a-component	Granulocyte-aggregometry [9]
Blood gas analysis	Acid Base Laboratory 2
$pO_2 \cdot pCO_2 \cdot pH$	(Radiometer, Copenhagen)

Granulocyte aggregometry according to Craddock [5] and Hammerschmidt [9] is performed by adding aggregated – i.e., C5a-containing – plasma to a suspension of test granulocytes [11].

A conventional thrombocyte aggregometer measures the intensity of a light transmission through the suspension of cells. The change in transmission is proportional to the particle count. Since the suspension contains fewer particles if more granulocytes aggregate, the change in transmission can be used as a measurement of the effect of the added plasma on the aggregation, and its content of C5a 10^{-5} formyl-methionyl-leucyl-phenylamine solution (FMLP) produces a pronounced aggregation of granulocytes [6] and was used as a standard.

Aggregation caused by patient plasma is given in percent of this aggregation standard.

The effect of hemoconcentration by fluid removal on leukocyte counts and complement concentrations was eliminated using hematocrit values for calculation of a correcting factor.

Changes in leukocyte counts, complement concentrations, and blood gases are given in percent changes of the initial values prior to onset of hemofiltration.

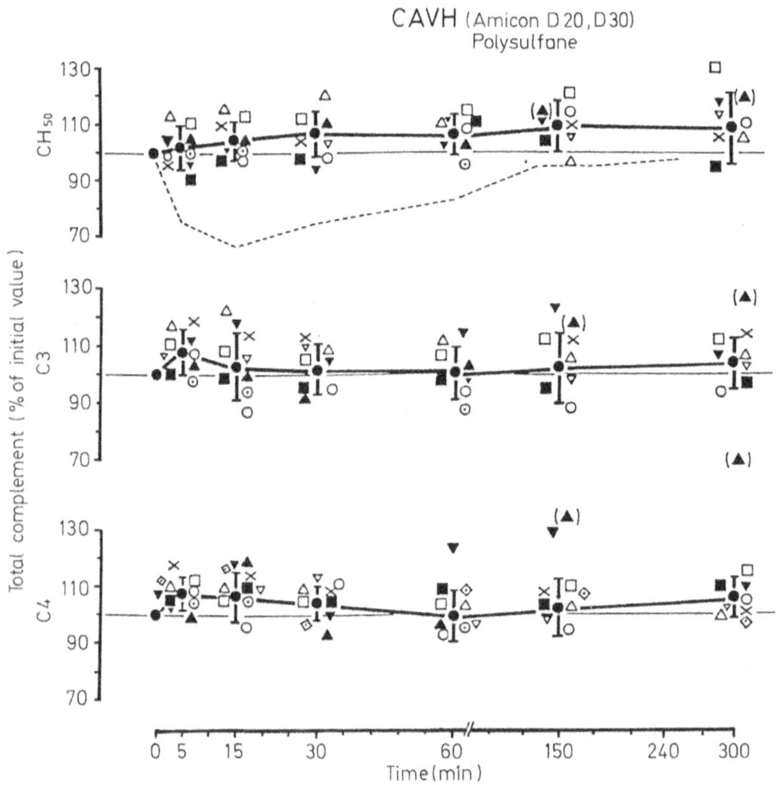

Fig. 4. Complement concentrations during CAVH (polysulfone capillaries). CH_{50}, hemolytic total complement. C3 and C4, determined immunologically by nephelometry. Results are given in percent of initial level. *Dotted line*, cuprophane dialysis (from [1], shown for comparison)

Results and Discussion

There was no significant change in leukocyte counts during either mechanical hemofiltration or CAVH. These results are in contrast with the findings of other authors who used cuprophane membranes for hemodialysis [1, 3, 11]. They found a significant decrease in leukocyte counts (70%–80% less than the initial counts) during the first 20 min of dialysis, which normalized within 1 h and then increased significantly above the normal range [2, 18].

With hemolytic complement determination (CH_{50}) according to Kabbat and Mayer, complement activation was not detectable during CAVH (Fig. 4), or HF (Fig. 5), contrary to the results during dialysis with cuprophane membrane [1].

Although the CH_{50} values were unchanged, the C3 and C4 components of complement were also determined separately to dectect any possible reduction of these components by means of nephelometry.

The C3 determination is of particular interest because C3 plays a central role in both the classical and alternate pathway of complement activation. As shown in Figs. 4 and 5, none of these parameters decreased during CAVH and conventional hemofiltration compared with prefiltration values, indicating that activation of the complement system was beyond the range detectable using this method.

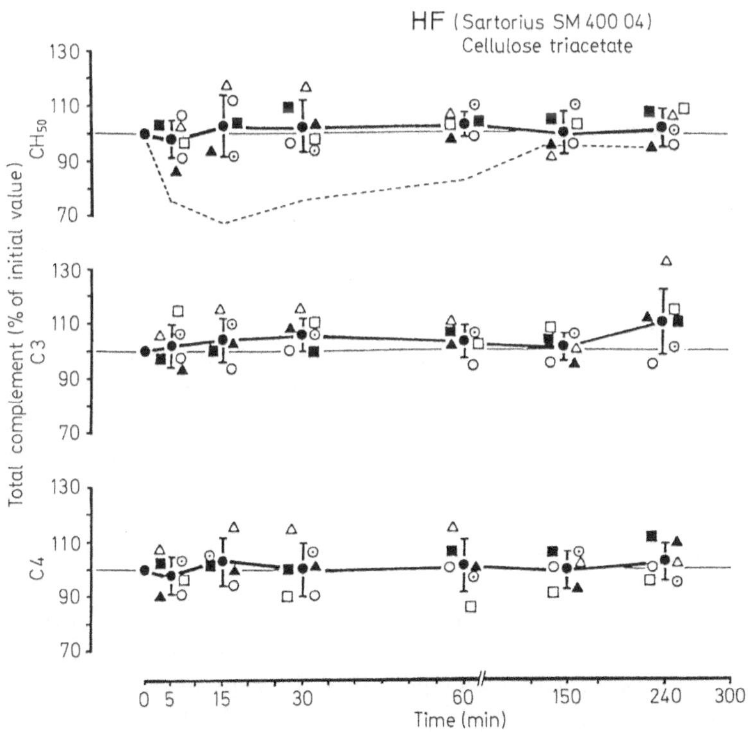

Fig. 5. Complement concentrations during HF (cellulose triacetate). Results are given in percent of initial levels. *Dotted line*, cuprophane dialysis (from [1], shown for comparison)

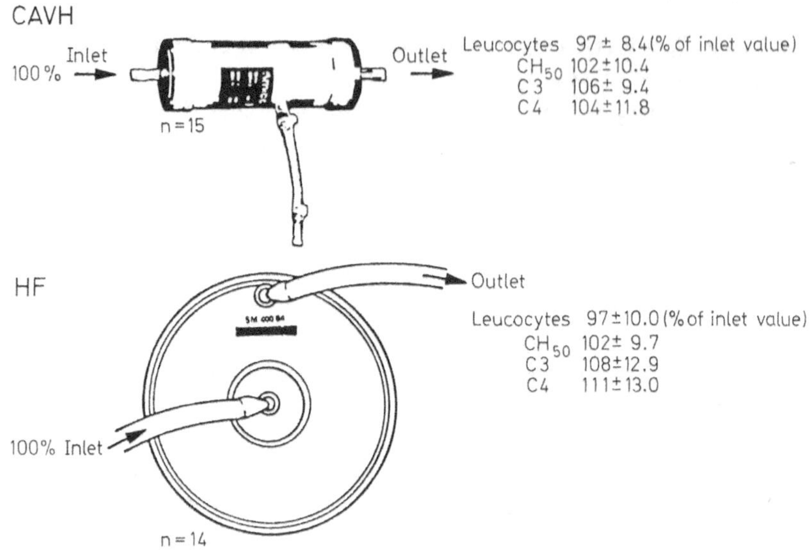

Fig. 6. Leukocyte counts and complement levels. Comparison of inlet levels (= 100%) with filter outlet levels

In order to exclude the possibility that trace amounts of complement, insufficient to produce leukopenia or concentration changes detectable by these methods, may have been activated in the extracorporeal circuit, blood samples where also taken from the blood line behind the hemofilter, i.e. before undergoing multifold dilution in the whole blood pool. As shown in Fig. 6, no differences could be detected between pre- and postfilter values.

The samples were tested for their C5a content by means of granulocyte aggregometry (described by Craddock et al. [5, 6] and Hammerschmidt et al. [9]).

This method of determining the activation of the complement system is highly sensitive, since it is based on the measurement of a complement only detectable in the blood when the whole system has been activated. Figure 7 (bottom) shows the results of aggregometry of blood samples taken from the inlet and the outlet of the filter and compared with prehemofiltration values. Neither in CAVH nor in HF was there a significant change of C5a content of samples at the filter outlet compared with prefiltration samples.

Since C5a, if any should have formed inside the filter, may quickly bind to granulocytes there, it might not be detectable by granulocyte aggregometry in the plasma behind the filter.

To trace even minimum activation of complement, the plastic materials (polysulfone and cellulose triacetate) were incubated at 37 °C for 60 min, in vitro, with heparinized plasma. Contrary to plasma incubated with cuprophane material, no C5a activity was found in these samples (Fig. 7 top and middle).

Arterial blood gases were analyzed in order to detect an impairment of the patient's pulmonary function due to exposure of their blood to the plastic surfaces.

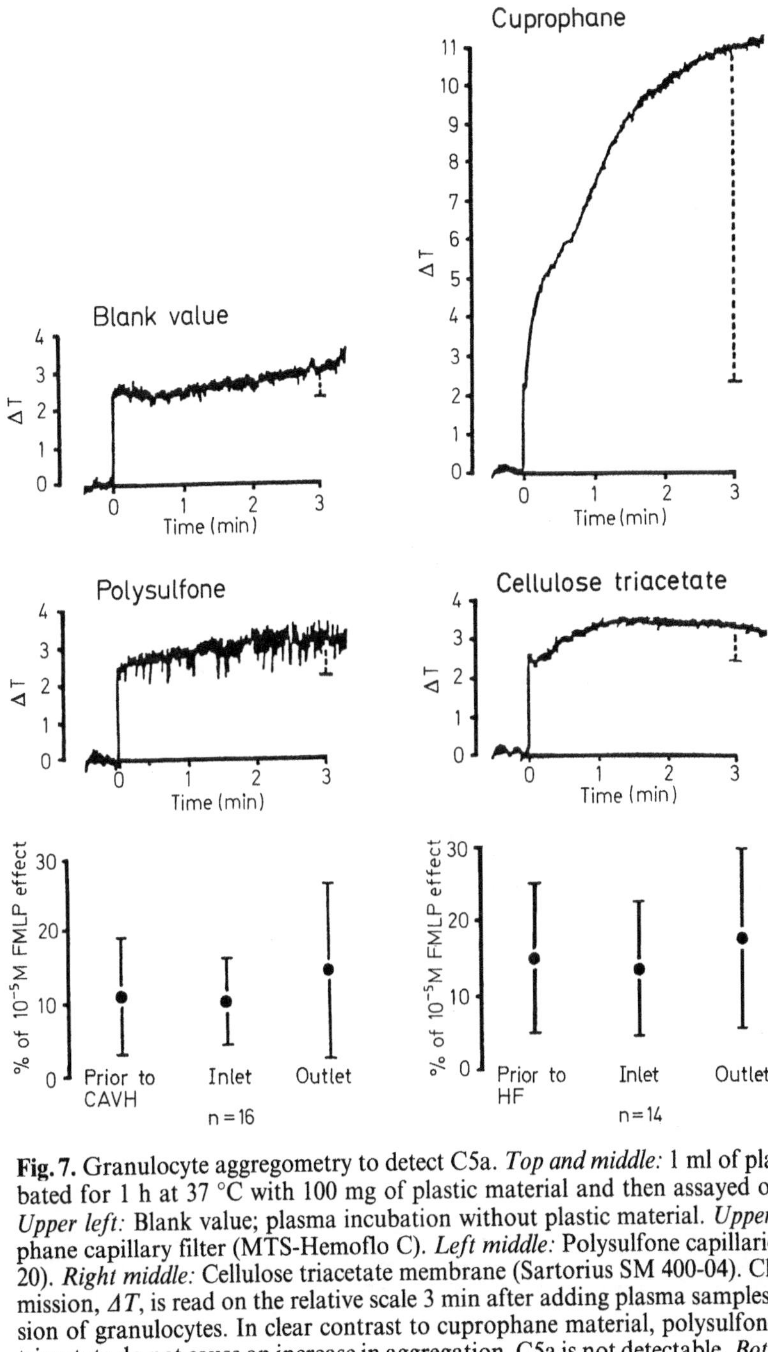

Fig. 7. Granulocyte aggregometry to detect C5a. *Top and middle:* 1 ml of plasma was incubated for 1 h at 37 °C with 100 mg of plastic material and then assayed of C5a content. *Upper left:* Blank value; plasma incubation without plastic material. *Upper right:* Cuprophane capillary filter (MTS-Hemoflo C). *Left middle:* Polysulfone capillaries (Amicon D-20). *Right middle:* Cellulose triacetate membrane (Sartorius SM 400-04). Change in transmission, ΔT, is read on the relative scale 3 min after adding plasma samples to the suspension of granulocytes. In clear contrast to cuprophane material, polysulfone and cellulose triacetate do not cause an increase in aggregation, C5a is not detectable. *Bottom:* Comparison of aggregation of patient plasma after filter passage (outlet) with aggregative prior to CAVH/HF and during filtration at the inlet of the filter. Values are given in percent of the standard aggregation of a 10–5 M FMLP solution

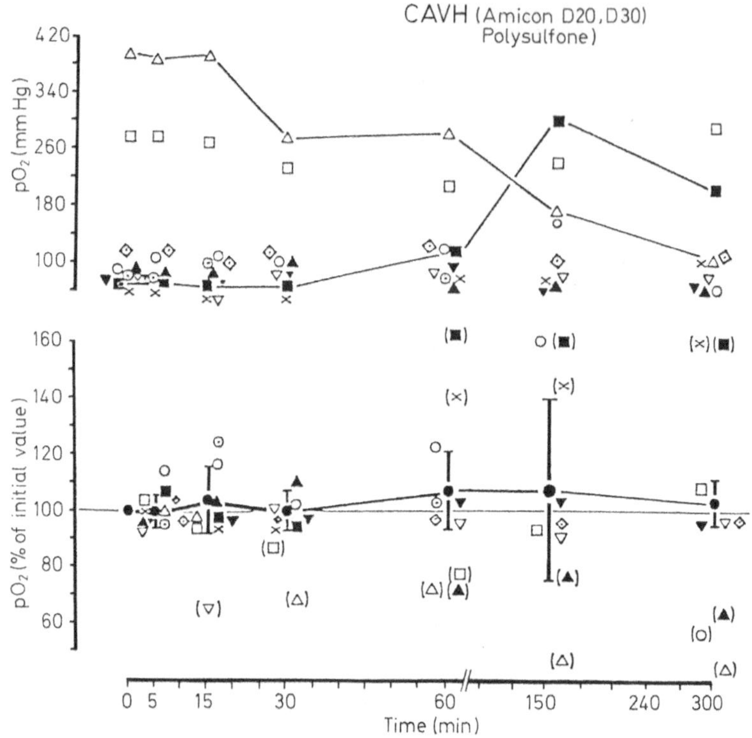

Fig. 8. Arterial PO_2 during CAVH (polysulfone capillaries). *Top:* Absolute PO_2 values (mmHg), pronounced shifts of PO_2 are seen in some patients caused by changing artificial respiration. *Bottom:* Arterial PO_2, changes given in percent of initial values. Results influenced by respirator changes are excluded and shown in parentheses

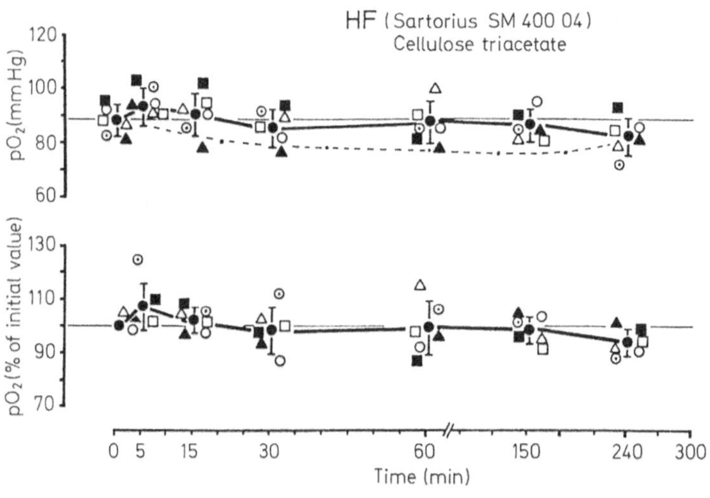

Fig. 9. Arterial PO_2 during HF (cellulose triacetate). *Top:* Absolute PO_2 values; all patients breathing spontaneously (room air). *Dotted line*, cuprophane dialysis (from [3]). *Bottom:* Arterial PO_2; results given in percent of initial values

In CAVH the results of blood gas analyses are difficult to interpret: All our CAVH patients needed artificial respiration before hemofiltration treatment. During the 5 h of our study in some patients the respirator had to be adjusted to the actual needs of the patients. Therefore some of our blood gas analyses reflect rather the mode of the artificial respiration than the effect of hemofiltration. Figure 8 (top) shows the absolute PO_2 values. The symbols of two patients are connected with lines in order to illustrate this problem. The respirator of the patient who started with a prefiltration PO_2 of 380 mmHg was adjusted consecutively to a more physiological level. Thus, the PO_2 decreased by 70%. The PO_2 of the other patient increased by 300% compared with the initial value due to respirator changes.

Figure 9 shows an unchanged arterial PO_2 during pump-driven HF. In hemodialysis with cuprophane, however, a drop in PO_2 of about 10–15 mmHg was observed by others [3].

In order to evaluate the effect of CAVH on blood oxygenation, all results were excluded which were influenced by respirator changes. The remaining data (Fig. 7, bottom) do not indicate a significant change of PO_2 after onset of CAVH.

References

1. Aljama P, Bird PAE, Ward MK, Feest TG, Walker W, Tanboga H, Sussman, M, Kerr DNS (1978) Haemodialysis-induced leukopenia and activation of complement: effects of different membranes. Proc Eur Dial Transpl Ass 15:144
2. Brubaker LH, Nolph KD (1971) Mechanisms of recovery from neutropenia induced by hemodialysis. Blood 38:623
3. Craddock PR, Fehr J, Brigham KL, Kronenberg RS, Jacob HS (1977) Complement and leukocyte-mediated pulmonary dysfunction in hemodialysis. N Engl J Med 296:769
4. Craddock PR, Fehr J, Dalmasso AP, Brigham KL, Jacob HS (1977) Hemodialysis leukopenia, pulmonary vascular leukostasis resulting from complement activation by dialyzer cellophane membranes. J Clin Invest 59:879
5. Craddock PR, Hammerschmidt D, White JG, Dalmasso AP, Jacob H (1977) Complement (C5a)-induced granulocyte aggregation in vitro, a possible mechanism of complement-mediated leukostasis and leukopenia. J Clin Invest 60:260
6. Craddock PR, White JG, Weisdorf DJ, Hammerschmidt DE (1980) Digital integration of granulocyte aggregation responses. A simple and reproducible method for the quantification of granulocyte adhesiveness. Inflammation 4:381
7. Dumler F, Levin NW (1979) Leukopenia and hypoxemia unrelated effects of hemodialysis. Arch Intern Med 139:1103
8. Graf H, Stummvoll HK, Haber P, Kovarik J (1980) Pathophysiology of dialysis related hypoxemia. Proc Eur Dial Transpl Ass 17:155
9. Hammerschmidt DE, Bowers TK, Lammi-Keefe CJ, Jacob HS, Craddock PR (1980) Granulocyte aggregometry: a sensitive technique for the detection of C5a and complement activation. Blood 55:898
10. Hammerschmidt DE, Harris PD, Wayland JH, Craddock PR, Jacob HS (1981) Complement-induced granulocyte aggregation in vivo. Am J Pathol 102:146
11. Hjorth R, Jonsson AK, Vretblad P (1981) A rapid method for purification of human granulocytes using Percoll. A comparison with dextran sedimentation. J Immunol Methods 43:95
12. Jacob AI, Gavellas G, Zarco R, Perez G, Bourgoignie JJ (1980) Leukopenia, hypoxemia, and complement function with different hemodialysis membranes. Kidney Int 18:505

13. Kaplow LS, Goffinet JA (1968) Profound neutropenia during the early phase of hemodialysis. JAMA 203:1135
14. Kramer P, Kaufhold G, Gröne HJ, Wigger W, Rieger J, Matthaei D, Stokke T, Burchardi H, Scheler F (1980) Management of anuric intensive-care patients with arteriovenous hemofiltration. Int J Artif Organs 3:225
15. Mahajan S, Gardiner H, DeTar B, Desai S, Muller B, Johnson N, Briggs W, McDonald F (1977) Relationship between pulmonary functions and hemodialysis induced leukopenia? Trans Am Soc Artif Intern Organs 23:411
16. O'Flaherty JT, Kreutzer DL, Ward PA (1977) Neutrophil aggregation and swelling induced by chemotactic agents. J Immunol 119:232
17. Sacks T, Moldow CF, Craddock PR, Bowers TK, Jacob HS (1978) Oxygen radicals mediate endothelial cell damage by complement-stimulated granulocytes. An in vitro model of immune vascular damage. J Clin Invest 61:1161
18. Skubitz KM, Craddock PR (1981) Reversal of hemodialysis granulocytopenia and pulmonary leukostasis: A clinical manifestation of selective down-regulation of granulocyte responses to C5a. J Clin Invest 67:1383
19. Toren M, Goffinet JA, Kaplow LS (1970) Pulmonary bed sequestration of neutrophils during hemodialysis. Blood 36:337

Puncture and Long-Term Cannulation of the Femoral Artery and Vein in Adults

H. J. Gröne and P. Kramer

For the treatment of acute renal failure (ARF) with hemodialysis or hemofiltration, vascular access can be achieved by external arteriovenous shunts [32] or by percutaneous catheterization of large vessels. Percutaneous catheterization of the femoral vessels for hemodialysis was described by Shaldon et al. in 1961 [34]. Several groups have reported their extensive experiences with short-term catheterization of the femoral vessels for hemodialysis [6–8, 13–15, 25].

We also use the percutaneous puncture of the femoral artery and vein for arteriovenous hemofiltration [33].

The catheters remain in the vessels during continuous treatment that lasts many days.

Methods

Set of Instruments for Puncture (Fig. 1)

The puncture cannula is cut lanceolate. It, as well as the guide wire, are siliconized to increase their sliding capability.

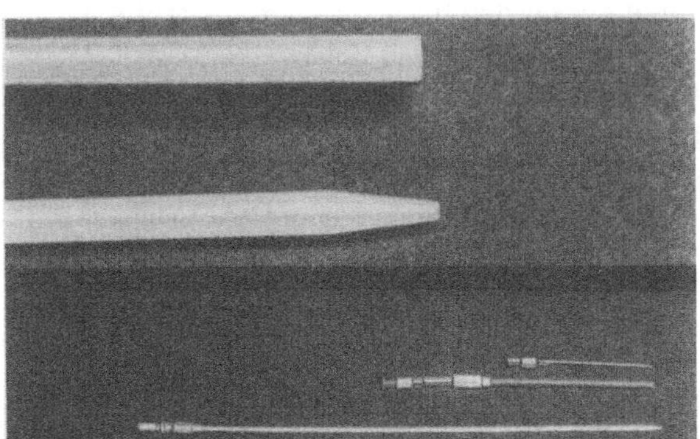

Fig. 1. Set of instruments for continuous arteriovenous hemofiltration: "dry-siliconized" puncture needle and guide wire (length 53 cm, flexible tip 4 cm), dilating catheter with conical, rounded tip, indwelling catheter (intravasal length 11 cm) with internal diameter of 8 CH. Dilating and indwelling catheters are made of Rilsan

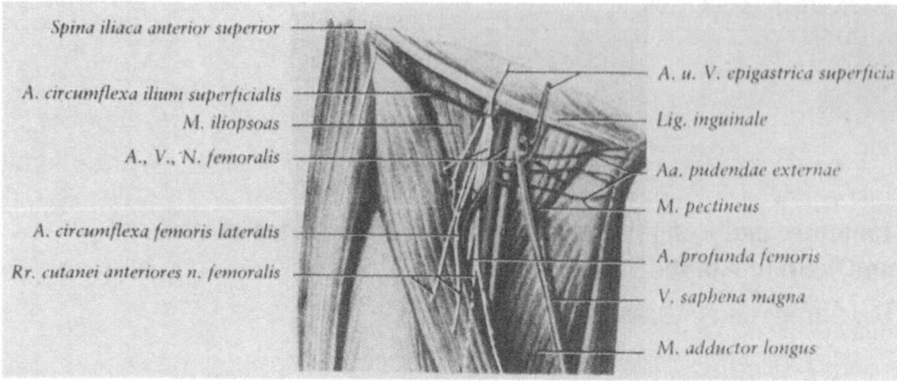

Fig. 2. Anatomy of the femoral triangle (Waldeyer A., *Human Anatomy*, Walter de Gruyter, Berlin 1969, p. 408)

The guide wire has a 4 cm long flexible tip. Dilating and indwelling catheters (intravascular length 11 cm) consist of Rilsan, a mixture of teflon and polypropylene. The catheters have a smooth surface and slide easily. The dilating catheter has a conical, rounded tip to avoid potential trauma to the endothelium. The high flexibility of the indwelling catheter is substantially reenforced by two metallic, X-ray-positive strips. The outside of the catheter is of uniform structure, since the metallic contrast strips are covered externally with plastic. The indwelling catheter has a single opening at the end and no side perforations. Its internal diameter is 8 CH.

Topography of the Femoral Artery and Vein (Fig. 2)

The femoral vein runs medially to the femoral artery; the femoral nerve runs laterally to the artery. The femoral artery puts out strong branches within the femoral triangle, i.e., the arteriae circumflexae and the arteria femoris profunda. The arteria femoris profunda travels dorsally at the lower third of the triangle and laterally from the arteria femoralis. Puncture and attempted cannulation of one of these arterial side branches can result in perforation of the vessel and severe femoral bleeding. Therefore, it is preferable to puncture the arteria femoralis in the upper third of the triangle. Since the vena saphena magna joins the vena femoralis in a steep angle, a catheter can be advanced from the vena saphena magna into the vena femoralis.

Puncture and Cannulation (Fig. 3)

Vessel puncture and catheter insertion are performed by means of the modified Seldinger technique [33, 43]. Sterile drapes and sterile gloves are used. The skin is punctured only after thorough disinfection. The inguinal region is exposed by supporting the sacral vertebra. The thigh is abducted and slightly rotated outwardly.

The course of the arteria femoralis is determined by palpation. The puncture site is to lie 2–3 cm below the ligamentum inguinale at the area of strong pulsation of the artery.

Skin and subcutaneous tissue are infiltrated with a local anesthetic caudally to the proposed puncture site of the vessel. While the arteria femoralis is securely held in place between the index and middle fingers of one hand, the other hand carefully pushes the puncture cannula, held at a 45° angle to the thigh, in a cranial direction [12, 25].

Once blood spurts from the cannula, it should be held level with the thigh, to prevent injury to the posterior wall of the artery and advanced only a few more millimeters. The cannula is now blocked with the index finger. The guide wire, flexible tip first, is inserted through the cannula until the extravasal length slightly exceeds that of the dilating catheter. The guide wire should slide in without effort; if it can only be pushed into the vessel against a resistance, an exact intravasal position is not guaranteed and catheterization should not be continued [44]. Directly cranially to the puncture cannula, the skin is incised for approximately 0.5 cm with a scalpel. The puncture cannula is then retracted over the guide wire while compressing the puncture site with a sponge. The dilating catheter is now moved forward, over the guide wire, into the artery with a constant circular motion. The mobility of the guide wire should be verified several times during insertion of the dilating catheter to prevent its jamming on a kink in the guide wire and cutting into the vessel.

After the insertion of the dilating catheter, until the silicon portion of the catheter rests on the skin, the indwelling catheter is pushed into the artery with constant turning. The indwelling catheter is then securely sewn to the skin. The guide wire and the dilating catheter are removed. At this point, the silicon portion of the indwelling catheter is compressed with the fingers to prevent loss of blood. A three-way stop cock is screwed on; the catheter is rinsed and filled with 10 ml heparinized saline.

The vena femoralis is catheterized the same way, preferably on the same side, to make patient care easier.

Arterial and venous catheters are connected to the tubing of the hemofilter after injecting 20–30 IU of heparin/kg in 20 ml of physiological saline solution into the femoral vein.

Careful puncture technique and thorough care of the catheters, the hemofiltration system, and the surrounding skin are necessary to avoid infections [26]. Both puncture sites are carefully and thoroughly covered with polyvidone-iodine ointment. The ointment adheres tightly to skin and catheters. Infection can occur through any opening in the system, valves, syringes, and the infusion set [38].

Direct blood pressure measurements via the arterial catheter, blood sampling, and administration of infusion solution through the venous catheter should only be done under strictly sterile conditions. In our experience, blood for laboratory tests, necessary to make therapeutic decisions, is often obtained through the femoral catheters. We like to point out again, however, that sterile conditions must be maintained when manipulating the catheter/hemofiltration system [19].

The flexibility of the catheters allows the thigh to bend up to 45°. The catheters remain in the femoral artery and vein during the entire continuous arteriovenous

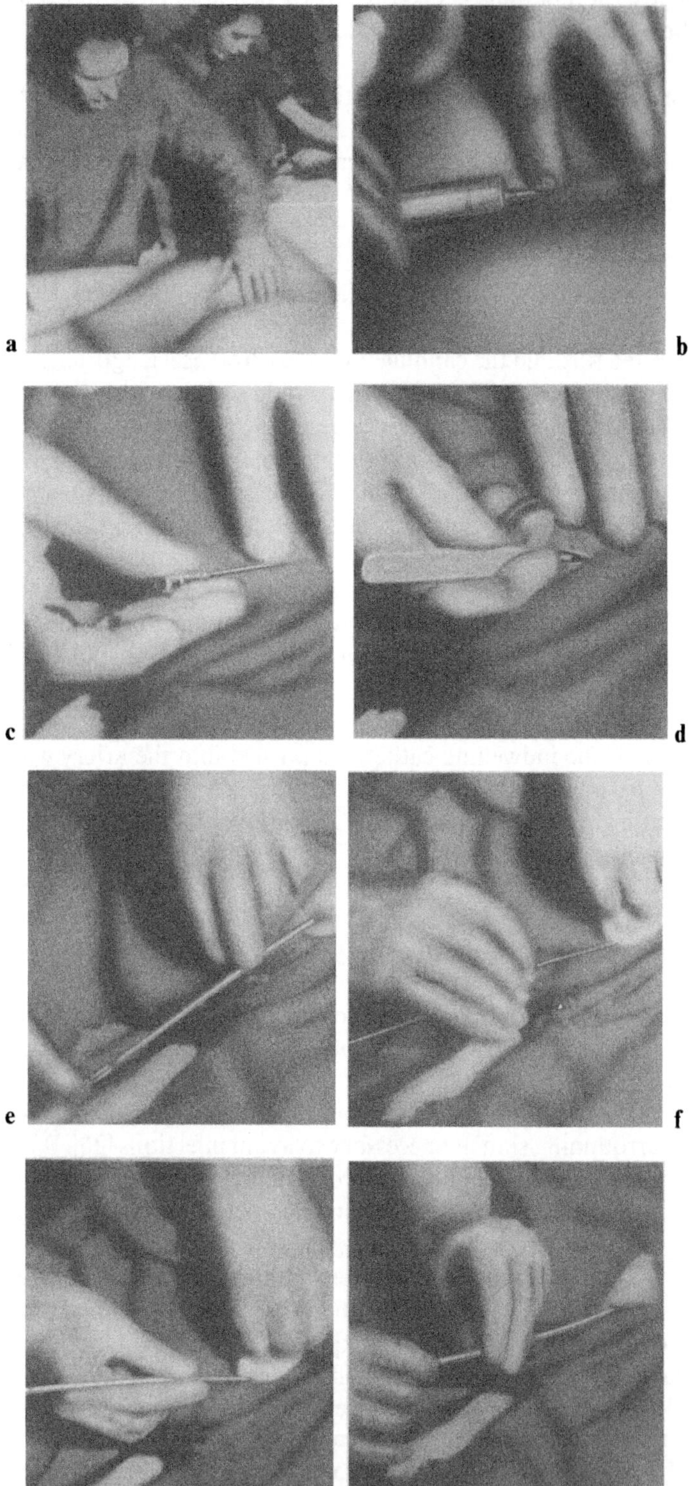

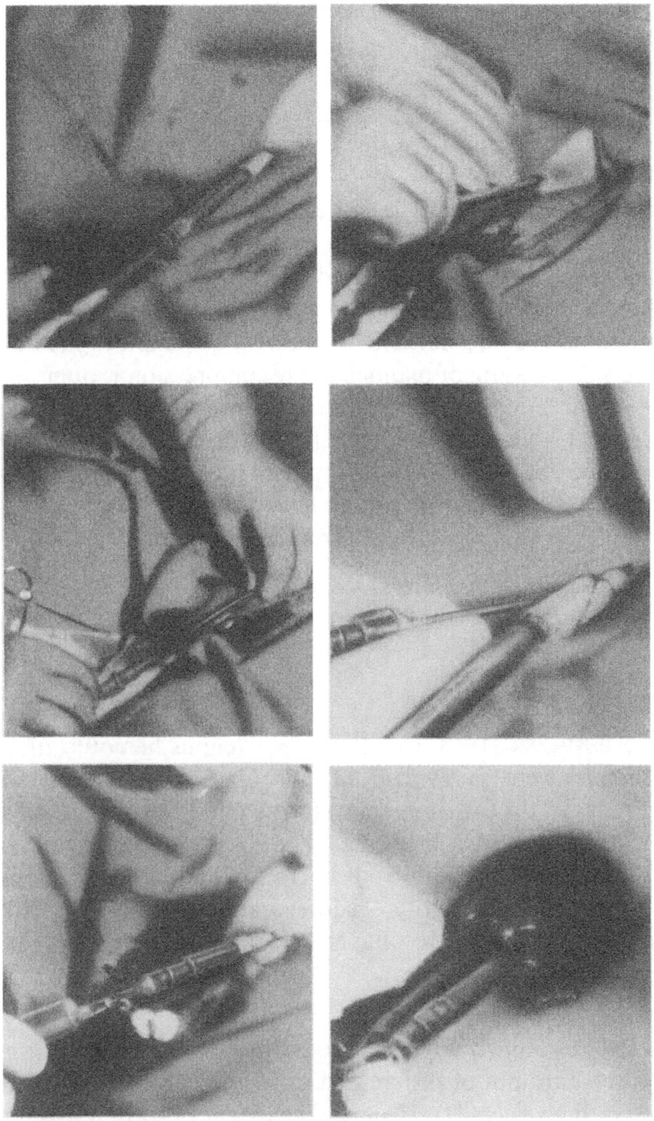

i j k l m n

Fig. 3 a–n. Puncture and cannulation of the arteria and vena femoralis. **a** Palpation of the artery with index and middle finger tips. **b** Subcutaneous infiltration with local anesthetic. **c** Puncture of the vessel. **d** After insertion of the guide wire, a 0.5 cm long incision is made directly above puncture needle. **e** Adjustment of the extravasal length of the guide wire to that of the dilating catheter. **f** Withdrawal of the puncture needle while compressing the puncture site with a sponge. **g** Insertion of the dilating catheter. **h** Once the dilating catheter makes contact with the puncture site, compression with the sponge can be stopped. Insertion of the dilating catheter followed by insertion of the indwelling catheter into the vessel with circular movement. **i** Inserted dilating and indwelling catheters and positioned guide wire. **j** The indwelling catheter is securely sewn to the skin. **k** Guide wire and dilating catheter are withdrawn; the silicon cuff of the indwelling catheter is compressed to avoid loss of blood. **l** After rinsing (10 ml heparinized 0.9% NaCl solution) and shutting-off the arterial indwelling catheter, the femoral vein is punctured. **m** Administration of approximately 2000 IU of heparin solution into the venous catheter. **n** Disinfection and application of a polyvidone-iodine ointment

hemofiltration treatment. Indwelling times of up to 3 weeks have been achieved without complications.

Removal of the Catheters

At the end of arteriovenous hemofiltration, the catheters are withdrawn. They should not be further used as a convenient blood withdrawal site for blood gas determinations or other laboratory tests. The catheters are pulled carefully while maintaining heparinization [31]. The puncture site of the artery is located caudally to the skin incision and is compressed manually for 30 min. The pulsations of the arteria dorsalis in the foot should be clearly palpable during compression. The necessary compression pressure is far less for the venous puncture site than for the arterial site. The side pressure of manual artery compression is often sufficient to compress the venous puncture. After 30 min, the puncture sites are compressed with a sandbag for 3 h. Continued administration of heparin is indicated for most bed patients to prevent formation of thrombi at the endothelial lesions. If thrombi are attached to the catheter, the patient has to be carefully monitored in order to recognize clinically significant local thrombi, arterial lung emboli, or peripheral arterial emboli in time.

Results

Rate of Complications

During the period Jan. 1981–Dec. 1983 over 150 arteriovenous hemofiltrations through femoral catheters were performed at the University Hospital of Göttingen. Indwelling times of the catheters ranged from a few hours to 50 days. Severe clinical complications occurred in two cases out of 300 catheterizations, approximately 0.7%. This number takes into consideration only catheterizations performed according to the recommended procedure, and in which the catheter/hemofiltration system was connected as recommended.

Thrombosis

Femoral vessels (n = 16), examined after arteriovenous hemofiltration during autopsy, regularly showed thrombi of different sizes in the catheter area. The catheters had remained in the vessels 1.5–14 days. The extent of thrombosis was independent of the time the catheter had remained in place [23]. Fibrin-rich thrombi, partially or completely surrounding the catheters, were observed (Fig. 4).

A thrombus that closed the lumen of the vena iliaca externa was found after a 14-day-long continuous arteriovenous hemofiltration, in this case of a 72-year-old woman, hemofiltration was performed because of postoperative, acute renal

Fig. 4. Thrombi in the arteria and vena femoralis and iliaca externa of a 77-year-old man with atherosclerosis, after 8 days of continuous arteriovenous hemofiltration. The arterial catheter is completely surrounded by thrombi; nonoccluding thrombus in the vena femoralis; arterial lung embolism was not documented

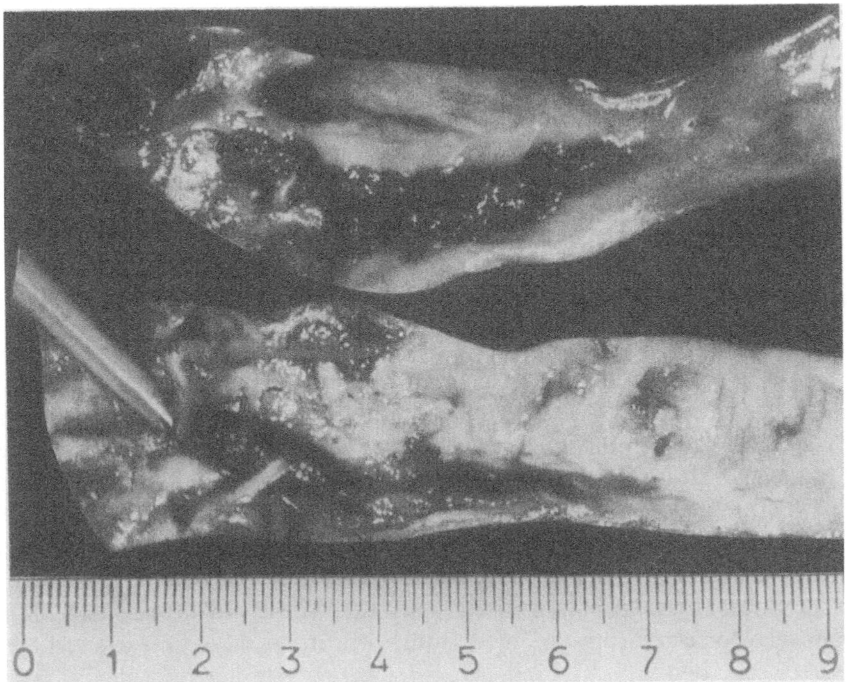
0
1
2
3
4
5
6
7
8
9

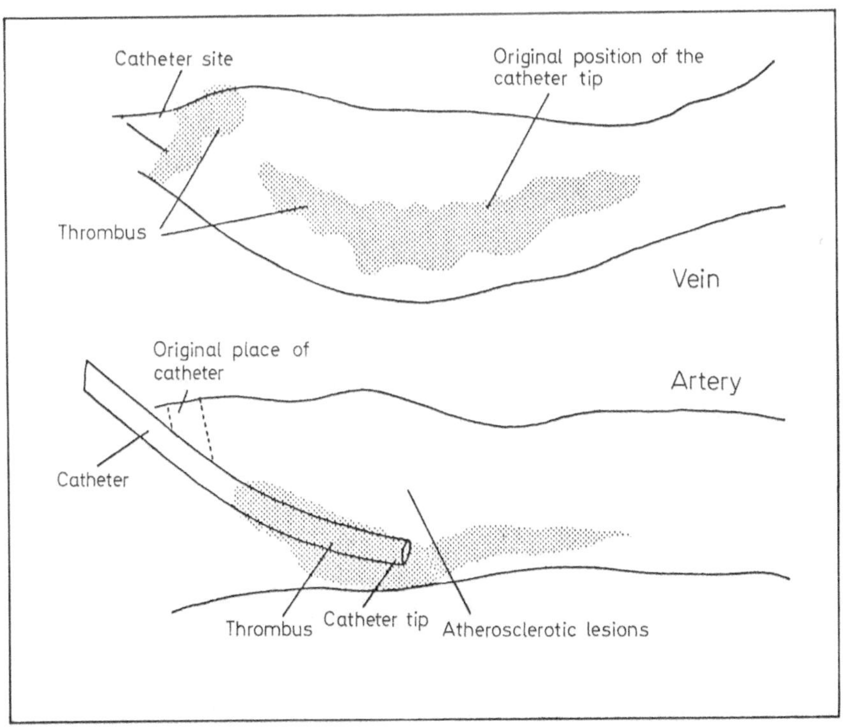
Catheter site
Original position of the catheter tip
Thrombus
Vein
Original place of catheter
Artery
Catheter
Thrombus
Catheter tip
Atherosclerotic lesions

failure, but without heparin. Heparin was not given because of severe bleeding tendency and good filtration rate.

Arterial lung emboli were not diagnosed clinically and not noticed in autopsied patients.

A peripheral arterial thromboembolus closed off the arteria poplitea 12 h after the start of arteriovenous hemofiltration in a 77-year-old man. The patient suffered from diuretic- and vasodilator therapy-resistant cardiac failure and progressively declining kidney function. He died 24 h later from protracted failure of the left ventricle.

Bleeding

A retroperitoneal hematoma was noticed in a 55-year-old female patient, whose left venous femoral catheter was exchanged with one of unrecommended design. The guide wire could only be inserted with force, but finally, blood was successfully aspirated through the indwelling catheter with perforations along the sides and at the end. (It is our opinion that these catheters are unsuitable for femoral cannulation.)

Due to a perforation of the vena iliaca externa caused by the catheter exchange, the tip of the catheter was placed extravasally, the side perforation intravasally. Retroperitoneal bleeding of more than 3 l resulted. The hypovolemic shock of this patient was corrected, but she died from myocardial infarction a short time later.

Periarterial hematoma at the puncture site could not be confirmed clinically. In the autopsied cases, only slight bleeding into the periarterial and perivenous fatty tissue was noted.

Infections

Infections around the puncture site and in the insertion canal were not found. There was no evidence of catheter-induced bacteremia and sepsis.

In the histologically examined vessel sections ($n = 16$) lined with thrombotic material, no bacteria were seen.

Discussion

The described puncture and catheterization of the femoral artery and vein are a simple method that can be implemented within a short time (5–15 min) [7, 15, 34]. This is most advantageous in an emergency situation. Preparation of peripheral vessels necessary for external arteriovenous shunts may be difficult to perform on intensive care patients (i.e., polytraumatized patients) is not needed. Ligature of vessels can be avoided with femoral catheterization. Since it is possible that some patients may end up with chronic kidney failure, it is important to preserve the peripheral arteries for future shunt sites.

Complications

The incidence of severe complications with prolonged cannulation of the femoral artery and vein corresponds with the rate reported by other study groups for short-term catheterization of the femoral vein (0.1% to 1.0%) [6–8, 14].

Thrombosis

Every vessel puncture causes trauma to the endothelium and therefore constitutes a possible site for thrombosis [11]. Although the synthetic material of which catheters are made will probably always be thrombogenic, the material we recommend is regarded as promoting thrombosis to a relatively lesser degree [30].

Ultrastructural examination of catheters revealed wall defects and coarse surface areas which can contribute to thrombosis inside and outside the lumen of the catheter [22, 24]. Wettability, electrical charge, and flexibility are additional characteristics of the catheters that determine the chance of thrombosis [5, 24]. Inflexible catheters push specifically against the vessel wall with their tips and cause additional lesions of the endothelium [11]. Factors that increase the risk of thrombosis iatrogenically should be avoided: i.e., multiple puncture attempts, lesions of the opposite vessel wall caused by the puncture cannula, hasty or jerky insertion of the guide wire and dilating catheter.

To date we have not found a clinically apparent venous thrombosis or arterial lung embolus [17, 18], probably also because the continuous heparin administration into the arterial tubing causes high heparin concentration in the hemofilter and in the venous part of the system, including the vena iliaca externa. The blood flow in the vein at the tip of the catheter is increased by arteriovenous hemofiltration. Careful puncture technique, construction of the tip of the dilating catheter which lessens the risk of injury to the endothelium, the conciseness and kink-resistance of the indwelling catheter with a small thrombogenic surface area may all explain the overall low incidence of thrombi as compared with the experience of others [23].

Reported rates of venous thrombi for short duration hemodialysis are only partially comparable with our results for prolonged cannulation. They are briefly discussed.

Fuchs et al. reported no thrombosis [7] for 5306 punctures of the femoral vein, the catheter remaining in the vein for the duration of hemodialysis. The risk of thrombosis increases if the catheter remains in the vessel after completion of hemodialysis. Kjellstrand et al. observed three cases of thrombosis of the femoral vein with one fatal arterial lung embolus, out of 700 catheter punctures of the femoral vein [14]. In these three cases the catheters remained in the vein 24–72 h without constant dialysis. A similar experience was reported by a Spanish study group. For 356 catheterizations of the femoral vein, venous thrombi were diagnosed in cases where the catheters remained in the vessel for a prolonged period after dialysis [8].

The media of the femoral artery consists predominantly of muscle cells. Wall dissections are less likely to occur during vessel puncture than during puncture of large vessels with a predominantly elastic media structure (i.e., aorta, proximal parts of brachiocephalic vessels). Arterial catheterization, however, can result in the rupture of atheromatous plaques. Atheromatous or thrombotic embolism can occur [35]. Thrombi in peripheral vessels such as the arteria iliaca externa and the arteria femoralis are subject to relatively fast organization and can reinforce preexsisting stenoses [37]. One occluding arterial thromboembolus was diagnosed in a patient with severe general atherosclerosis and decompensated cardiac insufficiency.

For patients with severe artherosclerotic changes, continuous arteriovenous hemofiltration should be restricted as a measure of last resort. In patients with low-to-medium grade atherosclerosis, the arterial thrombosis rate has not been reported to be higher than for other patients [2, 21].

Thromboses of the femoral artery were described in children, catheterized for cardiac symptoms: in some cases, reduced growth of the catheterized extremity was noted [10]. In this respect, continuous arteriovenous hemofiltration is problematic for children, but was performed by us without acute complications several times.

Thrombi and arterial peripheral, or central venous emboli can occur after strong and prolonged compression of the femoral artery and vein [21]. Especially patients with soft, easily compressible arteries, reduced cardiac output, and elevated blood viscosity are in danger of arterial thrombosis [21]. Femoral pulsations and pulsations of the feet have to be checked regularly during cannulation and after the catheters have been pulled. The circumference of the leg should be measured at regular intervals. Immediate surgical therapy of arterial thrombi and thromboemboli is recommended. The success rate is favorable, according to several reports [2, 4, 9].

The results of other studies regarding arterial cannulations are briefly presented. The rate of thrombotic complications by percutaneous retrograde arteriography was less than 0.16% [16]. The rate of all complications, for femoral arterial punctures of intensive care patients with a high mortality rate (36%), was reported to be 14% [28].

Bleeding

Retroperitoneal bleeding presents a rare, however potentially fatal, complication of femoral artery and vein puncture [6, 7, 14]. If the dilating or indwelling catheters rupture the vessel, retroperitoneal bleeding can occur. Pointed and inflexible catheters can penetrate soft vessels during rebedding of the patient or spontaneous movement of the lower extremities [27] and are, therefore, not recommended. Catheters with end opening and side perforations make it impossible to determine whether or not the catheter tip is positioned extravascularly; blood may easily be aspirated through the perforations on the side, which would be inside the vessel, while bleeding can continue unnoticed through the extravascularly positioned catheter tip. The risk of bleeding increases with an improper catheterization procedure and an improper connection of the catheters to the tubing systems. Disconnections of catheter and connecting tube were only noticed when the tubing was not screwed tightly to the catheter, i.e., tubing systems without luer lock.

One patient died from severe arterial bleeding caused by improper connection devices. Catheters that are not sewn securely to the skin can slide out of the vessels, leading to pronounced femoral bleeding. We want to emphasize that catheters must always be sewn securely to the skin, that catheters and tubing must be connected with luer-lock fittings, and that one should always leave catheter tubing and hemofilter exposed to full sight and not covered by a bed sheet.

Puncture of the arteria iliaca externa above the ligamentum inguinale does not allow adequate compression of the puncture site after the catheters are pulled out, since the iliac artery travels dorsally and usually is not compressible manually [3, 21]. This causes retroperitoneal bleeding. Retroperitoneal hematoma can also occur spontaneously with clotting disorders, chronic and acute kidney insufficiency, vascular and tumorous disease of the kidney and adrenal glands [1, 20, 39, 41, 42].

Signs of retroperitoneal bleeding may consist of sudden highly exacerbating pain of the abdomen, the hip, the buttocks and back, swelling and tension of the abdomen. Bowel movements may stop. The hematocrit can drop. Usually the heart rate increases and blood pressure drops. The psoas shadow loses its clear demarcation. Abdominal sonography can aid in diagnosis of suspected retroperitoneal bleeding. Caused by the bleeding, elevation of amylases through lesions of the pancreas, cholestatic jaundice, simulation of a strangulation hernia, and pleural effusions were described with retroperitoneal hematoma [29]. Therapy for catheter-provoked retroperitoneal bleeding consists of administration of blood and normalizing clotting parameters. Surgical intervention is indicated when the bleeding cannot be stopped with intensive conservative therapy.

The rate of perivenous and periarterial hematoma with the prescribed puncture technique [14, 15] is reported as low. Nevertheless, we experienced persistent arterial bleeding of the puncture site in a 34-year-old male, chronic dialysis patient, who was hemodialyzed intermittently through an inflexible femoral catheter (not recommended by us) because of a rethrombosed, infected arteriovenous shunt of the forearm and who walked around with the catheter in place. Although improved flexible catheters are available we will, for the time being, use prolonged cannulation of the femoral artery and vein only for bed patients.

Infections

Local infections of the skin and the puncture site reported for percutaneous puncture of the femoral vein [15] could not be confirmed by us. This absence can most likely be attributed, besides other factors, to the application of polyvidone-iodine ointment.

Other Possible Complications

The following are possible complications of the puncture and catheterization of the femoral artery and vein [18, 36], while only thrombosis, arterial embolism, and bleeding have been observed by us to date:

1. Thrombosis
2. Thrombophlebitis
3. Embolism, arterial (peripheral vessel occlusion) and venous (arterial lung embolus)
4. Sepsis
5. Bleeding, femoral and retroperitoneal
6. Arterial pseudoaneurysm
7. Arteriovenous fistula
8. Nerve damage
9. Cellulitis

Summary

Percutaneous puncture of the femoral artery and vein according to Seldinger presents a quick and simple vessel access, if done by an experienced person. The indwelling catheter of the set especially developed for continuous arteriovenous hemofiltration exhibits relatively low thrombogenicity and high flexibility. Based on continuous heparin administration into the catheter system, high heparin concentrations are achieved in the venous outflow; the risk of venous thrombosis is, therefore, significantly reduced. Prolonged cannulation, performed with strictly sterile handling and sufficient heparinization, is associated with only a minimal risk of bleeding, and infection. Since severe complications can occur, arteriovenous hemofiltration should only be resorted to with consideration of the risk/benefit ratio.

References

1. Bhasin HK, Dana CL (1978) Spontaneous retroperitoneal hemorrhage in chronically hemodialyzed patients. Nephron 22:322
2. Bouhoutsos J, Morris T (1973) Femoral artery complications after diagnostic procedures. Br Med J 3:396
3. Christian CM, Naraglin M (1978) A complication of femoral arterial cannulation in a patient undergoing cardiopulmonary bypass. Anesthesiology 49:436
4. Cormier JM, Lagneau P (1972) Complications sévère des artériographies rétrogrades percutanées (a propos de 69 observations). J Chir 104:395
5. Durst S, Leslie J, Moore R, Amplatz K (1974) A comparison of the thrombogenicity of commercially available catheters. Radiology 113:599
6. Erben J, Kvasnicha J, Bastecky J, Groh J, Zahradnik J, Rozsival V, Bastecka D, Fixa P, Kozak J, Herout V (1979) Long-term experience with the technique of subclavian and femoral vein cannulation in hemodialysis. Artif Organs 3:241
7. Fuchs HJ, Jenett G, Klehr U, Richter G, Wilbrandt und Frotscher U (1977) Die perkutane Punktion der Vena femoralis zur Hämodialysebehandlung. Dtsch Med Wochenschr 102:1280
8. Gomez PN, Alvarez Otero MJ, Garcia de Lomana T, Coronel Diaz F, Sierra Barcena E, Prats Sanchoz D (1980) Complicaciones de la cateterizacion percutanea de la vena femoral para hemodialisis, a proposito de tres casos. Rev Clin Esp 151:325
9. Hall R (1971) Vascular injuries resulting from arterial puncture of catheterization. Br J Surg 58:513
10. Hawker RE, Palmer J, Bury RG, Bowdler JD, Celermajer JM (1973) Late results of percutaneous retrograde femoral arterial catheterization in children. Br Heart J 35:447
11. Hecker JF, Fisk GG, Farrell PC (1976) Measurement of thrombus formation on intravascular catheters. Anaesth Intens Care 4:225
12. Hekster REM (1971) Vascular lesions at the puncture site in percutaneous catheterization. Radiol Clin Biol 30:39
13. Hocken AG (1979) Percutaneous femoral veincatheterization for hemodialysis, a single needle technique. Clin Nephrol 12:93
14. Kjellstrand CM, Meriono GE, Mauer SM, Casali R, Buschmeier TJ (1975) Complications of percutaneous femoral vein catheterizations for hemodialysis. Clin Nephrol 4:37
15. Küppers H, Risler T, Krian A, Königshausen Th, Hofmann K, Schnurr E, Grabensee B (1976) Perkutaner Zugang zu den Femoralgefäßen mittels Seldinger-Technik bei der Akutdialyse. Nieren- und Hochdruckkrankheiten 1:43
16. Lang EK (1963) A survey of the complications of percutaneous retrograde arteriography: Seldinger technic. Radiology 81:257
17. Lynn KL, Maling TM (1977) A major pulmonary embolus as a complication of femoral vein catheterization. Br J Radiol 50:667

18. McGoon MD, Benedelto PW, Greene BM (1979) Complications of percutaneous central venous catheterization: a report of two cases and review of the literature. Johns Hopkins Med J 145:1
19. Meakins JL (1979) Infection associated with radial artery catheters. Can Med Assoc J 121:1564
20. Milutinovich J, Follette WG, Scribner BH (1977) Spontaneous retroperitoneal bleeding in patients on chronic hemodialysis. Ann Intern Med 86:189
21. Morris T, Bouhoutsos J (1975) The dangers of femoral artery puncture and catheterization. Am Heart J 89:260
22. Müller KM, Blaschke R, Steinmaier F (1977) Oberflächenstrukturen von Venenkathetern. Med Welt 28:2055
23. Müller KM, Bleaser B (1976) Tödliche thromboembolische Komplikationen nach zentralem Venenkatheter. Dtsch Med Wochenschr 101:411
24. Nachnani GH, Lessin LS, Motomiya T, Jensen WN (1972) Scanning electron microscopy of thrombogenesis on vascular catheter surfaces. N Engl J Med 286:139
25. Nidus BD, Matalon R, Katz LA, Cabaluna C, Tan C, Eisinger RP (1974) Hemodialysis using femoral vessel cannulation. Nephron 13:416
26. Ryan JA, Abel RM, Abbott WM, Hopkins CC, Chesney T McC, Colley R, Phillips K, Tischer JE (1974) Catheter complications in total parenteral nutrition. N Engl J Med 290:757
27. Otteni JC, Grandhaye N, Dupeyron JP, Gauthier-Lafaye JP (1971) Deux complications fréquentes des cathéters veineux les fausses routes et les perforations vasculaires. Anesth Anal 28:149
28. Puri VK, Carlson RW, Bander JJ, Weil MH (1980) Complications of vascular catheterization in the critically ill. A prospective study. Crit Care Med 8:494
29. Salah MW (1972) Retroperitoneal hemorrhage simulating a strangulated inguinal hernia. Br Med J 4:403
30. Schlossmann D (1973) Thrombogenic properties of vascular catheter materials in vivo. The differences between materials. Acta Radiol Diagn 14:188
31. Schrader J, Bohnsack W, Kaiser H, Eisenhauer T, Kramer P, Köstering H (1982) Antikoagulation bei kontinuierlicher arterio-venöser Hämofiltration (CAVH). In: Kramer P (Hrsg) Arterio-venöse Hämofiltration. Vandenhoeck und Ruprecht, Göttingen, S 67
32. Scribner BH, Buri R, Caner JEZ, Hergstrom R, Burnell JM (1960) The treatment of chronic uremia by means of intermittent hemodialysis. A preliminary report. Trans Am Soc Artif Intern Organs 6:114
33. Seldinger S (1953) Catheter replacement of needle in percutaneous arteriography new technique. Acta Radiol 39:368
34. Shaldon S, Chiandussi L, Higgs B (1961) Hemodialysis by percutaneous catheterization of the femoral artery and vein with regional heparinisation. Lancet 1:857
35. Shah A, Gnoj J, Fisher VJ (1975) Complications of selective coronary arteriography by the Judkins technique and their prevention. Am Heart J 90:353
36. Silverman JF, Wexler L (1976) Complications of percutaneous transfemoral coronary arteriography. Clin Radiol 27:317
37. Sinapius D, Pini J (1973) Über die Lysierbarkeit arterieller Verschlüsse und Stenosen. Vasa 2:139
38. Stamm WE, Colella JJ, Anderson RL, Dixon RE (1975) Indwelling arterial catheters as a source of nosocomial bacteremia. N Engl J Med 292:1099
39. Swift DL, Lingeman JE, Baum WC (1980) Spontaneous retroperitoneal hemorrhage. A diagnostic challenge. J Urol 123:577
40. Thompson JE (1974) Acute peripheral arterial occlusions. N Engl J Med 290:950
41. Vanichayakornkul S, Cioffi RF, Harper E, O'Connell JMB, Shalhoub RJ (1974) Spontaneous retroperitoneal hematoma, a complication of hemodialysis. JAMA 230:1164
42. Vaz AJ (1979) Spontaneous retroperitoneal bleeding during acute hemodialysis. South Med J 72:1631
43. Wappenschmidt J (1966) Retrograde Arteriographie des Vertebraliskreislaufes. Röntgenblätter 19:293
44. Yonker JE (1965) Prevention of complications during vascular opacification studies. Radiol Clin North Am 3:453

Venovenous Ultrafiltration and Hemofiltration Via the Internal Jugular Vein Using a Double-Head Pump – A Simple Emergency Procedure

R. Bambauer and G. A. Jutzler

Despite technical improvements in treatment with hemodialysis, the transient vascular access is not yet solved satisfactorily. With subcutaneous implantation of heterologous and synthetic vascular grafts, besides the Cimino-shunt, very useful connections can be made. However, their life span is curbed by complications that could occur such as thrombosis, formation of aneurisms, bleeding, infections, etc.

Temporary vascular access still involves considerable problems. We therefore investigated new methods of access and introduced the catheterization of the v. cava superior through the v. jugularis interna, using a large-bore catheter [1]. In the area of intensive care medicine, an increasing number of diseases are encountered involving severe cardiac and pulmonary insufficiency accompanied by acute hyperhydration, with or without electrolyte imbalances, rhythm disorders, and cardiovascular shock. Rapid but careful dehydration is required when all known conservative methods of treatment, such as diuretics, fail. Further medical treatment seems reasonable only after successful fluid removal.

With the method of percutaneous puncture of the internal jugular vein and insertion of a large-bore catheter, a simplified venovenous ultrafiltration/hemofiltration may be started under emergency conditions utilizing a double-head pump according to the "single needle" method.

Method

The v. jug. int. runs from the base of the cranium in close proximity to the a. carotis into the truncus brachiocephalicus. Ventrally it is covered by the m. sternocleidomastoideus; dorsomedially it is adjacent to the vasomotor nerve trunk. Vein, artery, and nerve are enveloped by the fascia media colli (Fig. 1) to which they are fused, causing the v. jug. int. to be spread out in the fascia and the lumen to be always open. It runs subcutaneously between the two lobes of the m. sternocleidomastoideus only in the lower part. The diameter in adults is approximately 15 mm and expands caudally. The right jugular vein is somewhat larger than the left one and forms an almost straight connection to the right atrium.

Since Hermoshura et al. [9] first described percutaneous puncture of the v. jug. int. in 1965, 17 different methods of puncturing this vessel have been reported to

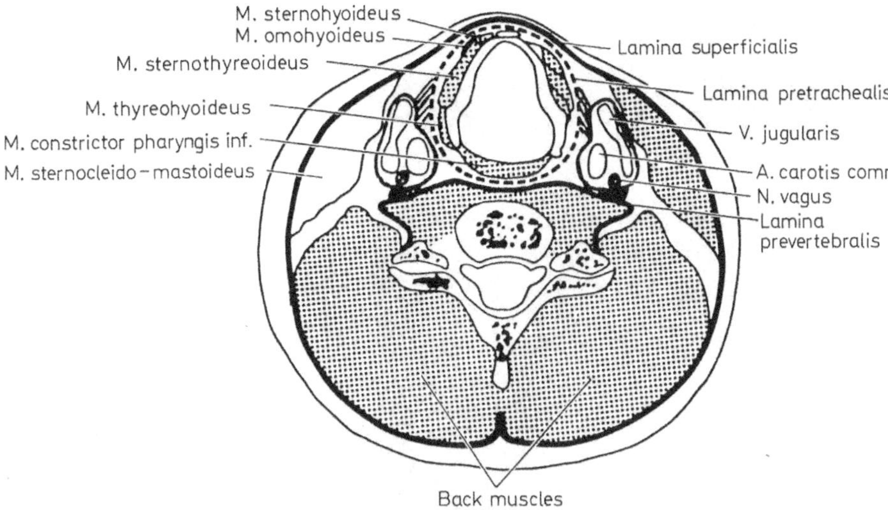

Fig. 1. Schematic cross section of the neck (from Born, P; *Topographic Anatomy*, Gustav Fischer, Stuttgart 1972)

date [3]. They are all distinguished by high success and low complication rates. We preferred to use the right vein; on the left side, the ductus thoracicus and the higher situated pleural dome could entail additional complications. Catheterization has to be performed under aseptic conditions (thorough disinfection of the neck area, sterile draping, sterile gown, and gloves). The patient rests in slight "Trendelenburg" position (20°) in order to increase venous pressure and thereby minimize the likelihood of an air embolus.

After local anesthesia and a small incision in the skin we proceed percutaneously through the upper tip of the triangle formed by the caput sternale and caput claviculare of the m. sternocleidomastoideus.

A "Braun cannula" is pushed at a 30° angle to the skin surface to the medial edge of the caput claviculare after palpation of the course of the carotid artery. The v. jugularis interna is found at a depth of approximately 3–4 cm. Often aspiration of blood is only possible after the needle is slowly pulled back since the vessel walls of the jugular vein collapse when the cannula is pushed in. After successful puncture, the Seldinger technique is used for insertion of the indwelling catheter. When the catheter is pushed in, the resistance of the fascia media colli has to be often overcome with slight force. The location of the catheter tip should be confirmed by X-ray (Fig. 2). In order to avoid radiation exposure, the catheter tip may be located with an intraatrial electrocardiogram fed through the catheter [2, 7, 12, 15–17].

Ultrafiltration/hemofiltration is performed with a double-head pump over a hollow fiber diafilter. One pump draws the venous blood from the catheter and pushes it through the diafilter into an adjacent air trap. Once this is filled with the predetermined volume of blood, the pump shuts off and the second pump moves this blood through the venous line through Y-tubing back to the patient

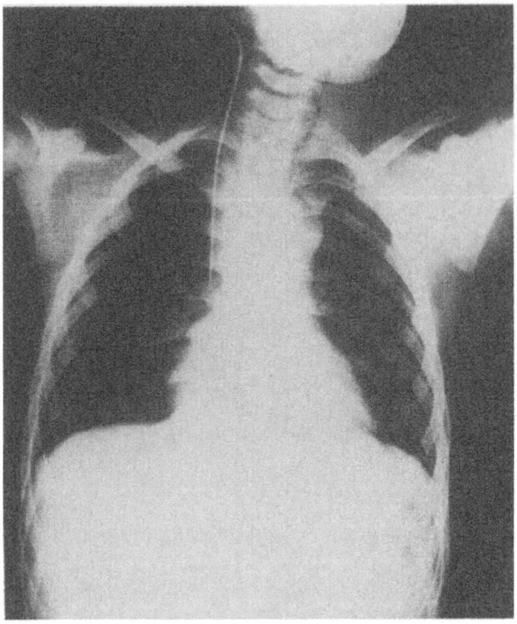

Fig. 2. X-ray of the positioned Shaldon catheter

(Fig. 3). The double-head pump works according to the principle of pressure and volume control. The system is safeguarded by a combined air and blood level detector and a volumetric control. The discontinuous mode of operation of both pumps causes a constant variation in flow and pressure. The pressure of the venous back flow is controlled by the second pump. This means that high pressure in the hollow fiber membrane, which would otherwise be needed for blood back flow, can be avoided. The main advantages of the double pump system are:

1. A rather large volume flows through the diafilter without the maximum pressure exceeding the safety limits.
2. The mean pressure in the diafilter can be adjusted to each required condition.

For venovenous "single needle" ultrafiltration/hemofiltration, the determinants of the filtration rate are: speed of the roller pumps or pressure inside the capillaries (+150–+350 mmHg) and negative pressure on the filtrate side (0–150 mmHg).

In this way the system can be regulated individually and adapted to every situation. The desired filtrate volume is determined prior to each treatment. The clinical situation determines the filtration rate. Consequently, the duration of treatment varies; depending on filtration rate and volume, treatment in our patients lasted from 30 min to 4 h. In case of hypotensive circulatory conditions already prior to onset we fill the diafilter and tubing system with 5% human albumin solution or substitute with a commercial hemofiltration solution by means of a third pump, usually at a substitution rate of 15–20 ml/min less than the fil-

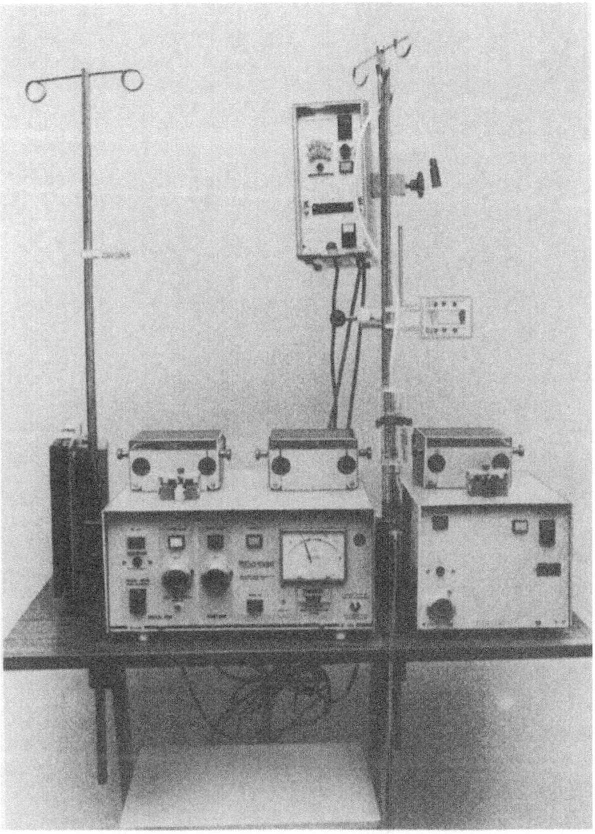

Fig. 3. Simplified ultrafiltration/hemofiltration system consisting of double-head pump and substitution pump

tration rate. This allows gentle removal of as much plasma water from the patient as necessary.

As a rule, heparin is administered intermittently. We inject a bolus of 1000–2000 IU heparin and monitor the coagulation time after 30–60 min. If necessary, an additional 500–1000 IU heparin are given; 2000–3000 IU are usually sufficient for one treatment. Low dose heparinization (100–300 IU heparin/h) is used to keep the catheter open between treatments.

Our Observations

Puncture of the right v. jug. interna and insertion of a Shaldon catheter was performed on 182 patients for acute dialysis. Puncture was necessary for 95 patients because of acute exacerbation of chronically compensated kidney insufficiency and for 87 patients because of acute renal failure.

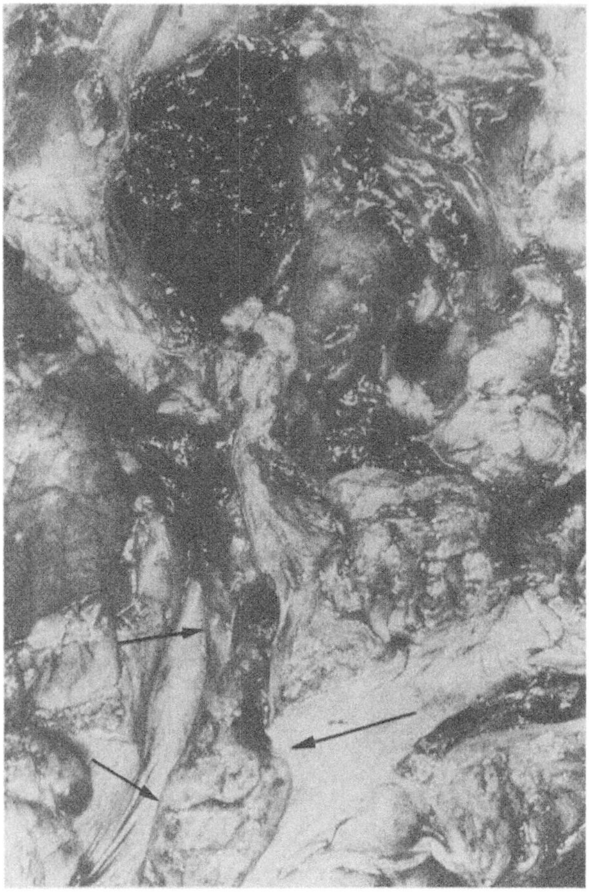

Fig. 4. Thrombosis in the v. subclavia and v. jugularis interna in a 79-year-old female patient

With regard to the catheter, we observed the following complications: The a. carotis was punctured inadvertently in four patients. Through immediate compression, significant bleeding was avoided.

At indwelling times in excess of 14 days we saw infected skin at the puncture site in 15 cases. In four patients the catheter was removed because they developed fever. For the remaining 11 patients local use of antibiotics was sufficient to heal the infection; therefore the catheters were left in place. In four other patients the catheter had to be removed prematurely also because of a temperature between 38.5 and 39.5 °C. The puncture sites, however, were not infiltrated and the skin smears confirmed no pathogens.

Thrombosis was observed in the area of the neck and the subclavian veins in a 74- and a 79-year-old female patient. Both patients had an indwelling peripheral subclavian catheter on the right side, which presumably initiated the thrombosis that eventually advanced through the Shaldon catheter into the jugular vein. In

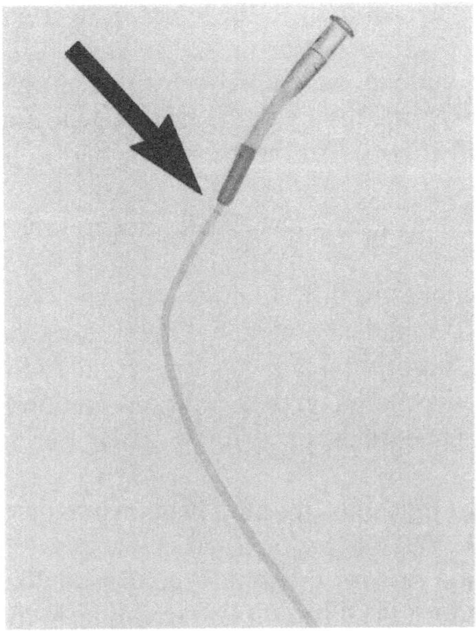

Fig. 5. Shaldon catheter pinched off at the entrance

Table 1. Veno-venous hemofiltration: Therapy and course

Age/ year	Diagnosis	Vascular access		No HF	Diafilter Amicon	Filtrate volume/HF (ml)	Course
		V. jug. i.	v. subcl.				
63	AH, LE	+		7	30	2000–3000	+
51	AH by CRF	+	–	8	30	1000–1500	+
72	AH by ARF	+	–	7	20	500–3100	+
24	ARF, DIC	–	+	5	20	1000–2500	–
30	ARF by Sepsis	+		4	20	1000–1500	+
30	ARF, postop.	+	–	3	30	1500–2000	–
53	ARF, postop.	+	–	7	20	500–2500	–
28	ARF, postop.	+	–	4	20	1000–1500	+
25	ARF by Sepsis	–	+	2	20	1500–2300	+
64	ARF, postop.	+	–	3	30	1000–1500	+
26	PCC, LE	+	–	1	40	3000	–
27	ARF, DIC, postop.	+	–	6	30	500–1500	–
67	ARF, postop.	+	–	6	30	500–1500	+
28	ARF, LE	+	–	6	20	1200–3500	–
38	AH by CRF	+	–	6	40	1400–6900	+
59	LE, AHF	+	–	1	30	2500	–
49	ARF, postop.	+	–	2	30	1500–2000	–
41	AH by CRF	+	–	6	30	1500–2000	+
62	AH by CRF	+	–	4	30	1000–2000	+
45	AH by CRF	+	–	6	20	800–2000	+

AH: acute hyperhydration, LE: lung edema, CRF: chronic renal failure, ARF: acute renal failure, DIC: disseminated intravascular coagulation, PCC: decompensated primary congestive cardiomyopathy, AHF: acute hepatic failure

both patients the Shaldon catheters indwelled only 7 days, and the lumen of the right v. jug. int. was not occluded completely, contrary to the lumen of the right v. subclavia (Fig. 4).

Problems caused by defective catheter material were observed with eight patients. There were five cases of defective silicone tubing at the entrance site and in three cases the catheter was pinched off (Fig. 5). All these catheters had to be removed or exchanged.

The Luer connection slipped off the venous catheter in a female patient, resulting in low-degree air embolism.

In 18 of the 182 patients simple venovenous ultrafiltration/hemofiltration was performed using a double-head pump. In two patients, an indwelling v. subclavia catheter was used. Between one and eight filtration treatments were required for removal of 500–6900 ml of plasma water, depending on the hydration conditions of these patients. In five cases the blood pressure dropped 70–90 mmHg during hemofiltration (Table 1).

By immediately reducing and balancing fluid substitution, this pressure drop could quickly be corrected.

No significant variations in the filtration rate for different hematocrit values were observed. It was always possible to adjust the filtration rate according to the clinical situation. If it was necessary to remove more than 1.5 l per treatment the filtration was kept below 18 ml/min.

Discussion

Based on various publications [3–5, 10] and on our own experiences obtained from 182 patients, we have reached the following conclusion:

Because of the low complication rate and the favorable puncturing possibilities, the access route through the v. jug. int. seems to be the safest access to the v. cava superior and it is distinctly superior to the puncture of the femoral artery [6, 11, 13, 14] and also the subclavian vein [8, 18]. According to Burri et al. [3] the most dangerous complication is the puncture of the a. carotis; the frequency of this complication is 0.61%. If this occurs inadvertently compression for 5 min is usually sufficient to stop the bleeding.

In our patient population inadvertent puncturing of the a. carotis occurred four times (2.2%). No cases of embolism, thrombosis, septicemia, or death were reported in the literature. Perforations, hydro- or pneumothorax are only mentioned in particular cases.

Particular attention should be paid to the fact that the v. jug. int. is always filled with blood and can be punctured even during shock.

Therefore the method is suitable also for high-risk patients. After-bleeding and hematomas caused by puncture are rare since the blood pressure in the vein is lower than in the surrounding tissue. The size of the vessel permits easy insertion of large-bore catheters. Indwelling times of 8–10 weeks and more are not rare.

Since thrombosis was only experienced with two elderly patients, we recommend indwelling times for such patients of less than 4 weeks.

In contrast to this, more complications are seen with the catheterization of the femoral vein [6, 11, 13, 14], particularly with repeated punctures of the same patient, which certainly causes more injury to the vessel wall. Also, the patient has to remain immobile because of the danger of perforation; but patients with v. jug. int. catheters are free to move.

The above-described percutaneous puncture of the v. jug. int. for catheterization of the superior vena cava with a Shaldon catheter proved to be a suitable, rapid method of connection for hemodialysis, hemofiltration, hemoperfusion, or plasma filtration treatment. This access is particularly suited for simplified hemofiltration via a diafilter and double-head pump. Simplified venovenous ultrafiltration/hemofiltration is indicated by acute overhydration resistant to high doses of furosemide caused by (a) acute renal failure, (b) severe congestive heart failure, and (c) hemodilution after cardiopulmonary bypass. In cases of circulatory collapse, the described vascular access has the advantage that the lower third of the catheter lies at the transition of the superior vena cava to the atrium, where sufficient blood supply allows a mean blood-flow rate as high as 400 ml/min by means of the double-head pumps.

If the patient already has an indwelling central venous catheter, it can be used as a splint for the insertion of a Shaldon catheter without new puncture.

Between hemofiltrations the Shaldon catheter can be used for infusions, transfusions, and for measurements of central venous pressure.

Considering the described precautions for puncture such as sterility, as little injury to the vessel wall as possible, and correct positioning of the catheter tip, this method is very successful when performed by a physician experienced in catheterization. In our opinion only in cases of infection at the point of entry, or uncertain anatomical conditions such as expanded struma or tumors in the neck area, should alternative access routes such as the subclavian vein or the femoral vein be considered.

References

1. Bambauer R, Jutzler GA (1981) Jugularis-interna Punktion zur Shaldon-Katheterisierung. Ein neuer Zugang für akute Hämodialysen. Nieren- und Hochdruckkrankh 9:109
2. Bambauer R, Jutzler GA (1980) Lagekontrolle großlumiger zentraler Venenkatheter mittels Elektrokardiographie. Intensivmed Prax 17:312
3. Burri C, Henkemeyer H, Pässler HH (1976) Technik und Gefahren des Cava-Katheters. Infusionsther 3:174
4. Daily PO, Pandall P, Griepp RB, Sumway NE (1970) Percutaneous internal jugular vein cannulation. Arch Surg 101:534
5. Defalque RJ (1974) Percutaneous catheterization of the internal jugular vein. Anesth Analg 53:116
6. Fuchs HJ, Jenett G, Klehr U, Richter G, Wildbrandt R, Frotscher U (1977) Die perkutane Punktion der Vena femoralis zur Hämodialysebehandlung. Dtsch Med Wochenschr 102:1280
7. Götz E (1979) Stellungnahme zum Beitrag von F.-J. Loers: Erfahrungen mit dem intrakardialen EKG zur Lagekontrolle des Cava-Katheters. Anaesth Intensivmed 20:68
8. Hennemann H (1978) Die Vena subclavia – Akutdialysezugang der ersten Wahl? Intensivmed Prax 15:235
9. Hermoshura B, Vanagsand L, Dickey MW (1965) Measurement of pressure during intravenous therapy. JAMA 181:1965

10. Jernigan WR, Gardner WC, Mohr MM, Milburn JL (1971) The internal jugular vein for access to central venous system. JAMA 97:97–98
11. Kjellstrand OM, Merino GE, Mauer SM, Casali R, Buselmeier TJ (1975) Complications of percutaneous femoral vein catheterization for hemodialysis. Clin Nephrol 4:38
12. Klinnert U (1977) Transvenöse Elektrodenkatheter als Hilfsmittel zur Diagnostik. Diagnostik 10:127
13. Kramer P, Langescheid C, Matthaei D, Rieger J (1977) Behandlung der diuretikaresistenten Überwässerung mit arterio-venöser Hämofiltration. Dustri, München
14. Lederle RM, Portmann HJ, Wermuth G (1979) Erfahrungen mit einem modifizierten Femoraliskatheter zur Hämodialysebehandlung. Intensivmed Prax 16:258
15. Loers FJ (1978) Erfahrungen mit dem intrakardinalen EKG zur Lagekontrolle des Cavakatheters. Anästh Intensivmed 19:495
16. Niemann W, Koch D (1976) Lagebestimmung zentralvenöser Katheter durch intrakardinale EKG-Ableitung. Prak Anästhesie 11:31
17. Urthaler F, Halter J (1971) Central venous catheter used recording intracardiac electrocardiagram. Br Heart J 33:275
18. Wetzels E, Musselmann L (1980) Dialysebehandlung des akuten Nierenversagens. Intensivmed Prax 17:34

Comparison Between Scribner Shunt and Femoral Catheters as Vascular Access for Continuous Arteriovenous Hemofiltration

C. J. Olbricht, H. J. Schurek, S. Tytul, C. Müller, and H. Stolte

Introduction

The treatment of patients with postoperative acute renal failure (ARF) by hemodialysis still bears major problems. Especially in the increasing number of patients with postoperative ARF accompanied with failure or impaired function of other organ systems, the duration of hemodialysis and fluid withdrawal are often limited by severe hypotension. In addition, the rapid changes of serum parameters and fluid balance due to intermittent hemodialysis are unphysiologic and may be detrimental to these severely ill patients [9].

The more physiologic continuous arteriovenous hemofiltration (CAVH), a method recently developed by Kramer and co-workers [11–13] may offer an alternative and improved method of treatment for patients with postoperative ARF. Therefore, the first goal of the present study was to evaluate the quality and efficiency of CAVH in patients with postoperative ARF.

As the standard vascular access, Kramer and co-workers introduced the percutaneous catheterization of the femoral artery and vein with special large-bore catheters without lateral perforations [7]. With appropriate technique of catheterization and with proper handling, the rate of complications was as low as 0.7%, even during long-term continuous catheterization of up to 50 days [7], provided the patients were strictly immobilized. However, in several patients the vascular access by femoral artery and vein cannulas is limited or impossible. In a substantial number of patients subjected to open-heart surgery the arterial input catheter of the cardiopulmonary bypass is placed in the femoral artery and the other femoral artery may be reserved for a postoperative insertion of the intraaortic balloon pump. In elderly patients with femoroiliac occlusive disease and in patients after aortofemoral bypass surgery, the cannulation of the femoral artery is also not possible. Patients of both postoperative groups have a high incidence of ARF [1, 3, 8, 19] and treatment by CAVH may be indicated. Therefore, we applied Scribner shunts as vascular access for CAVH and the second goal of this study was to evaluate the efficiency of CAVH with Scribner shunt as vascular access in comparison with femoral artery and vein catheters.

Methods

Patients and Clinical Background

Forty-one patients with postoperative ARF and multiorgan failure were included in this study. All were treated at least 48 h and exclusively by CAVH to allow an assessment of the method; 34 patients had a Scribner shunt as vascular access (group A) and in 7 patients percutaneous catheters in femoral vein and artery were used as vascular access (group B). As shown in Table 1 the clinical background of both groups was similar. All patients had undergone major surgery and/or polytrauma.

Technique of CAVH

In 28 patients, the vessel tips of the Scribner shunt were implanted in the posterior tibial artery and the vena saphena. Because of occlusive arterial disease on the lower leg in six patients the vessel tips were implanted in the radial artery and in a lower arm vein. Since no differences were found in both groups, all 34 patients were referred to one group. In the remaining seven patients the femoral artery and vein were catheterized with special large-bore cannulas (Vygon, Aachen, FRG) as recently described by Gröne and Kramer [7]. The technique of CAVH was performed according to Kramer and co-workers [11–13] with slight modifications. Amicon-30 filters were used (Amicon, Lexington, MA). The anticoagulation was started with 15 IU heparin/kg body weight and was maintained with individual doses of heparin of between 250 and 1250 IU/h to keep the whole-blood partial thromboplastin time (PTT) 50% above baseline values. The whole-blood PTT was measured at the bedside using the method of Farrell and co-workers [5].

The filtrate was collected and measured in intervals of 30–60 min. The fluid balance was maintained by continuous infusion of substitution fluid into the venous line of the hemofilter. The substitution fluid contained (in mmol/l): Na^+ 142, Ca^{++} 2.0, Mg^{++} 0.75, Cl^- 103, and lactate 44.5. CAVH was continued until recovery of renal function.

Table 1. Clinical background of 34 patients with Scribner shunt (Group A) and of seven patients with femoral artery and vein catheters (Group B)

	Number of patients			
	Total	On respirator	Hypercatabolic[a]	Adrenergic support[b]
Group A Scribner shunt	34	33	26	34
Group B Femoral catheters	7	7	5	7

[a] Daily net production of urea >0.36 g per kg body weight [4]

[b] Continuous need for dopamine and/or dobutamine to maintain systolic blood pressure at or above 100 mmHg

Measurement of Blood Pressure and Blood Flow

In eight patients of group A (Scribner shunt) and in the seven patients of group B (femoral artery and vein catheter) the mean arterial blood pressure was measured repeatedly by intraarterial catheters using a Statham pressure transducer (Statham Gould P 23 DB). Simultaneously in the same patient the blood-flow rate into the hemofilter was measured at the arterial tube with a directional Doppler ultrasonic device (DelaLande Electronics, type DU 01000). The calibration of the device revealed a standard deviation of $\pm 5\%$. During the measurements of blood pressure and blood flow the filtration rate was determined.

Analytical Methods

Serum K^+, Na^+, Cl^-, creatinine, and urea were measured daily by routine methods using a multichannel Technicon autoanalyzer (SMAC). Protein was determined using Lowries method [15]. Standard bicarbonate was calculated by routine blood gas analysis. The hematocrit was measured daily.

Statistics

The results were given as mean values $\pm$ standard deviation. The significance of differences was tested using Student's *t*-test or a Wilcoxon rank-sum test when appropriate. *P* values of less than 0.05 were considered significant.

Results

Course of Treatment

The duration of treatment ranged from 53 to 1375 h with a total treatment time of 279 days in group A, and ranged from 72 to 168 h with a total treatment time of 31 days in group B. Included in this time were minor interruptions for surgery, resuscitation, and filter change. The average running time of one filter was 43 h in group A and 44 h in group B. Nine patients of group A survived and had a recovery of renal function. In group B, two patients had a recovery of renal function but finally only one patient survived. No death was related to uremia, hypervolemia, or hyperkalemia. Gastrointestinal bleeding, which was the major complication, occurred in seven patients of group A and in three patients of group B. However, interruptions of CAVH were necessary only in two patients for two days.

Course of Creatinine, Urea, Potassium, and Bicarbonate

Group A

In the majority of patients (30) a steady-state serum creatinine slightly below 500 μmol/l was achieved after 72 h of CAVH (Fig. 1). The steady-state serum urea concentration was about 38 mmol/l (Fig. 1).

As shown in Table 2, serum potassium and standard bicarbonate were in the normal range during more than 90% of all treatment days.

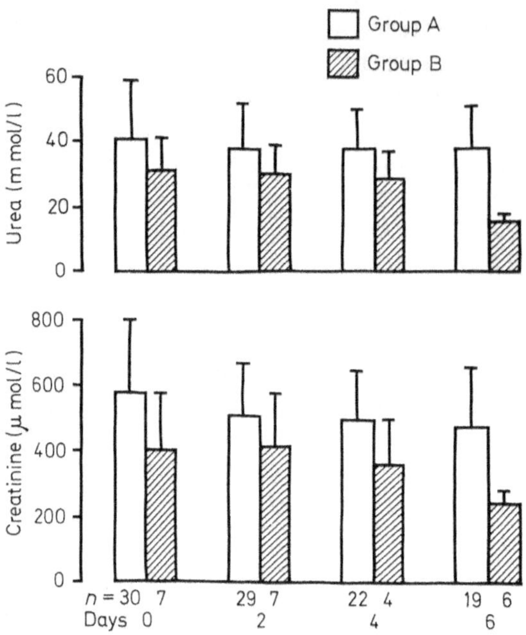

Fig. 1. Course of serum creatinine and serum urea during the first 6 days of CAVH. The values are means ± standard deviation; *n* denotes the number of patients. *Open bars* represent the values of 30 patients with Scribner shunt (group A) with sufficient treatment of ARF and a filtration rate of 14.2±4.6 l/24 h. *Hatched bars* represent the values of the seven patients of group B with femoral artery and vein catheters. The filtration rate was 16.6±6.9 l/24 h

Table 2. Serum concentrations of potassium and standard bicarbonate during CAVH

	Days of treatment	
Serum concentration mmol/l	Group A[a]	Group B[b]
K^+		
<6	236	31
6–7	20	0
>7	2	0
HCO_3^-		
14–20	16	6
20–27	237	18
28–32	5	7

[a] The 30 patients of group A with a filtration rate of 14.2±4.6 l/24 h; total treatment time was 258 days
[b] All seven patients of group B; total treatment time was 31 days; filtration rate was 16.6±6.9 l/24 h

In these 30 patients the filtration rate was 14.2±4.6 l per 24 h (= 9.8 ml/min).

In a minority of patients (4) the serum concentrations of creatinine and of urea increased continuously to above 500 μmol/l and above 40 mmol/l, respectively. Serum potassium was elevated above 6 mmol/l in all four patients during 10 days.

The total treatment time of these four patients was 21 days and the filtration rate was 9.9±3.2 l per 24 h (6.8±2.2 ml/min). This filtration rate was lower than the 14.2 l/24 h observed for the majority of patients ($P<0.01$). The treatment course for these four patients was characterized by frequent interruptions due to repeated surgery, resuscitation, and numerous filter changes.

Group B

The course of creatinine and urea in serum during the first six days of CAVH is depicted in Fig. 1. The mean values of both parameters were markedly lower than in patients with CAVH and Scribner shunt as vascular access. No patient had increasing concentrations of urea and creatinine. The filtration rate was 16.6±6.9 l/24 h (11.5±4.8 ml/min). This is slightly but not significantly higher than the 14.2 l/24 h observed for 30 patients of group A. As shown in Table 2, the serum concentration of potassium was within the physiologic range during all treatment days. The standard bicarbonate was higher than 20 mmol/l during more than 80% of all treatment days (Table 2).

Blood Pressure, Blood Flow, and Filtration Rate

CAVH with appropriate fluid substitution did not influence the blood pressure of the patients. As shown in Fig. 2, the relationship between mean arterial blood pressure up to 90 mmHg and filter blood flow was linear in both groups. The *X*-intercept of both lines was close to 20 mmHg. The slope of the regression line of group B was 1.88 times higher than the slope of regression line A. In practical terms, this means that at a given blood pressure the blood flow into the filter was almost twice as high in patients with femoral artery and vein cannulas than in patients with Scribner shunts.

The relationship between blood flow and filtration rate was linear in both groups with very similar regression lines (Figs. 3 and 4).

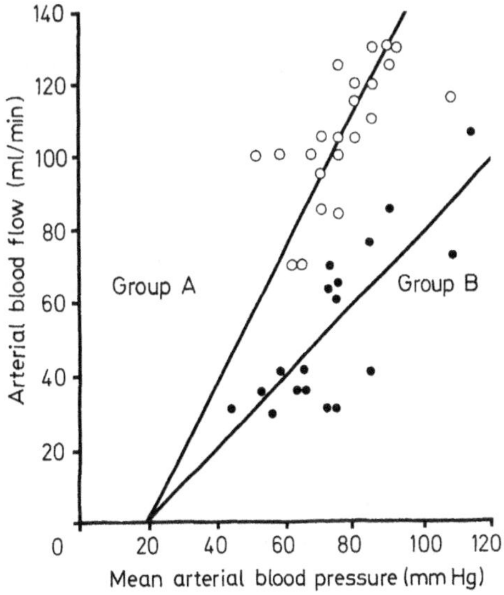

Fig. 2. Blood flow into the hemofilter (Amicon-30) in relation to mean arterial blood pressure of patients in groups A and B. Regression line A was calculated from 18 measurements in eight patients with Scribner shunt. Slope = 0.99; intercept = −19.2; correlation coefficient = 0.64. Regression line B was calculated from 22 measurements in the seven patients with femoral artery catheter. Slope = 1.86; intercept = −37.1; correlation coefficient = 0.84

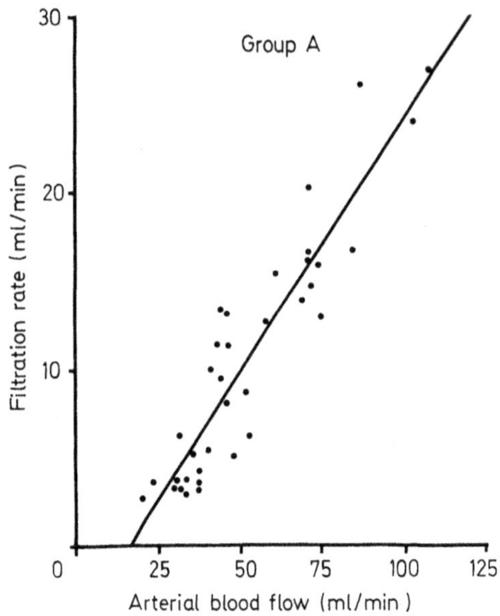

Fig. 3. Filtration rate in relation to blood flow into the hemofilter (Amicon-30) during CAVH with Scribner shunt (group A). The regression line was calculated from 38 measurements in eight patients. Slope = 0.29; intercept = −4.6; correlation coefficient = 0.93

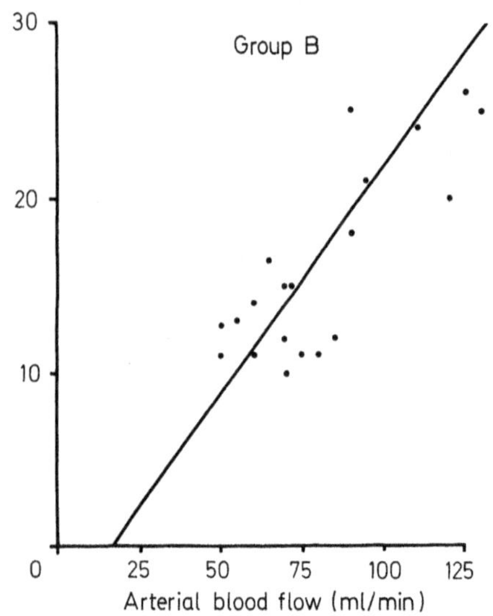

Fig. 4. Filtration rate in relation to blood flow into the hemofilter (Amicon-30) during CAVH with femoral artery and vein catheter (group B). The regression line was calculated from 22 measurements in seven patients. Slope = 0.26; intercept = −4.2; correlation coefficient = 0.84

The hematocrit ranged from 27% to 42% in group A and from 29% to 42% in group B. The mean serum protein was 55 ± 5 g% in group A and 57 ± 5 g% in group B.

Discussion

The routine vascular access for CAVH is the percutaneous large-bore cannula in femoral artery and vein. However, in several patients after open-heart surgery, in patients after aortofemoral bypass surgery, and in patients with femoroiliac occlusive disease, the cannulation of the femoral artery is not feasible. Both groups of postoperative patients have a high incidence of ARF, mostly associated with failures of other organ systems and unstable hemodynamics. ARF in these patients is a typical indication for CAVH since a sufficient intermittent hemodialysis frequently is not possible [11–13, 17]. Therefore, we performed the CAVH with Scribner shunts in lower leg and forearm as an alternative to femoral artery and vein catheters. The results of the present study clearly demonstrate that a sufficient treatment of patients with ARF is possible with CAVH and Scribner shunts as vascular access. In 30 of 34 patients in group A, a steady-state creatinine was achieved at about 500 μmol/l. This corresponds to a creatinine clearance of about 10 ml/min and is an acceptable value. Serum urea was comparatively higher with a mean value of 38 mmol/l after the first 2 days of CAVH. However, more than 70% of the patients were hypercatabolic according to the definition of Cameron et al. [4] with a daily urea production exceeding 0.36/kg body weight (Table 1). Taking this into consideration, the steady-state concentration of urea is reasonable even in comparison with results of intermittent hemodialysis. In addition, the constant values of serum urea and other serum components during CAVH at steady state may be less harmful to the patient, even at somewhat higher concentrations, than are the rapid changes of serum parameters and fluid balance during intermittent hemodialysis [9].

Serum potassium was within the normal range for >90% of the treatment days by CAVH alone and additional measures to lower serum potassium had to be applied during 22 days only. This represents a remarkably good control of serum potassium despite the high rate of release of intracellular potassium in most hypercatabolic patients.

Standard bicarbonate was measured to characterize the acid-base balance. Again, during >90% of all treatment days a normal standard bicarbonate was maintained. This allows two important conclusions. First, the infused lactate was converted into bicarbonate at a rate sufficient to compensate the bicarbonate loss with the continuous filtration. Second, the filtration rate was sufficient to remove the fixed acid which results from the metabolic production at a rate of 50–100 mEq/day [18] (or even more) in hypercatabolic patients.

In the majority of patients (30) of group A, the mean filtration rate was 14 l/day. This seems to be a sufficient filtration rate to control azotemia in ARF, whereas in the minority of patients (4) a daily filtration of 10 l was insufficient to control azotemia. However, in both groups, the continuous high daily fluid turnover allowed the daily infusion of 3–5 l caloric solutions for total parenteral nutrition without hemodynamic problems or hyperhydration. Especially in the hypercatabolic patients a high parenteral calorie intake is one of the main preconditions for survival [2]. During intermittent hemodialysis or hemofiltration, fluid withdrawal in patients with unstable hemodynamics and multiorgan failure may be limited by severe hemodynamic reactions and sufficient parenteral nutrition may be impossible.

The complication rate was remarkably low. In spite of continuous heparinization, only five minor and two serious bleedings occurred during CAVH. During the serious bleedings CAVH had to be interrupted for 2 days, but no emergency surgery was necessary to stop these gastrointestinal bleedings.

The complication rate was not higher, as far as bleeding is concerned, than reported by others for ARF and hemodialysis [6, 10, 14, 16]. Another complication was shunt thrombosis, which occurred in three patients without signs of pulmonary embolism.

We conclude that in the majority of our patients a sufficient treatment of ARF was possible by CAVH with Scribner shunt. The comparison of CAVH with Scribner shunt and CAVH with femoral artery and vein catheters is somewhat limited in the present study, since group B comprises seven patients only. However, the data regarding the relation of blood pressure, arterial blood flow, and filtration rate are drawn from similar numbers of patients (A, 8; B, 7) in both groups and are worth comparing. In both groups the relationship between filter blood flow and filtration rate was linear. The regression lines had the same *X*-intercept and very similar slopes. This has two implications. First, at a given blood flow, the filtration fractions were not very different. The filtration fraction in this discussion means the relation of filtration rate to blood flow. Second, the filtration fraction increases with higher blood flow in a hyperbolic function with an asymptotic approach to the maximum filtration fraction. The maximum filtration fraction is the slope of the regression lines.

In both groups, the relationship between blood pressure and blood flow was linear, too. However, the different slopes clearly demonstrate that, at a given mean arterial blood pressure, the blood flow into the filter was almost twice as high in group B (with femoral artery catheters) compared with group A (with Sribner shunts). The fact that the relation between blood flow and filtration rate was linear and very similar in both groups, implies that during CAVH with femoral artery and vein cannulas, a much higher filtration rate can be expected at a given blood pressure than during CAVH with Scribner shunt. The explanation for this difference is a lower flow resistance of the femoral artery catheter and the higher blood flow in the arteria femoralis, especially under the infusion of catecholamines.

As expected for group B the mean daily filtration rate was higher than in group A, but the results were not significantly different. The steady-state serum concentrations of creatinine and urea were about 25% lower in group B (Fig. 1).

According to the higher blood flow/blood pressure relation of the femoral cannulas, one would have expected an even higher filtration rate than the measured filtration rate in group B. However, the mean arterial blood pressure was lower in group B. Hence, in patients with lower mean arterial blood pressure one should prefer the femoral catheter technique.

Conclusions and Recommendations

The study clearly demonstrated that CAVH with Scribner shunt as vascular access is an efficient method for treatment of patients with ARF. The major therapeutic goals in treatment of ARF were achieved, namely, control of fluid balance and sufficient fluid withdrawal to allow parenteral hypercaloric nutrition; control of azotemia; control of serum potassium and control of metabolic acid-base balance.

The precondition for a sufficient treatment of ARF with CAVH is an average daily filtration rate of 14 l. The specific patient may need somewhat lower or considerably higher filtration rates, depending on body weight, on extent of hypercatabolism, and on initial serum levels of urea and potassium.

The vascular access by femoral artery and vein catheters should be the first choice whenever possible. The catheters can be easily inserted without time lag and the complication rate is low with appropriate handling [7]. The expected filtration rate and hence the efficiency of treatment is higher at a given blood pressure. This may be important in patients with low blood pressure and instable hemodynamics. However, when the vascular access by femoral vessels is not feasible, one should not hesitate to start CAVH with a Scribner shunt as vascular access. In the overwhelming majority of the patients a sufficient treatment of ARF can be expected. Scribner shunts on both lower leg and forearm are as efficient as vascular access. Three groups of patients should be considered primarily for Scribner shunt: patients after aorta-femoral bypass surgery, patients after open-heart surgery with cardiopulmonary bypass via femoral artery, and patients with iliacofemoral occlusive disease. The management and the precautions during CAVH with Scribner shunt are the same as described in this book for CAVH with femoral vascular access.

References

1. Abel RM, Buckley MJ, Austen WG, Barnett GO, Beck CH, Fischer JE (1976) Etiology, incidence and prognosis of renal failure following cardiac operations. J Thorac Cardiovasc Surg 71:323
2. Abel RM, Beck CH Jr, Abbott WM, Ryan JA Jr, Barnett GO, Fischer JE (1973) Improved survival from acute renal failure after treatment with intravenous essential L-amino acids and glucose. N Engl J Med 28:695
3. Bhat JG, Gluck MC, Lowenstein J, Baldwin DS (1976) Renal failure after open-heart surgery. Ann Intern Med 84:677
4. Cameron JS, Ogg C, Trounce JR (1967) Peritoneal dialysis in hypercatabolic acute renal failure. Lancet I:1188
5. Farrell PC, Ward RA, Schindhelm K, Gotch FA (1978) Precise anticoagulation for routine hemodialysis. J Lab Clin Med 92:164
6. Fischer RP, Polk HC Jr (1975) Changing etiologic patterns of renal insufficiency in surgical patients. Surg Gynecol Obstet 140:85
7. Gröne H-J, Kramer P (1982) Punktion und Langzeitkanülierung der Arteria und Vena femoralis beim Erwachsenen. In: Kramer P (ed) Arterio-venöse Hämofiltration. Nieren- (Ersatz)- Therapie im Intensivpflegebereich. Vandenhoeck und Ruprecht, Göttingen, S 31–46
8. Hilbermann M, Myers BD, Carrie BJ, Derby G, Jamison RL, Stinson EB (1979) Acute renal failure following cardiac surgery. J Thorac Cardiovasc Surg 77:880
9. Kjellstrand CM, Evans RL, Petersen RJ, Shideman JR, von Hartitzsch B, Buselmeier TJ (1975) The "unphysiology" of dialysis: a major cause of dialysis side effects? Kidney Int 7:30
10. Kleinknecht D, Ganaval D (1973) Preventive hemodialysis in acute renal failure: its effect on mortality and morbidity. In: Friedman EA, Eliahou HE (eds) Conference on acute renal failure. DHWE publ (NIH), Washington DC, No. 74, pp 608–616
11. Kramer P, Seegers A, DeVivie R, Matthaei D, Scheler F (1979) Therapeutic potential of hemofiltration. Clin Nephrol 11:145
12. Kramer P, Schrader J, Bohnsack E, Grieben G, Gröne HJ, Scheler F (1981) Continuous arterio-venous hemofiltration (CAVH) – a new kidney replacement therapy. Proc Eur Dial Transplant Assoc 18:743

13. Kramer P, Böhler J, Kehr A, Gröne HJ, Schrader J, Matthaei D, Scheler F (1982) Intensive care (IC) potential of continuous arteriovenous hemofiltration (CAVH). Trans Am Soc Artif Intern Organs 28:28
14. Linton AL (1980) Diagnostic criteria and clinical course of acute renal failure. In: Chapman A (ed) Acute renal failure. Livingstone, London, pp 33–34
15. Lowry OH, Rosebrough NJ, Farr AL, Randall RJ (1951) Protein measurement with the Folin phenol reagent. J Biol Chem 193:265
16. Lunding M, Steiness I, Thaysen JH (1964) Acute renal failure due to tubular necrosis: immediate prognosis and complications. Acta Med Scand 176:103
17. Olbricht C, Müller C, Schurek HJ, Stolte H (1982) Treatment of acute renal failure in patients with multiple organ failure by continuous spontaneous hemofiltration. Trans Am Soc Artif Intern Organs 28:33
18. Relman AS (1964) Renal acidosis and renal excretion of acid in health and disease. Adv Intern Med 12:295
19. Yeboah ED, Petrie A, Pead JL (1972) Acute renal failure and open-heart surgery. Br Med J 1:415

Coagulation – Anticoagulation – Heparin Dosage

Alterations of Blood Coagulation in Patients with Acute Renal Failure

J. Schrader, P. Kramer, H. Köstering, and F. Scheler

Problems of blood coagulation in patients undergoing continuous arteriovenous hemofiltration (CAVH) often complicate the clinical course because the acute illness which leads to acute renal failure (ARF) may induce disseminated intravascular coagulation or consumption coagulopathy [2, 3, 6, 11].

Since fibrin deposits and hyaline thrombi were demonstrated in the kidney by several authors, disseminated intravascular coagulation (DIC) has been attributed to pathogenesis and progression of ARF [6–8, 14].

Further, importance of coagulation disturbances in patients with ARF result from bleeding complications and from problems with anticoagulation.

This chapter considers coagulation disturbances in patients with acute oligoanuric renal failure.

Blood coagulation studies were carried out in 28 patients with acute oligoanuric renal failure. Septicemia, multiple trauma, and abdominal surgery were the most frequent causes of renal failure. Blood samples were taken from the cubital vein in the first 2 days after onset of CAVH. All 28 patients received a mean heparin dose of 10 IU/kg/h. The results of the coagulation and fibrinolysis pa-

Table 1. Coagulation and fibrinolysis parameters in ARF patients and normal persons (mean values ±SD)

	ARF		NP	
PTT (s)	52.9	±12.1	37.3	± 2.9
Thrombin time (s)	22.3	± 4.0	19.2	± 1.5
Heparin (IU/ml)	0.25	± 0.07	< 0.1	
Fibrinogen (mg %)	487.3	±146.3	342.3	±56.4
Fibrin monomers (%)	1.7	± 0.6	< 0.1	
Quick's test (%)	68.6	± 18.8	100,0	± 5.8
Factor VII (%)	63.2	± 14.4	89.2	±12.4
Factor VIII (%)	288.0	± 78.0	122.3	±17.4
Factor XIII (%)	78.0	± 22.0	116.6	±19.9
Antithrombin-III (%)	68.7	± 18.7	105.1	±15.9
Plasminogen (mg %)	7.4	± 2.4	12.4	± 1.4
α_2-Antiplasmin (%)	131.0	± 24.4	106.2	± 6.6
α_2-Antiplasmin/plasminogen	1.7		1.0	
α_1-Antitrypsin (mg %)	408.0	± 52.0	231.2	±41.2

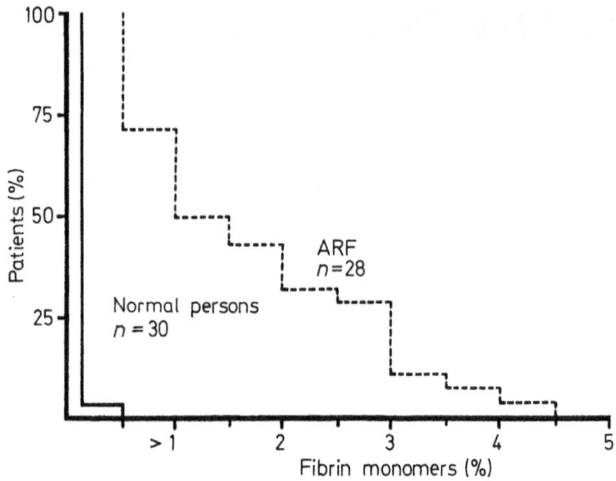

Fig. 1. Fibrin monomers in ARF patients and healthy persons (protamine sulfate test)

rameters are displayed in Table 1 as mean values ± SD, and compared with a control group of normal persons.

As a result of heparin treatment, partial thromboplastin time (PTT) and thrombin time were slightly prolonged. The mean heparin concentration was 0.25 IU/ml. Fibrinogen was elevated distinctly as compared with the control group. Fibrin monomer complexes – measured by protamine sulfate test – demonstrated a massive rise as a result of an increased thrombin generation. The distribution of the single values of all 28 patients is shown in Fig. 1. In 75% of patients fibrin monomers were elevated. Quick's test and factor VII were lowered possibly by consumption or by vitamin K deficiency. Factor VIII was highly elevated as a sign of hypercoagulability or endothelial changes.

The mean value of factor XIII was lowered, which may partly explain the bleeding in some patients.

Antithrombin (AT) III, the most important thrombin inhibitor and heparin cofactor, was diminished due to enhanced consumption. In $^2/_3$ of the patients AT-III activity was found to be below the normal range and in ¼ of the patients even below 55% of AT-III activity (Fig. 2). This acquired AT-III deficiency leads to diminished protection against intravascular coagulation processes and therefore possibly to progression of the underlying disease. Moreover, the necessary heparin therapy would not have been effective in some of these patients. Additionally, this may be the cause of repeated filter clotting. Substitution of AT-III concentrate is a new treatment of this deficiency.

Besides the alterations of coagulation, these patients had lowered plasminogen and an elevated α_2-antiplasmin determined with chromogenic substrates (Fig. 3). The increase of the ratio of α_2-antiplasmin/plasminogen indicates a reduced fibrinolytic activity.

In summary, a severe hypercoagulability and a diminished fibrinolysis was demonstrated in 28 patients with acute oligoanuric renal failure. Thus, it may be speculated that the deposition of fibrin in the kidney may be an important mechanism in the pathogenesis of ARF [2, 6–8, 14, 16]. But DIC does not lead automatically to fibrin deposits in the microcirculation. After the activation of the co-

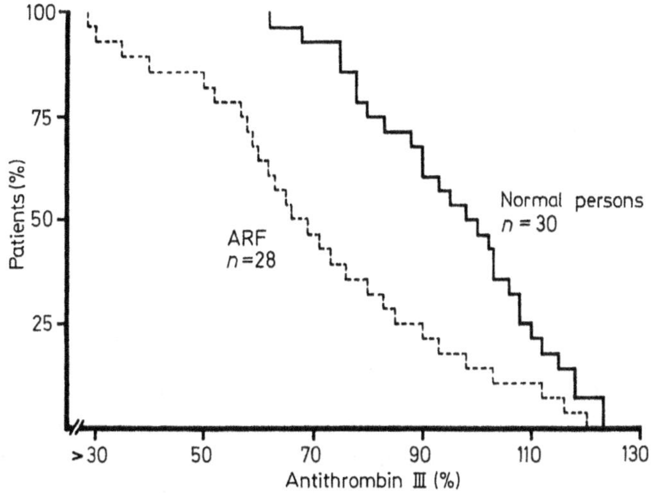

Fig. 2. Antithrombin-III activity in ARF patients and healthy persons (chromogenic substrate S-2238)

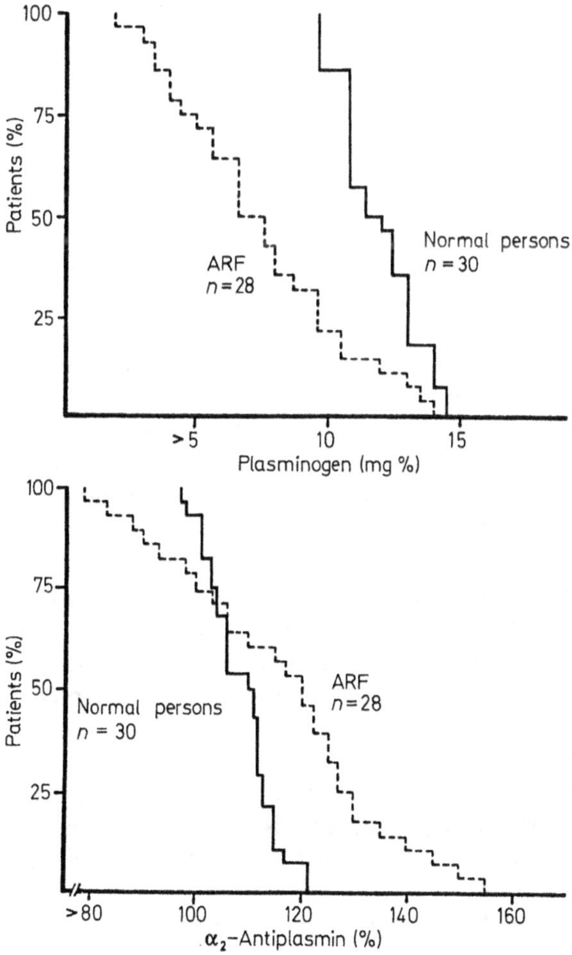

Fig. 3. Plasminogen and α_2-antiplasmin in ARF patients and healthy persons (chromogenic substrate S-2251)

agulation cascade, local factors seem to determine whether or not thrombi develop in the microvessels. Together with the quantity and potency of procoagulants entering the circulation, a diminished fibrinolysis and a blockade of the reticuloendothelial system the two most important defense mechanisms, play an important role in the development of fibrin deposits [2, 8, 9, 14, 16–18].

Deposition of fibrin in the kidney can be mediated through a stimulation of α-adrenoreceptor sites or an action of the renin-angiotensin system [8, 9, 17, 18]. Hoie and Schenk [4] concluded from their experiments that thrombin has a vasoconstrictive activity independent of the glomerular fibrin embolization.

Whitaker et al. [17] demonstrated that angiotensin-II increased the severity of renal damage due to DIC. Further studies have shown that the administration of epinephrine or norepinephrine enhances renal glomerular thrombosis after inducing intravascular clotting [8, 9, 16, 18]. But it is important to note that stimulation of the α-adrenoreceptor sites or the renin-angiotensin system (RAAS) by itself does not cause glomerular thrombosis; the clotting mechanisms must be triggered systemically before [8, 18].

On the other hand, it was shown that fibrin deposits could be prevented by blocking the α-adrenoreceptor sites or by sodium chloride loading [8–10, 17, 18].

Conclusion

Fibrin deposition in the kidney might be inhibited or even prevented by stimuli which interfere with any phase in the complicated sequence of the following reactions:

1. Beginning with the entry of procoagulants into the blood stream through acute illness leading to renal failure
2. processing through the platelet-coagulation-kallikrein-kinin system, thrombin generation, and fibrin formation and ending with
3. fibrin deposition in the microcirculation.

An inhibition of fibrin formation by heparin may prevent renal fibrin deposits. Thus, prophylactic heparin treatment before soluble fibrin is formed, possibly together with a substitution of diminished antithrombin-III, may be advantageous in these patients [4, 12–14, 18]. In the future, perhaps plasminogen and C_1-esterase-inhibitor substitution may gain clinical importance.

Another problem is that critically ill patients with acute renal failure die after an initial recovery as a consequence of multiple organ failure, often after a longlasting course. It has been reported recently that measurements of the coagulation cascade, of the fibrinolysis, and of the kallikrein-kinin system may help to predict the prognosis for these patients [1, 5, 15].

Several reports have focused on low antithrombin-III, low plasma levels of prekallikrein, kinin inhibition, low plasminogen, and low factor XII as indicators of fatal outcome in intensive care patients [1, 5, 15]. This is supported by our own results: None of our patients with an antithrombin-III below 60% and a plasminogen level below 5 mg/dl survived.

In addition, disturbances of blood coagulation may complicate the clinical course through bleeding complications caused by consumption coagulopathy. In addition to DIC, uremic thrombopathy and (in some patients) a lowered factor XIII may promote bleeding in patients with acute renal failure.

Further alteration of the coagulation system may occur by the extracorporeal circulation of the CAVH. Therefore, a comprehensive analysis of the coagulation system and necessary specific substitution therapy should be carried out before starting CAVH. In this way an effective heparin treatment is achieved and the danger of bleeding complications diminished.

References

1. Aasen AO, Ruud TE, Kierulf P, Vaage J, Strömme JH, Aune S (1983) Monitoring of critically ill patients using automated chromogenic petide substrate assays. Thromb Haemost 50:181
2. Clarkson AR, Mac Donald MK, Fuster V, Cush JD, Robson JS (1970) Glomerular coagulation in acute ischaemic renal failure. Q J Med 39:585
3. Crisnic I, Cucuianu M, Manasia M, Uza G (1971) Disseminated intravascular coagulation and acute renal failure. Thromb Haemost 26:332
4. Hoie J, Schenk WG (1972) Experimental intravascular coagulation: impairment of renal blood flow following thrombin infusion in the dog. J Trauma 12:302
5. Kierulf P, Aasen AO, Aune S, Godal HC, Ruud TE, Vaage J (1982) Chromogenic peptide substrate assays in patients with multiple trauma. Acta Chir Scand [Suppl] 509:69
6. Kincaid-Smith P (1972) Coagulation and renal disease. Kidney Int 2:183
7. Kincaid-Smith P (1973) The role of coagulation in the obliteration of glomerular capillaries. Perspect Nephrol Hypertens 1 PT2:877–890
8. Mc Kay DG (1973) Blood coagulation and renal disease. Perspect Nephrol Hypertens 1 PT2:771–807
9. Mc Kay DG, Whitaker AN, Cruse V (1969) Studies of catecholamine shock. An experimental model of microangiophatic hemolysis. Am J Pathol 56:177
10. Rammer L, Gerdin B (1975) Protection against the impairment of renal function after intravascular coagulation in the rat kidney by increased ingestion of sodium chloride. Nephron 14:433
11. Schrader J, Köstering H, Kaiser H, Kramer P, Scheler F (1981) Blood coagulation disturbances during oliguria and polyuria of acute renal failure in man. Thromb Haemost 46:352
12. Schrader J, Köstering H, Kramer P, Scheler F (1982) Antithrombin III substitution in dialysis dependent renal insufficiency. Dtsch Med Wochenschr 48:1847
13. Schrader J, Köstering H, Scheler F (1983) Clinical relevance on determination of Antithrombin III. Laboratoriumsblätter 33:87
14. Schuster HP, Long MW, Blair J, Sedensky JA, Mammen EF (1980) The influence of disseminated intravascular coagulation on renal function after experimental hemorrhagic shock. Resuscitation 8:3
15. Smith-Erichsen N, Aasen AO, Amundsen E (1982) Treatment of sepsis in the surgical patient evaluated by means of chromogenic peptide substrate assays. Acta Chir Scand [Suppl] 509:33
16. Wardle EN (1976) The functional role of intravascular coagulation in renal disease. Scot Med J 21:83
17. Whitaker AN (1973) Interaction of angiotensin with disseminated intravascular coagulation. Am J Pathol 72:1
18. Whitaker AN, Mc Kay DG, Csavossy J (1969) I. Disseminated intravascular coagulation. Am J Pathol 56:153

Anticoagulation in Continuous Arteriovenous Hemofiltration

J. Schrader, H. Kaiser, T. Eisenhauer, P. Kramer, H. Köstering, and F. Scheler

Anticoagulation is as necessary for continuous arteriovenous hemofiltration (CAVH) as for pump-driven hemofiltration, in order to prevent clotting in the filter. The difference in anticoagulation between arteriovenous hemofiltration and conventional hemodialysis and hemofiltration results from the considerably lower blood-flow rate due to the absence of pumps and due to the longer duration of continuous treatment. Also, patients treated with CAVH to date usually suffered from an acute illness, and polytraumatized and surgical patients especially could not be endangered by unnecessarily high doses of heparin.

Therefore, this chapter considers the problems and new treatment trends with regard to anticoagulation in CAVH.

Effect of a Minimum Dose (10 IU/kg Body Weight) on the Coagulation System

Finding a minimum heparin dosage for patients in danger of hemorrhaging, that would prevent filter clots and disseminated intravascular coagulation without causing bleeding, was of first importance. In a pretest, 17 healthy persons received 10 IU heparin/kg body weight i.v. and coagulation parameters were determined prior to and 5, 10, 15, 30, and 60 min after injection. Figure 1 shows the results of partial thromboplastin time (PTT) and thrombin time. After 5 min, PTT was significantly prolonged to 63 s and thrombin time to 23 s. Both parameters returned continuously to almost initial values after 60 min. With this minimum dosage, good anticoagulation was achieved without threat of bleeding.

No change was found in thromboplastin time according to Quick, or in the values of fibrinogen, fibrin monomers, plasminogen, α_1-antitrypsin, and α_2-macroglobulin. Only the level of antithrombin-III decreased slightly after 30 min (mean values), but had already returned after 60 min.

Measurements During CAVH

Based on these results patients were given an initial dose of 10 IU/kg body weight systemically for CAVH. As continuous infusion, about 10 IU heparin/kg body weight/h were administered into the arterial blood as soon as it entered the extracorporeal system before the hemofilter (see Kramer and Grieben, Fig. 1, this volume). Simultaneously, blood from the extracorporeal system and from the systemic circulation was tested for coagulation, taking sodium citrated blood

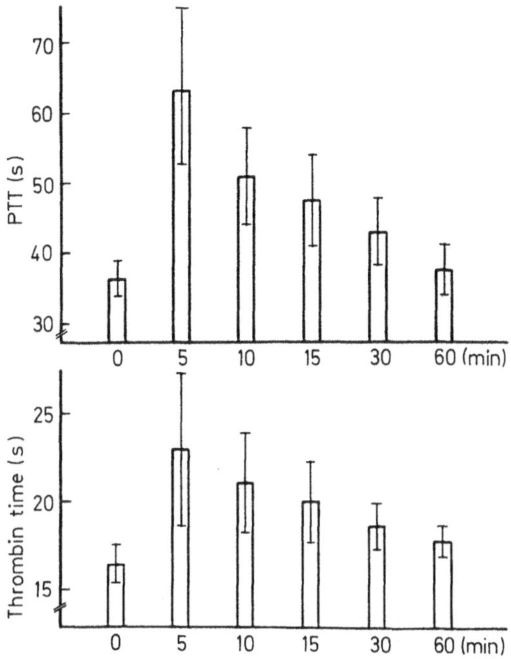

Fig. 1. PTT and thrombin time of 17 healthy persons after administration of 10 IU heparin per kg body weight (mean values ± SD)

samples from the venous line behind the hemofilter and from a cubital vein at the same time.

Clotting Parameters of Extracorporeal and Systemic Circulation

Figure 2 shows PTT, thrombin time, and heparin concentrations for 28 patients during arteriovenous hemofiltration. There are flow-dependent, marked differences between systemic circulation and extracorporeal circulation. The values for PTT and thrombin time were clearly prolonged in the extracorporeal system, and the heparin level was higher. Good anticoagulation was achieved in the extracorporeal system with the mean value for PTT of 89 s, thrombin time of 33 s, and heparin concentration of 0.6 IU/ml. In the systemic circulation, however, PTT

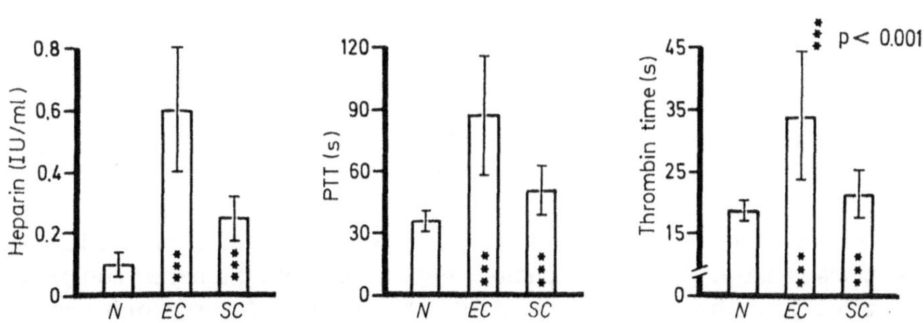

Fig. 2. PTT, thrombin time, and heparin concentration of patients during CAVH (mean values ± SD). *N*, normal persons ($n=30$); *EC*, extracorporeal circulation ($n=28$); *SC*, systemic circulation ($n=28$)

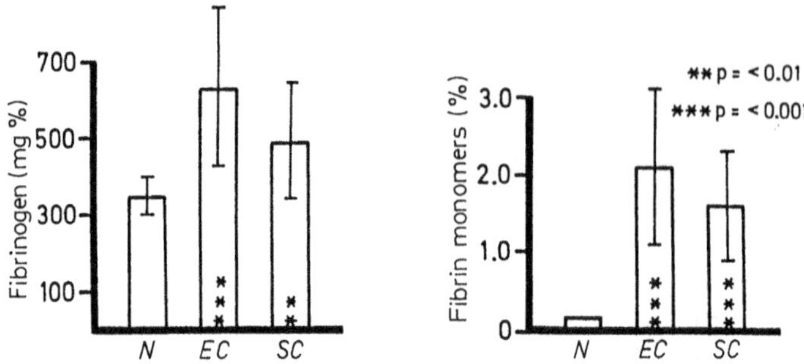

Fig. 3. Fibrinogen and fibrin monomer complexes of patients during CAVH (mean values ± SD). *N*, normal persons ($n=30$); *EC*, extracorporeal circulation ($n=28$); *SC*, systemic circulation ($n=28$)

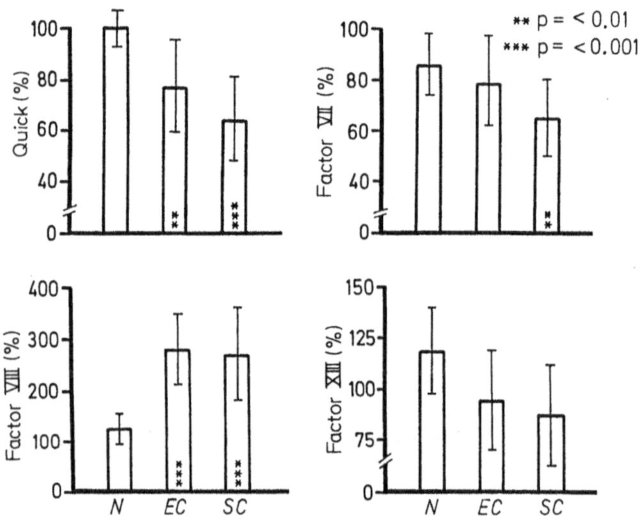

Fig. 4. Value of Quick, factor VII, factor VIII, and factor XIII of patients during CAVH (mean values ± SD). *N*, normal persons ($n=30$); *EC*, extracorporeal circulation ($n=28$); *SC* systemic circulation ($n=28$)

with a mean value of 51 s and thrombin time with a mean of 18 s were only slightly prolonged. The heparin concentration of 0.23 IU/ml was only slightly elevated and surely did not pose a threat of bleeding. With conventional pump-driven hemofiltration or hemodialysis with higher blood-flow rates (>150 ml/min), no significant difference was found between extracorporeal and systemic circulation.

Fibrinogen and fibrin monomer complexes were significantly elevated in the systemic and extracorporeal circulation (Fig. 3). The fibrin monomer complexes were already significantly elevated before onset of CAVH as a sign of hypercoagulability as reported [11]. But a significant activation of coagulation by the extracorporeal circuit with consecutive elevation of fibrin monomers or decrease of fibrinogen was not observed with this heparin dosage.

Heparin was of additional therapeutic value in the treatment of hypercoagulability. The values in the systemic circulation for Quick's test, factor VII, factor VIII, and factor XIII differed only slightly from those of the extracorporeal circulation (Fig. 4). This indicates that no additional activation of coagulation by CAVH occurred with this heparin dosage.

The levels of antithrombin-III were reduced to the same extent in the extracorporeal and systemic circulation, resulting possibly in a reduced protection against intravascular clotting. Furthermore, since antithrombin-III is a necessary heparin cofactor, a deficiency of this inhibitor must be considered when hemofilters are frequently thrombosized.

Summarizing the determinations of the clotting parameters of these 28 patients with acute oligoanuric renal failure, a minimum heparin dosage of about 10 IU/kg body weight effected sufficient anticoagulation in the extracorporeal circulation, while only slightly prolonging PTT and thrombin time in the systemic circulation.

With this heparin dosage the hemofilters were functional, on the average, 24–48 h, however, utilization of hemofilters for 1 week was not uncommon [8, 9].

Extracorporeal Blood Flow and Clotting Parameters

Blood-flow rate plays an important role in the heparinization of CAVH patients. Compared with pump-driven dialysis or filtration, blood-flow rates are considerably lower and fluctuate more.

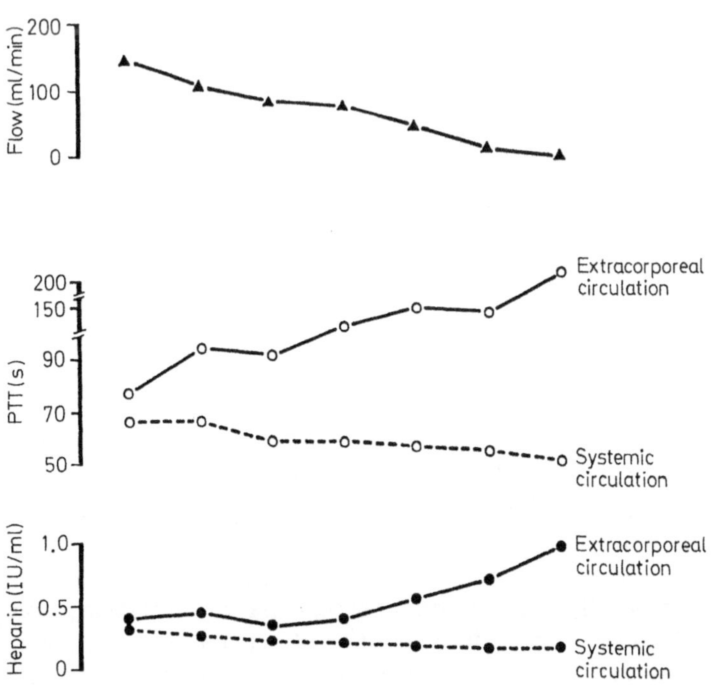

Fig. 5. PTT and heparin concentration of a female patient during successive reduction of blood-flow rate after each 20 min equilibration time

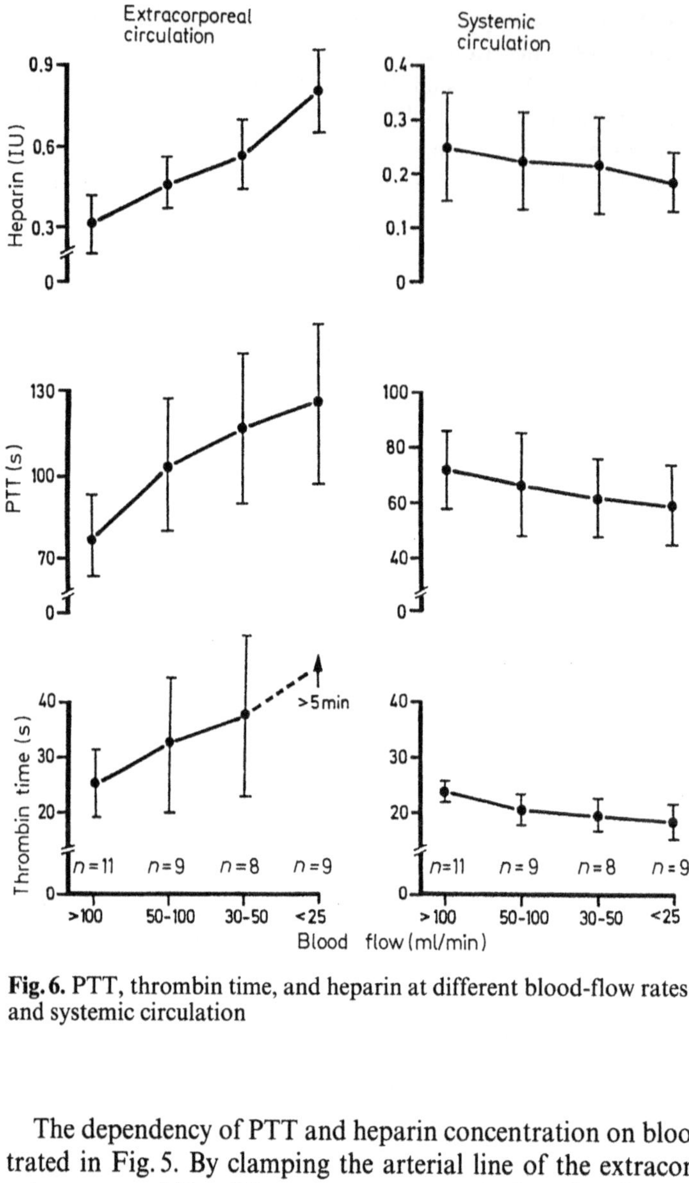

Fig. 6. PTT, thrombin time, and heparin at different blood-flow rates in the extracorporeal and systemic circulation

The dependency of PTT and heparin concentration on blood-flow rate is illustrated in Fig. 5. By clamping the arterial line of the extracorporeal system, the extracorporeal blood-flow rate was successively reduced every 20 min.

Extracorporeally, PTT was significantly prolonged and the heparin concentration was elevated with decreasing blood-flow rate. Systemically, PTT decreased somewhat during this time, possibly because of increased heparin consumption in the extracorporeal system. Continuous heparin administration, thus, seems to be self-regulating with this method: When blood-flow is reduced, quicker clotting is risked. The higher dose of heparin necessarily in the extracorporeal system now becomes available, because of the reduced dilution of heparin by the extracorporeal blood. For this reason continuous heparin administration into the arterial line of the extracorporeal system is superior to any other method of heparin application for CAVH. However, after prolonged poor flow rates, the risk of filter clotting with erythrocyte, leukocyte, and thrombocyte aggregates increases. At nearly complete stasis the applied heparin dose is not able to prevent clotting for any duration especially if too much water is drawn off the capillaries on the ultrafiltrate side by elevated negative pressure and the blood becomes highly concentrated. In Fig. 6 the mean values of heparin concentration, PTT, and thrombin time in the extracorporeal and systemic circulation can be seen of patients whose blood-flow rates were successively reduced after 30-min equilibration times. According to these values, also with decreasing blood-flow rates, PTT and thrombin time are prolonged and heparin concentration is elevated in the extracorporeal circuit. PTT and thrombin time are shortened and heparin concentration is decreased in the systemic circulation. At blood-flow rates of >150 ml/min, PTT and thrombin time are nearly equal in the extracorporeal and systemic circulation.

Monitoring of Anticoagulation

With chromogenic substrates direct determinations of heparin are possible, thus allowing reliable monitoring of anticoagulation [14, 16]. For practical purposes it was interesting to show that PTT and thrombin time correlated well with the directly measured heparin activity. The correlation coefficient between PTT and heparin was 0.95 (Fig. 7) and between thrombin time and heparin 0.89 (Fig. 8).

Monitoring of heparinization is, therefore, possible by monitoring thrombin time, or even better, by monitoring PTT, which is absolutely sufficient for clinical purposes. Prolonging PTT for about 15 s in the systemic circulation is sufficient to achieve good anticoagulation and does not significantly increase the danger of bleeding [4, 7, 11, 13, 15]. For PTT and thrombin time determination the blood withdrawal site is of great importance.

To check the effect of heparin on the coagulation system of the patient, blood has to be drawn from a body vein.

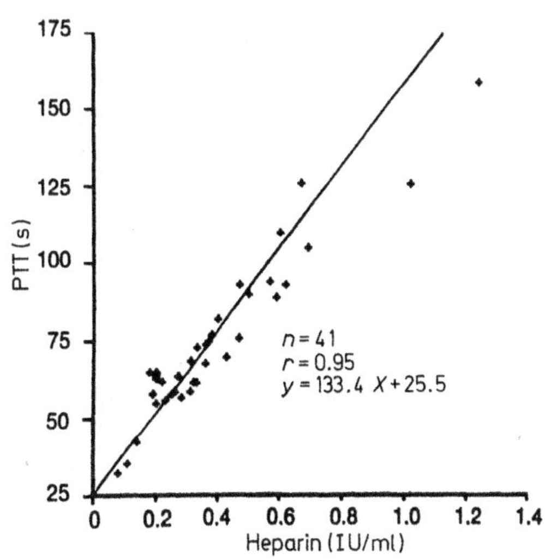

Fig. 7. Relationship between PTT and heparin activity (chromogenic substrate S-2222)

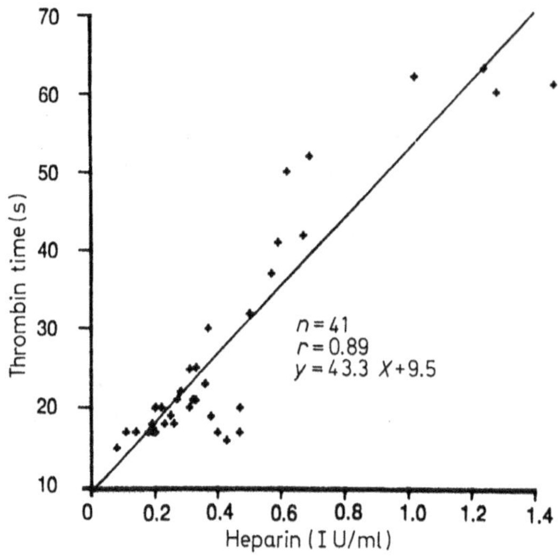

Fig. 8. Relationship between thrombin time and heparin activity (chromogenic substrate S-2222)

To determine anticoagulation in the extracoporeal system, blood has to be taken from the venous line of the extracorporeal circulation. It has to be considered that with decreasing blood-flow rates, the patient receives less heparin from the extracorporeal system, temporarily, until a new steady state is established.

New Trends: Low Molecular Weight Heparin

In order to maintain the antithrombotic properties and to reduce the anticoagulant effects, heparin fractions of different molecular weight have been investigated. It could be demonstrated that the anticoagulant activity depends upon the molecular weight of heparin. With decreasing molecular weight of heparin an increase in factor (F) Xa inhibition and a decrease in thrombin inhibition was observed. Low molecular weight (LMW) heparin with high affinity for antithrombin-III strongly inhibits F Xa, as well as F XIIa and kallikrein, but has only very little effect on thrombin as well as on F IX and F XI. In contrast to standard unfractionated (UF) heparin, LMW heparin caused only a slight prolongation of PTT and thrombin time. The increased anti-FXa activity, with only little effect on PTT and thrombocytes, of LMW heparin, should result in an improved ratio between antithrombotic activity and bleeding risk [1–6, 12].

LMW heparin was compared with standard, UF heparin in conventional hemodialysis and hemofiltration in our hospital. In particular, necessary doses and effects on coagulation system and lipoprotein lipase (LPL) were investigated in 49 patients [12]. At low doses, the amount of LMW heparin required to produce a similar blood heparin level as with UF heparin was half that of the UF heparin dose. At higher doses the blood heparin level rose more rapidly with UF than with LMW heparin. Highly significant differences were found in PTT and thrombin time between UF and LMW heparin. PTT was increased by 120 s on average, using UF heparin, whereas LMW heparin only produced an increase of 5–7 s. Thrombin time was increased by 230–250 s under UF heparin and 5–8 s under LMW heparin. No significant differences were found in factor VIII activity and

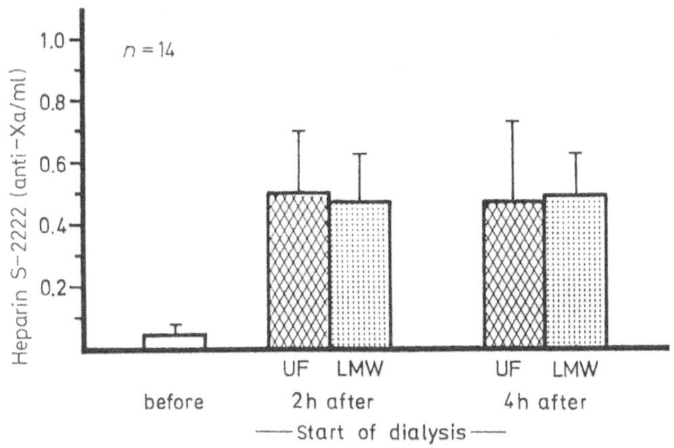

Fig. 9. UF- and LMW-heparin plasma activity in 14 hemodialysis patients under low doses of heparin

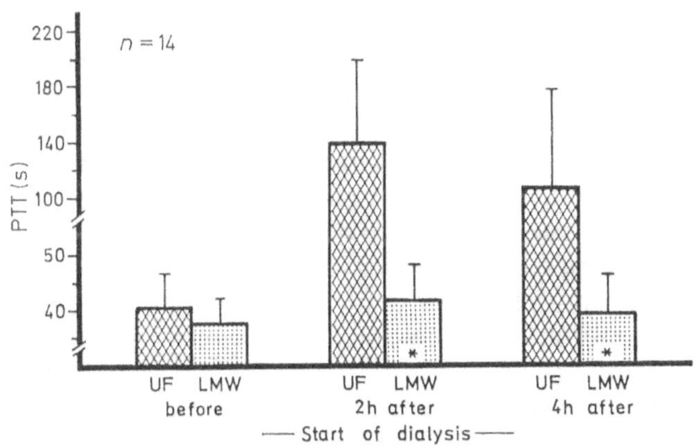

Fig. 10. PTT under treatment with UF- and LMW-heparin in 14 hemodialysis patients

fibrin monomers, ruling out a difference in the activation of the coagulation system by both heparins. Similarly, there were no changes in Quick's test, fibrinogen, antithrombin-III, plasminogen, and α_2-antiplasmin. LMW heparin also produced a significantly smaller activation of LPL, resulting in a reduced release of free fatty acids (FFA). This must be considered as an advantage of LMW heparin since FFA are involved in the development of arteriosclerosis, platelet aggregation, and displacement of protein-bound drugs in these patients.

Of 49 patients, 14 were treated with low doses of both heparins (UF heparin, initial dose 26.2 ± 6.8, dose/h 11.8 ± 1.8 IU/kg body weight; LMW heparin, initial dose 13.1 ± 3.4, dose/h 5.9 ± 0.9 anti-F Xa IU/kg body weight).

The results of heparin activity and PTT are shown in Fig. 9 and Fig. 10. In this group the same plasma heparin activity was achieved with both heparins, while the PTT was only minimally prolonged by LMW heparin. It is therefore obvious that the application of LMW heparin requires measurement of the anti-F Xa activity with chromogenic substrates.

In conclusion: On account of its slight influence on PTT and thrombin time, while retaining its antithrombotic effectiveness, it is probable that the bleeding risk with LMW heparin will be reduced. Further advantages of LMW heparin over UF heparin are to be found in the smaller effect on platelets. LMW heparin would appear to be indicated in dialysis patients with bleeding risk, with diabetic retinopathy, on anticoagulant or antiplatelet therapy, and in patients with thrombocytopenia.

Summary and Recommended Dosages

For continuous heparin administration about 10 IU/kg body weight/h are sufficient for good anticoagulation of the extracorporeal circuit with only insignificantly elevated clotting values of the systemic circulation. This heparin dosage proved adequate to maintain good blood flow and filtrate output increased risk of bleeding.

At this low dosage, heparin has to be administered continuously to the arterial line of the extracorporeal system. If heparin administration is discontinued (i.e., the heparin pump is changed), the patient has to be anticoagulated before interruption with 2000 IU heparin systemically. This dose lasts for about 30 min. At a continuous administration of 10 IU/kg body weight/h, anticoagulation of the extracorporeal system was noticeably dependent on blood-flow rate. At lower blood-flow rate, longer clotting times were observed in the extracorporeal circulation after some sort of autoregulation. The safest and simplest way to monitor and control heparin therapy is by determination of thrombin time, or better, of PTT. Most reliable is the measurement of heparin activity with a chromogenic substrate (for therapeutic range, see Fig. 2).

Heparin dosage is determined in clinical practice according to thrombin time or PTT, taking into consideration individually differing tolerance. The reaction to heparin can be especially affected by the antithrombin-III level, but also by beta-lipoproteins, platelet factors, thrombocytes, and vessel walls.

In considering dosages, it is useful to split the patients into three groups (Fig. 11):

Group I. Patients needing arteriovenous hemofiltration, with thromboembolic complications or disseminated intravascular clotting but with intact vessel system. Here, an initial dose of 50–70 IU/kg body weight and continuous infusion of 10–20 IU/kg body weight/h is recommended, where PTT should be prolonged to twice the normal value.

Group II. Patients with an intact vascular system or with controllable potential bleeding sites (surface wound, well-drained wound, easily controllable hematoma) should be treated relatively generously with heparin as prophylaxis against thromboembolic complications and as therapy for hypercoagulability of acute renal failure. Initially a dose of 15–25 IU/kg body weight and continuous infusion of about 10 IU/kg body weight/h are given with expected prolonging of PTT by about 15 s.

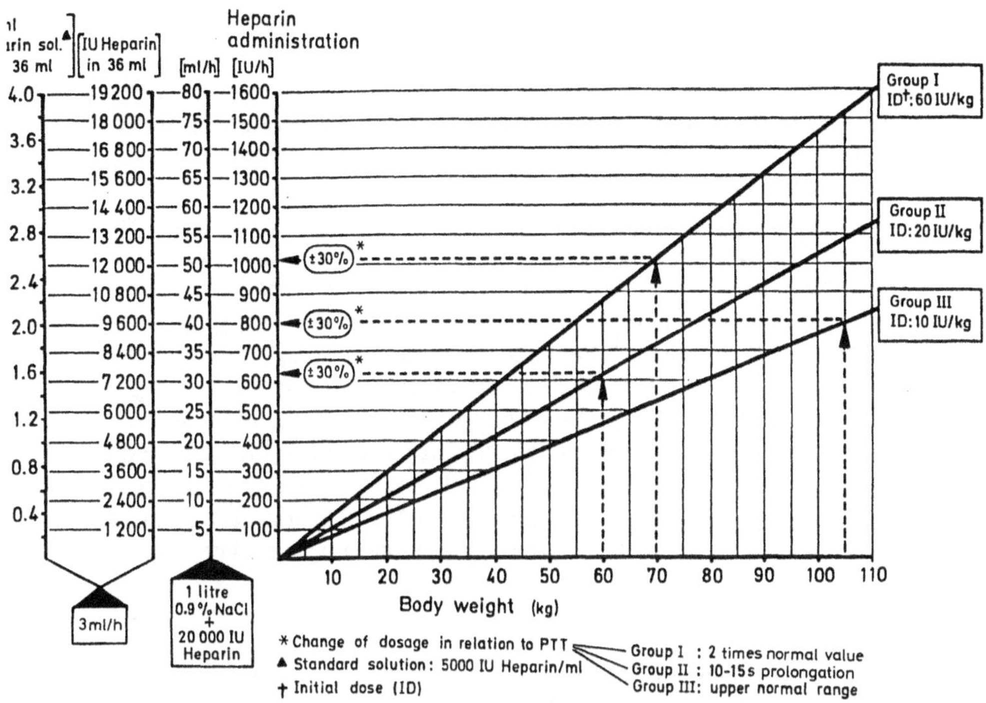

Fig. 11. Nomogram to determine individual initial and maintenance doses of heparin for three groups of patients with varying degrees of susceptibility to thrombosis and bleeding, and for administering a continuous supply of heparin (see text for details). One example is given for each group: a patient of group II weighing 60 kg would receive 1200 IU initially and 600 IU/h continuously (30 ml infusion solution containing 20000 IU heparin/l). At a constant administration rate of 3 ml/h, 7200 IU, or 1.5 ml heparin stock solution should be drawn up to 36 ml in a 50 ml syringe. The other two cases pertain to a patient weighing 105 kg (from group III) and a patient weighing 70 kg (from group I)

Group III. Patients susceptible to dangerous bleeding, particulary those suffering from polytrauma, and new surgical patients, should receive an initial dose of 10 IU/kg body weight, and 7–10 IU/kg body weight/h during continuous infusion, whereby the PTT should reach the upper limit of the normal range.

The nomogram (Fig. 11) serves for quick determination of individual dosages and practical heparin application. The physician has to decide to which group the patient belongs, and, with regard to the weight of the patient, determine an initial dose and then the rate of heparin administration. For the performance of continuous heparin administration two possibilities are shown in the nomogram: The first column shows how many ml infusion solution (1 l 0.9% NaCl+20000 IU heparin) have to be added to the arterial line of the extracorporeal system per h. Isoflux systems work best for this purpose (see nomograms in Schünemann and Kramer, Fig. 2, this volume), whereby the infusion bottle has to be hung at least 2 m above patient level to overcome the arterial pressure. The advantage of these methods of intake is that considerably larger volumes of transport fluid are used for heparin infusion and better than continuous mixing with blood is guaranteed;

besides that, no infusion pump is needed. The other two columns show the administration of heparin via an infusion pump at a constant infusion rate of 3 ml/h, using a 50 ml syringe pump. The two columns show how many IU heparin have to be dissolved in 36 ml and how many ml heparin stock solution have to be brought up to 36 ml with normal saline to achieve the desired heparin infusion.

With respect to varying reaction towards heparin, the determination of PTT is of great significance, especially for patients of group III. To achieve the desired change in PTT for the three different groups, the ascertained heparin administration rate will have to be varied by $\pm 30\%$. The quoted values for PTT, however, are often exceeded during the first 8 h after onset of heparin therapy and the anticipated PTT ranges are only achieved later under steady-state conditions. If the heparin therapy has no effect on the clotting system, or if the effect of heparin is waning despite increased dosage, lack of antithrombin-III should be suspected – which can be eliminated with a suitable substitution [10]. While it should be noted that the nomogram is not valid for use of LMW heparin (in this case monitoring of heparin activity is required), the use of LMW heparin may eventually become an indication for patients of group III with bleeding complications.

References

1. Barrowcliffe TW, Johnson EA, Eggleton CA, Kemball-Cook C, Thomas DP (1979) Anticoagulant activities of high and low molecular weight heparin fractions. Br J Haemetol 41:573–583
2. Bengtsson G, Olivesona R, Hook M, Riesenfeld J, Lindendahl U (1980) Interaction of lipoprotein lipase with native and modified heparin-like polysaccharides. Biochem J 189:625–633
3. Carter CJ, Kelton JG, Hirsh J, Santos AV, Gent M (1982) The relationship between the hemorrhagic and antithrombotic properties of low molecular weight heparin in rabbits. Blood 59:1239–1245
4. Hirsh J, O'Sullivan EF, Gallus AS (1970) The activated thromboplastin time in the control of heparin treatment. Aust Ann Med 46:334
5. Holmer E (1980) Anticoagulant properties of heparin and heparin fractions. Scand J Haematol Suppl 25:25–39
6. Holmer E, Mattson C, Nilsson S (1982) Anticoagulant and antithrombotic effects of heparin and low molecular weight heparin fragment in rabbits. Thromb Res 25:475–485
7. Köstering H (1981) Die Thromboembolien. Schattauer, Stuttgart
8. Kramer P (1982) Arterio-venöse Hämofiltration. Vandenhoeck and Ruprecht, Göttingen-Zürich, S 67–80
9. Kramer P, Schrader J, Bohnsack W, Grieben G, Gröne HJ, Scheler F (1981) Continuous arteriovenous hemofiltration (CAVH): a new kidney replacement therapy. Proc Eur Dial Transplant Assoc 18:743
10. Schrader J, Köstering H, Kramer P, Scheler F (1982) Antithrombin III – Substitution bei dialysepflichtiger Niereninsuffizienz. Dtsch Med Wochenschr 107:1847–1850
11. Schrader J, Bohnsack W, Kaiser H, Eisenhauer T, Kramer P, Köstering H (1982) Antikoagulation bei kontinuierlicher arterio-venöser Hämofiltration. In: Kramer P (Hrsg) Arterio-venöse Hämofiltration. Vandenhoeck und Ruprecht, Göttingen-Zürich, S 67–80
12. Schrader J, Rieger J, Müschen H, Stibbe W, Köstering H, Kramer P, Scheler F (1985) Anwendung von niedermolekularem Heparin bei Hämodialysepatienten. Klin Wochenschr 63:49–55
13. Swartz RD (1981) Hemorrhage during high-risk hemodialysis. Using controlled heparinization. Nephron 28:65–69

14. Teien AN (1979) Assay of heparin using factor Xa and a chromogenic substrate. In: Scully MF, Kakkar VV (eds) Chromogenic peptide substrates. Churchill Livingstone, Edinburgh, pp 196–205
15. Vogel GE, Kopp KF (1978) The conflict between anticoagulation and hemostasis during hemodialysis. Int J Artif Organs 1:181–186
16. Witt I (1977) New methods for the analysis of coagulation using chromogenic substrates. De Gruyter, Berlin

Activated Clotting Time for Heparin Dosage Monitoring in Continuous Arteriovenous Hemofiltration

K. Koorejian, R. H. Bartlett and J. London

The main purpose of heparinization in continuous arteriovenous hemofiltration (CAVH) is to prevent the hemofilter from clotting without having to systemically anticoagulate the patient. As with any extracorporeal circuit, when blood comes in contact with a foreign surface, protein is absorbed within milliseconds and platelet adhesion occurs. The more fibrinogen that attaches to the circuit, the greater the affinity for platelets. When platelets attach to the surface, they activate more platelet adhesion which leads to fibrin formation if there is no heparin in the system [1]. The anticoagulant heparin prevents clot formation by increasing the action of antithrombin-III, an inhibitor of thrombin, and therefore inhibits the conversion of fibrinogen to fibrin. Thrombin inhibition is dose related and heparin is rapidly metabolized, thus the heparin effect can be titrated to any desired level by adjusting a continuous infusion. Our approach to anticoagulation with CAVH is derived from the method of Kramer [2], combined with our experience with prolonged extracorporeal circuits like ECMO [3].

The patient is given a loading dose of heparin systemically 3 min prior to opening the blood lines to a new filter so that the initial blood flow exposed to the filter is anticoagulated. This initial blood contact event is important. Any fibrin formation will trap platelets and red blood cells, leading to capillary occlusion or total clotting. Once the filter has been exposed for several minutes to this initial blood flow, the prosthetic surfaces are coated with a molecular layer of proteins and less activation takes place. This is the reason we include albumin in the priming solution – to fill the binding sites [4].

The first few minutes of CAVH are critical in regard to clotting, as this flow of blood establishes the flow pattern for the life of the filter.

The heparin effect is measured to be sure that the patient has a normal response to the drug, – namely, slight systemic anticoagulation. If the heparin effect is excessive, the risk of bleeding is increased and the dose should be decreased, even if bleeding has not occurred. If the heparin effect is minimal even at high doses, an antithrombin-III deficiency should be suspected. If the patient is bleeding, the heparin dose should be decreased until the heparin effect is minimal, even if this results in filter failure.

Tests of Heparin Effect

Heparin therapy can be measured by a variety of methods. The ideal test as outlined by Congdon should (a) have a rapid end point, (b) be capable of being performed at the bedside, and (c) be reproducible through increasing heparin concentrations in and out of the therapeutic range [5].

Measurement of heparin concentration is not useful, because a given concentration (e.g., 0.5 units/ml) may anticoagulate one patient and have no effect in another. Hence, heparin *effect* must be measured.

The measurement of the heparin effect requires (a) a stimulus to activate the coagulation cascade, (b) a temperature and agitation control, and (c) a method to detect clot formation.

Heparin effects can be monitored in blood or plasma, but blood measurements are preferred because interactions between heparin, platelets, and white blood cells are not reflected in plasma measurements. Utilizing whole blood to monitor heparin therapy is more convenient and better suited to bedside methods of the measurement of heparin effects.

The standard test of coagulation has been the Lee-White whole blood clotting time test [6], first presented in 1913. Some disadvantages with this method include its variability, and also the length of time involved to obtain results. This test is not recommended for heparin monitoring.

The activated partial thromboplastin time (APTT) [7], and the thrombin time (TT) [8] tests, have been widely used as indicators of the heparin effect. The disadvantages of these tests are: centrifugation is required, measurements are made on plasma, a variety of commercial reagents are used, and there is considerable variation in sensitivity to heparin. In 1981, Brandt and Triplett [9] pointed out that standardization of the APTT as a method for monitoring heparin therapy would require standardization of individual reagent components.

The prothrombin time (PT) [10], is reflective predominantly of prothrombin activity, which is not affected by heparin. This method is more sensitive in oral anticoagulant control, rather than heparin activity.

The thrombin clotting time (TCT) ("thrombin time" assay on whole blood) has been used as a means to monitor heparin therapy. An automatic clot timer, the Fibrometer is used to determine the time from activation to clot formation. This test has proven sensitive to varying doses of heparin and can be performed at the bedside. In some hospitals the TCT is reported as "heparin units/ml," but this is simply determined from a nomogram after measuring the time. The results of any test of heparin effect should be reported in seconds, along with the normal range. For CAVH, this time should be approximately twice normal.

Measurements of coagulation on blood or plasma performed in the laboratory are done by drawing the blood into a calcium-chelating anticoagulant. When the activator is added, sufficient calcium is included to override the chelator, so the time to fibrin formation is similar to that observed at the bedside with fresh blood. The beside method is preferred, because variations in time, temperature, heparin breakdown, clotting factor, and platelet inactivation may all occur during the trip from the bedside to the laboratory.

Our method of choice is the activated clotting time (ACT), to determine the efficacy of heparin therapy in CAVH. In 1979, Baden et al. [11] described the BaSon test for monitoring heparin therapy. This test involves the use of Platelin Plus activator (General Diagnostics), a mixture of diatomaceous earth and rabbit thromboplastin. Distilled water and Platelin Plus reagent are combined in a ratio of 2.5:1, and 0.1 cc of this mixture is dispersed into test tubes and frozen. When ready for use, these tubes are thawed and brought to room temperature. The reagent is effective for 2 h after it has been thawed. Before blood is inserted into the test tube, the contents of the tube must be gently mixed. This is performed by gently rolling the tube between one's hands. Then, 0.2 cc blood is dispersed into the test tube along one edge and mixed with the reagent by inverting the tube once. The tube is then placed in the ACT tester, a machine that consists of a tilting heating device, and a sensor to detect clot formation. When a clot forms, an alarm sounds and the ACT (in seconds) is read on the digital display.

A normal ACT ranges from 80 to 120 s. The ACT in a patient on CAVH should be 100–250 s. The fresh reagent is essential for reproducible results. Using the ACT machine with a dry reagent is unsatisfactory.

The Hemochron device [12] (International Technidyne) is another method of agitation and clot detection. This system, as supplied, is not satisfactory in our experience, but the problem is probably due to the activating reagent. The Hemochron may be accurate if the BaSon reagent is used.

Heparin Management in CAVH

A preheparin baseline ACT is obtained from the patient, along with a PT, PTT, TT, and complete blood count with a platelet count. The heparin loading dose is given, and the infusion started on the arterial side of the circuit. The ACT is obtained every 2 h for the first 24 h of CAVH, then every 4 h, depending on the patient's clinical status. If the ACT is between 100 and 250 s, and the patient exhibits no systemic bleeding, then the heparin infusion can be maintained at 500 units/h. If the ACT is >250 s, the heparin infusion rate should be decreased even if there are no signs of systemic bleeding. With systemic bleeding the heparin drip should be decreased (or discontinued) even if the ACT is normal.

The use of the ACT to monitor heparin therapy in CAVH has proven to be a reliable test and convenient to perform at the bedside. We are able to obtain results quickly and therefore can make appropriate changes in heparin administration with the use of the hemofilter.

References

1. Bartlett RH, Andersen JC (1982) Blood-surface interactions: an overview. In: Stanley JC, Burkel WE, Lindenauer SM, Bartlett RH, Turcotte JC (eds) Biologic and synthetic vascular prostheses. Grune and Stratton, New York, pp 63–81
2. Kramer P, Schrader J, Bohnsack W et al. (1981) Continuous arteriovenous hemofiltration: a new kidney replacement therapy. Proc Eur Dial Transplant Assoc 18:743
3. Fong SW, Burns NE, Williams G, Woldenski C, Gazzaniga AB, Bartlett RH (1974) Changes in coagulation and platelet function during prolonged extracorporeal circulation in sheep and man. Trans Am Soc Artif Intern Organs 20:239–247

4. Roohk HV, Pick J, Hill R, Hung E, Bartlett RH (1976) Kinetics of fibrinogen and platelet adherence to biomaterials. Trans Am Soc Artif Intern Organs 22:1–7
5. Congdon JE, Kardinal CG, Wallin JD (1976) Monitoring heparin therapy in hemodialysis. JAMA 226:1529–1531
6. Lee RI, White PD (1913) A clinical study of the coagulation time of blood. Am J Med Sci 145:495–503
7. Basu D, Gallus A, Hirsh J, Cade J (1972) A prospective study of the value of monitoring heparin treatment with the activated partial thromboplastin time. N Engl J Med 287:324–327
8. Penner JA (1974) Experience with the thrombin clotting time assay for measuring heparin activity. Am J Clin Pathol 61:645–653
9. Brandt JT, Triplett DA (1981) Laboratory monitoring of heparin. Am J Clin Pathol 76:530–537
10. Quick AJ (1966) Hemorrhagic diseases and thromboses. Lea and Febiger, Philadelphia
11. Baden JP, Sonnenfield M, Ferlic RM, Sellers RD (1971) The BaSon test: a rapid bedside test for control of heparin therapy. Surg Forum 22:172–174
12. Kurec AS, Morris NW, Davey FR (1979) Clotting, activated partial thromboplastin and coagulation times in monitoring heparin therapy. Ann Clin Lab Sci 9:494–500

Setup and Fluid-Balancing Equipment

Preparation of the Setup for Performing Arteriovenous Hemofiltration

P. Kramer and G. Grieben

Description of the Blood- and Ultrafiltrate-Conducting System

Figure 1 realistically depicts the simple tubing system which is required to perform continuous arteriovenous hemofiltration (CAVH). By means of two femoral catheters, (Item number 1130.089, Vygon Aachen), blood is conducted through a capillary hemofilter (Diafilter-20, Amicon, or other products) with arterial inlet and venous return tubing.

Through the ultrafiltrate tubing included in the tubing set, ultrafiltrate runs into a measuring container (preferably a urimeter with a measuring volume of at least 500 ml) attached as low as possible to the frame of the patient's bed to achieve negative pressure of approximately 40 cm H_2O or, if possible, up to 100 cm H_2O.

Preparation of Hemofilter and Tubing System

Arterial blood and venous blood lines are pushed over the connection ports of the hemofilter, after washing them off with the usual skin disinfectant spray. The ultrafiltrate-conducting system, with the yellow connector at the side port, is attached in a like manner. Using a 1000 ml infusion bag (0.9 g/dl NaCl) previously mixed with 5000 IU heparin, the hemofiltration system is rinsed free of air bubbles. First the ultrafiltrate tubing remains closed off by a clamp until the arterial line, the capillaries of the hemofilter, and the venous line are filled, free of air bubbles. Then the ultrafiltrate tubing is opened while clamping off the venous tubing to remove air from the extracapillary space (surrounding the capillaries). Only when all spaces of the hemofilter are free of air bubbles and the ultrafiltrate tubing is filled with saline down to the collecting container, the ultrafiltrate tubing is clamped off again and the rinsing procedure continued through the hemofilter.

To remove small air bubbles from the capillaries, the hemofilter has to be held vertically during rinsing so that the rinse solution flows out of the upper end of the capillaries. Rinsing under high pressure is most effective in displacing air. To do this, the infusion bag is rolled up like a tube of toothpaste from the hanging point down and compressed with both hands.

Once the system is rinsed with 1000 ml and free of air bubbles, the arterial and venous tubing are clamped off and the connection fittings capped for protection

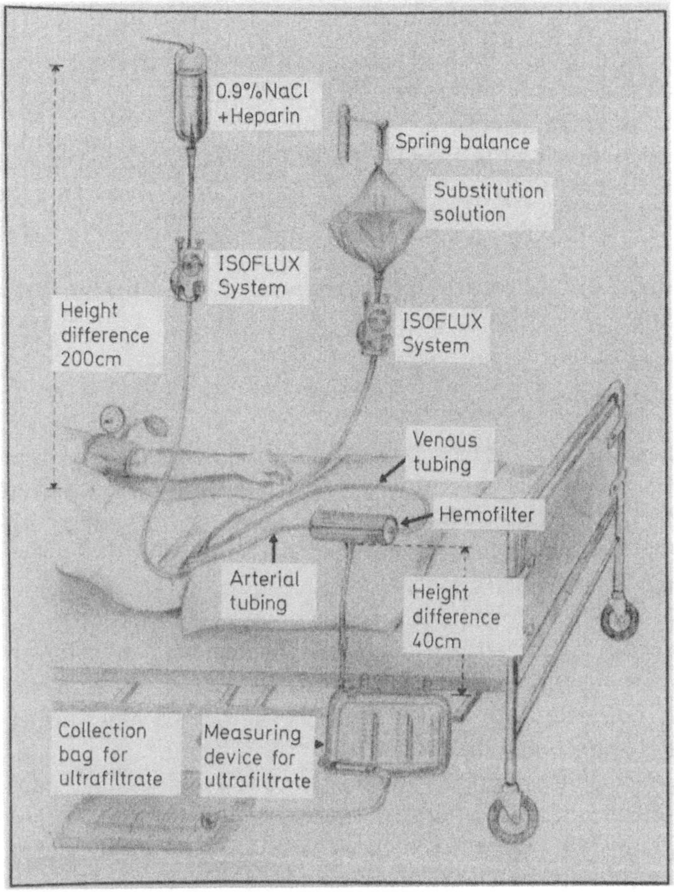

Fig. 1. Realistic illustration for performing arteriovenous hemofiltration. (For heparin administration, often a syringe infusion pump, and for the substitution solution, a volumetric pump, are also often utilized. Most recently, electronic flow balances, have been used for control of fluid balance)

or directly attached to the three-way valves of the femoral catheters. (Note: use only tubing systems with luer locks and do not use other three-way valves except those delivered with the set!)

Performance of Arteriovenous Hemofiltration [1]

Before opening the extracorporeal circulation, the patient receives systemically an initial dose of approximately 20 IU heparin per kg body weight. Then, continuous heparin supply is connected to the arterial three-way valve. The simplest way to achieve this is to use an Isoflux infusion device (disposable system by Van Leer Medical) which keeps the preset infusion rate constant, independent of pressure changes in the arterial tubing and in the infusion container. To overcome the arterial pressure, the infusion bottle (1000 ml 0.9% NaCl + 20 000 IU heparin) has to be positioned at least 2 m above patient level. Most intensive care units today use 50 ml syringe pumps for administration of heparin.

After starting continuous heparin administration, the blood flow is opened to the arterial tubing by turning the three-way valve and removing the tubing clamp so that arterial blood can be seen pulsating where the tubing begins. After the clamp and three-way valve are opened on the venous side, blood flows visibly through the hemofilter, following the pressure gradient, and through the venous return tubing back to the patient. (Caution: It is of utmost importance to use the proper three-way valves with large internal diameter, otherwise blood flow is disturbed.)

Now the clamp on the ultrafiltrate tubing is removed and the filtration rates measured for calculation of the substitution rate.

Ultrafiltrate Substitution

Commercially available for ultrafiltrate substitution are 4.5 l bags of potassium-free Ringer's lactate solution [Na 140, Ca 3.75, Mg 1.5, Cl 104.25, and lactate 42 meq/l (see Wigger, this volume)]. The weight change of the bags can be observed on a 5-kg spring balance on the infusion pole. An Isoflux infusion system is sufficient to regulate the infusion rate.

Many intensive care units use volumetric infusion pumps or the recently commercially available electronic flow balance (Sartorius) together with an Isoflux infusion system. Also the ultrafiltration may be accurately measured by an electronic flow balance. The rate of infusion is dependent on the rate of ultrafiltration, the desired fluid removal, and the rate of administrating other parenterals. *Example*: Filtration rate 500 ml/h, rate of administering 100 ml/h, desired effective fluid removal 100 ml/h, rate of ultrafiltrate substitution 300 ml/h. At these values, the patient will, in 24 h, filter off 12 l, lose a total of 2.4 kg weight and receive 7.2 l substitution solution and 2.4 l other parenterals.

References

1. Kramer, P, Tiffin MC (1981) Arteriovenous hemofiltration (video tape: Detailed illustration of mechanism and preparation of the system for performing CAVH). Institut für Entwicklungsplanung und Strukturforschung, Hannover

Simple Techniques for Accurate Fluid Balancing During Continuous Arteriovenous Hemofiltration

B. Schünemann and P. Kramer

Conceptually, continuous arteriovenous hemofiltration (CAVH) is a simple method that can be performed in every intensive care unit. Since large volumes of fluid are exchanged with this procedure – in special cases up to 1200 ml/h – exact fluid balancing requires much attention.

The following description suggests how balancing can be safely managed under simple conditions. It is not claimed to be comprehensive, since many users in intensive care medicine surely practise their own various proven methods of fluid balancing (see the devices of Dr. Schurek, Hannover and Dr. Mason, London).

Pragmatically speaking, one can distinguish between dosage of infusion solution and systems for measuring filtrate volume.

Contrary to mechanical hemofiltration, there will be less mention here of automated balancing equipment that regulates infusion volume according to predetermined fluid balance, taking filtrate flow rate into account.

Systems for Infusion Dosage

The method using graduated infusion bottles and adjusting dosage by drop rate regulated with a roller clamp is simple but cumbersome and time consuming for staff. Also, it is difficult to maintain a constant flow rate with such simple infusion systems since pressure variations in the infusion system can change the flow rate up to 30% [1].

It becomes particularly problematic when several infusions are controlled this way simultaneously because the infusions interfere with each other in the common tubing. It is therefore questionable whether or not exact dosage is possible considering the usual degree of attentiveness in an intensive care unit.

A new type of infusion system has gained acceptance for its reliabilty. The Isoflux system (van Leer Medical) makes dosage of an infusion volume possible via a proportioning valve (Fig. 1). The advantage of this system is that after the initial adjustment, the drop rate can be kept constant for a long time independent of pressure variations in the tubing system close to the patient and changes of the fluid level in the infusion container. In contrast to conventional infusion systems the drop rate here varies only 5% at maximum [1].

When setting the rate, the viscosity of the solution also has to be considered, as in the nomograms in Fig. 2. Through three-valve inlets, mixed infusions are

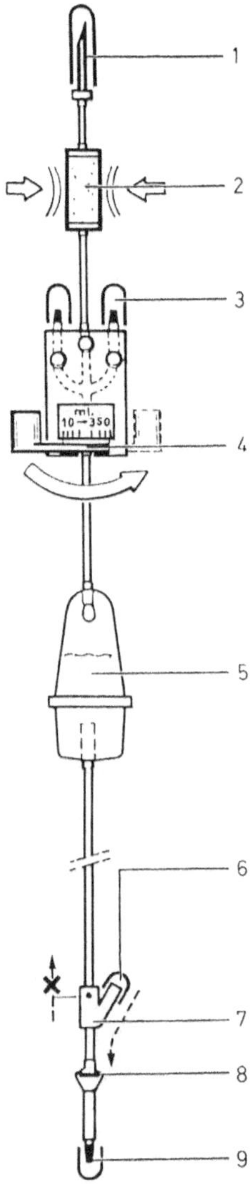

Fig. 1. Schematic illustration of Isoflux system. 1 Injection spike, also available as luer lock, 2 Flexible hand pump to fill the Isoflux system, 3 Connections for additional infusion container, 4 Control level for drop-rate setting, 5 Drop chamber, 6 Connection site for supplementary infusion, 7 Silicon nonreturn valve, 8 Latex adapter, 9 Luer connection (Note: for CAVH use only units supplied with luer lock)

Fig. 2 A, B. Nomograms for the determination of drop rate of infusion solutions, modified according to Jeanneret et al. [1], when the rate of infusion in ml/min of ml/h and different drop sizes are known. The Isoflux infusion system was the primary device in establishing the values for infusion of normal electrolyte solutions and viscous solutions like 40% glucose. The nomograms can also be used for any other infusion system to determine the rate of administration, provided drop size (drops/ml) are known. For extremely small (20/ml) and large (13/ml) drops the corresponding regression lines are drawn in. Examples for particular infusion rates with drop size 16/ml are drawn into the nomograms: infusion rate 480 ml/h or 8 ml/min = 120 drops/min, and infusion rate 37.5 ml/h or 0.62 ml/min = 10 drops/min

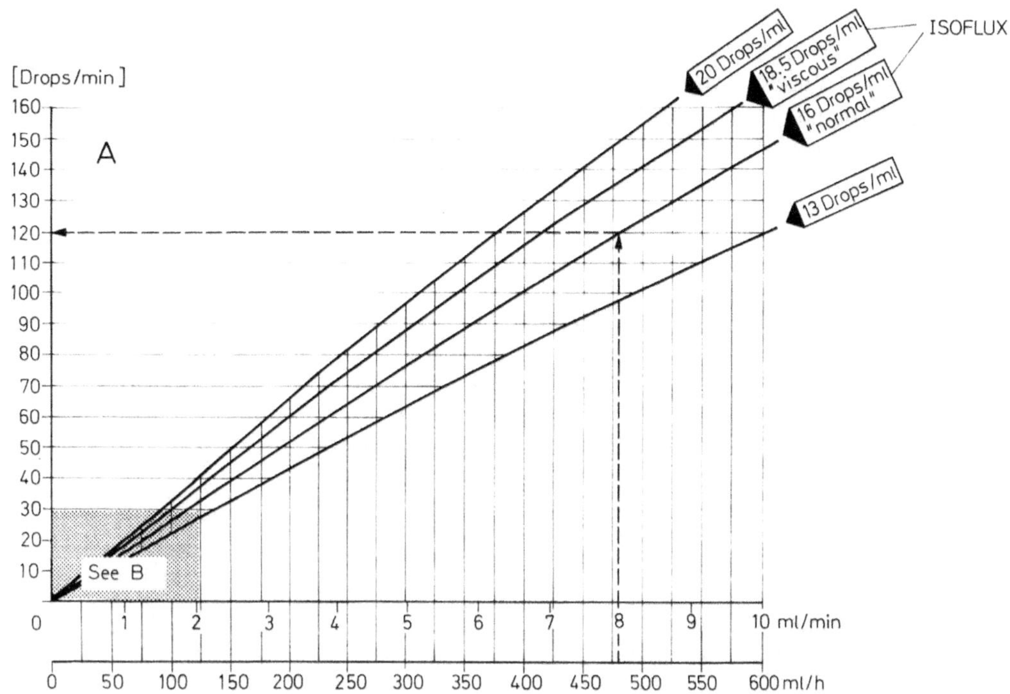
[Drops/min]
A
20 Drops/ml
18.5 Drops/ml "viscous"
16 Drops/ml "normal"
13 Drops/ml
ISOFLUX
See B
ml/min
ml/h

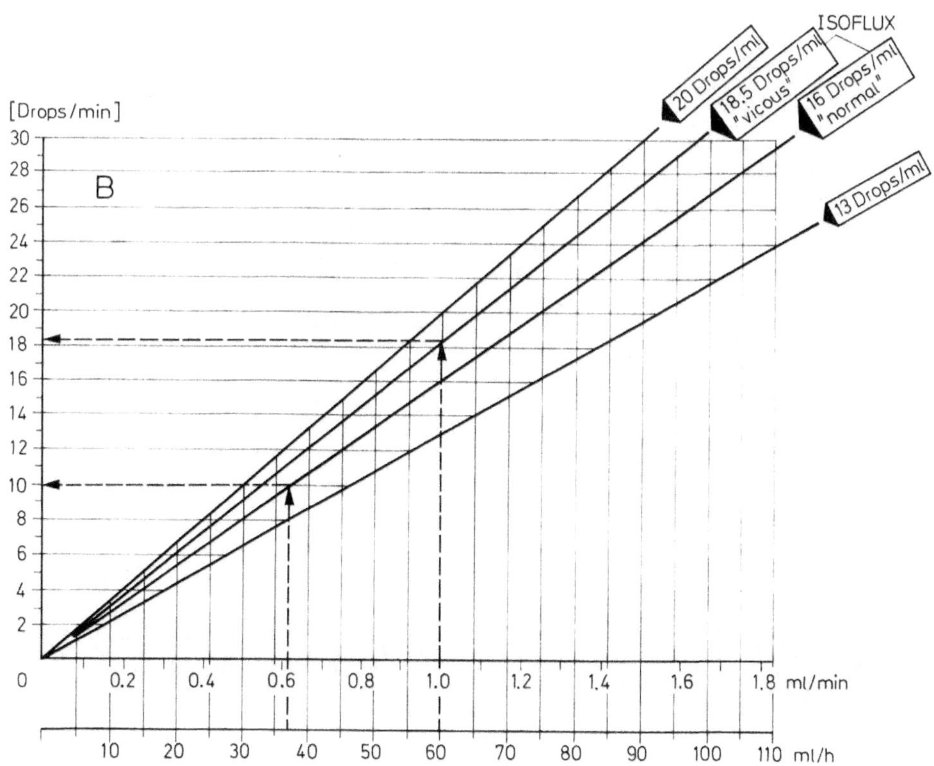
[Drops/min]
B
20 Drops/ml
18.5 Drops/ml "vicous"
16 Drops/ml "normal"
13 Drops/ml
ISOFLUX
ml/min
ml/h

possible which are of importance for parenteral nutrition. A silicone nonreturn valve protects from blood flow into the infusion system and in addition serves as protection against running empty, and therefore prevents air embolism.

The disadvantage is that the dosage setting only works accurately up to 400 ml/h, meaning that two of these systems have to be used in parallel at higher filtrate rates. Aside from the increase in cost, control of the system is affected as well. But there is still a savings in labor of approximately 61% [1] over using the simple infusion systems.

Spring Balance for Infusion Container

A 5-kg spring balance is suitable for the control of residual volumes of infusion bags and bottles (Fig. 3). It is not accurate enough for continuous control of infusion rate, but it permits suitable control of the infusion volume on an hourly basis.

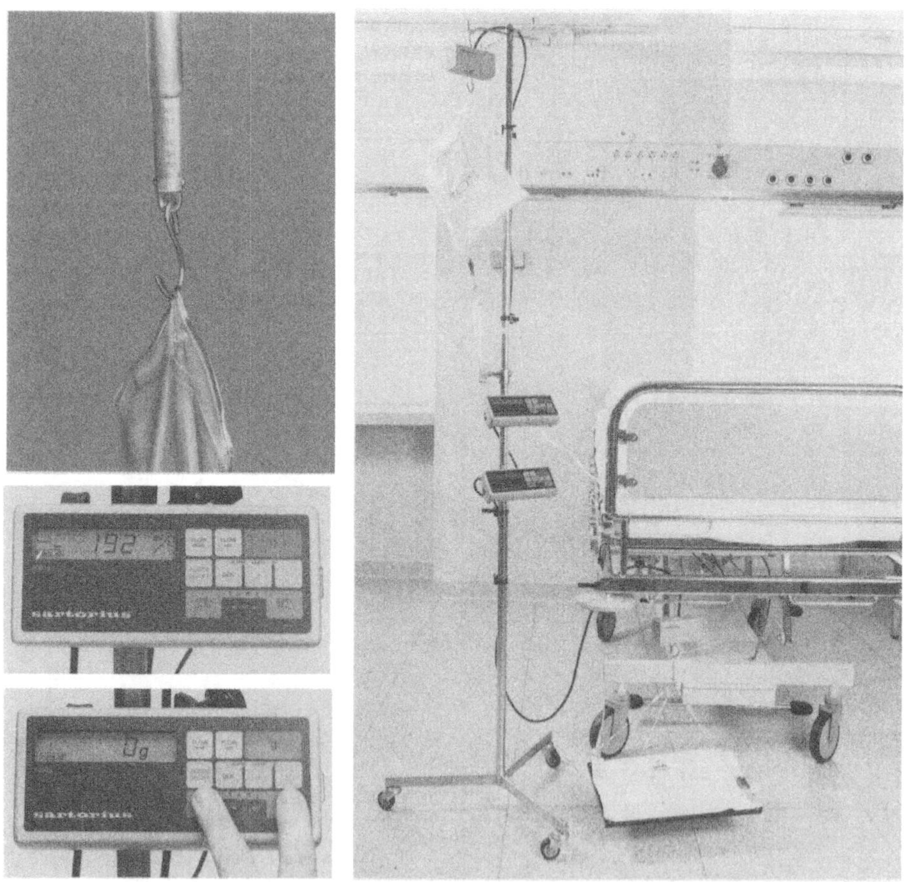

Fig. 3. A 5-kg spring balance and the first electronic flow balances. For details, see text

Figure 3 also demonstrates the first electronic flow balance (Sartorius), the digital readout not only showing the absolute weight, but also weight change per minute and per hour with an accuracy of ± 1.0 g. In combination with the Isoflux infusion system, this electronic flow balance offers for the first time exact setting and control of an infusion rate without a mechanically moved part with so-far unknown accuracy and at a reasonable price. The electronic flow balance is suited in the same way for measurement of the filtration rate: As shown in Fig. 3, the 4-l collecting bag is placed on a plate suspended by thin chains to the electronic balance. In clinical practice, the nurse first uses the flow rate display to adjust the substitution rate and the absolute weight display for the protocol of fluid balance. Every hour on the hour the weight change during the previous hour is written down. Calculations may be avoided by pressing the tare button every hour after the weight change is written down, setting the display to zero. If there are any doubts about the actual weight of the containers, this may be determined at any time.

Infusion Pumps

Infusion pumps seem to be suited for dosage of substitution solution, but are often subject to interference. With tubing roller pumps, inaccuracies with systematic deviations up to 1 l/day can occur due to pressure variations ahead of the pump when large volumes are exchanged. Volumetric pumps are apparently very precise and provide a digital readout of the infused volume at the same time. The disadvantage lies in the costly disposable infusion system.

Filtrate Measuring Systems

For the measurement of filtrate volume urine measuring bags with an hourglass, or a collection container working specifically on the overflow principle (as seen in Fig. 4), are usually suitable.

This measuring container holds 500 ml and therefore permits measurement of higher filtrate volumes. For cumulative balancing we also recommend 2-l graduated cylinders to precisely remeasure the filtrate volume in the urine bags, prior to discarding. The measurement of filtrate volume with electronic flow balances seems to be the solution for achieving error-free fluid balancing in the future.

Practical Execution of Exact Fluid Balancing

Basically, all dosage systems are practical but require different degrees of attention. The method of counting drops is simple and inexpensive, but needs constant monitoring and regulating unless the Isoflux system is used. Figure 5 is a summary of the scheme of manual fluid balancing. There the filtered and infused volumes have to be checked at least hourly and dosage setting adjusted accordingly. In the case of high filtration rates, balancing should be done half-hourly, especially if the ultrafiltration decreases and varies widely at the start of treatment. We recommend balancing control every 6 h. Cumulative balancing (addition of all hourly balancing steps) should not be done because of the chance of error. For

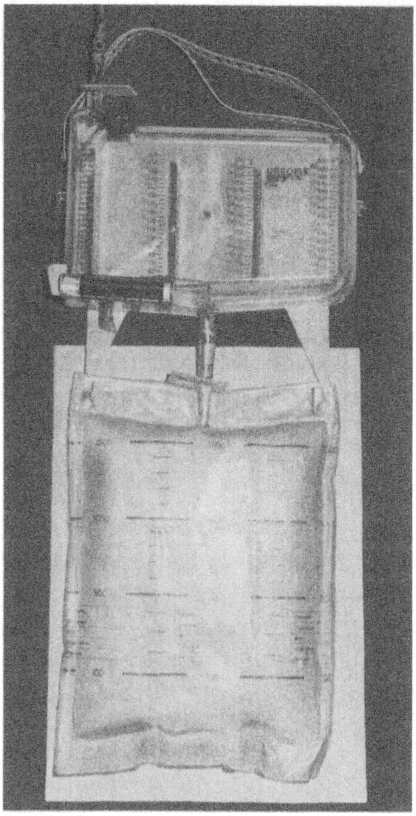

Fig. 4. Filtrate collection container with overflow system for exact measurement of minute and hourly volume

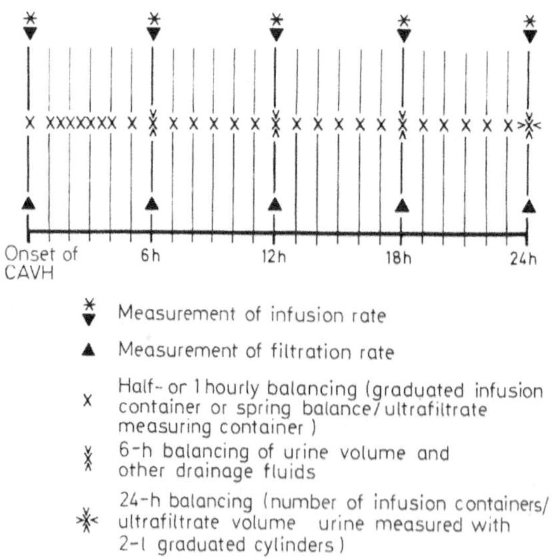

Fig. 5. Typical timetable for manual balancing

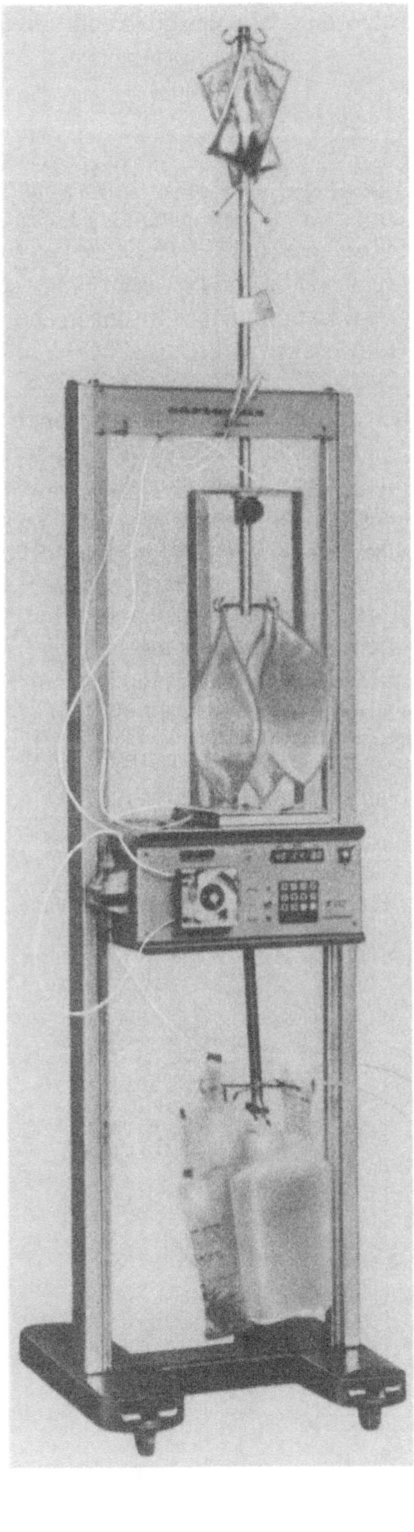

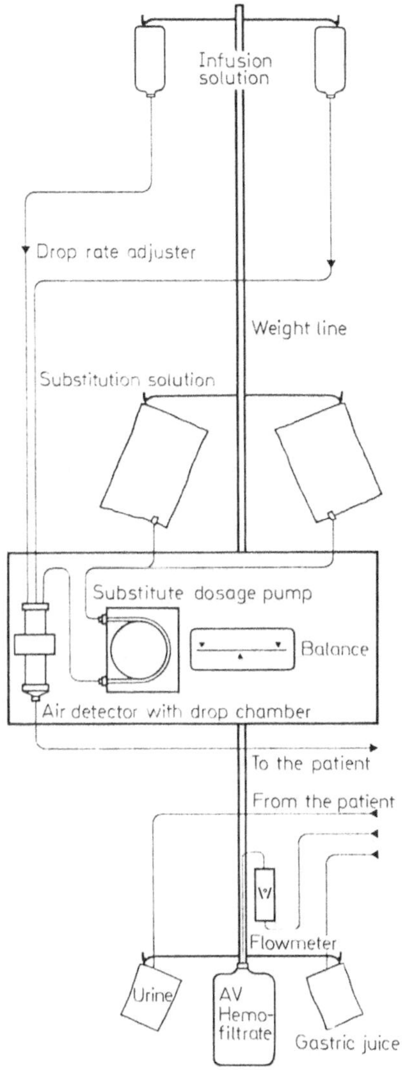

Fig. 6. Prototype of the fully automated balancing equipment Sartocare (Sartorius, Göttingen). Set-up and flow schematic

intermittent balancing, it is more important to consider the separately determined values of input and output during this time span. Aside from the 24-h balancing, weighing the patient daily or use of a bed scale would be a desirable additional control.

Causes for Errors and Measures for Their Prevention

Basically, errors can be divided into two categories: (a) those caused by the personnel, such as wrong readings of infusion containers (different reading levels), errors in maintenance, and poor protocol, and (b) those caused by inherent errors of the system, such as variation of the drop size depending on the viscosity of the solution, change of drop rate caused by pressure variations in the infusion system, fluid loss through leaks in the tubing system and dosage errors caused by the roller pumps.

It can be generally stated that the incidence of misbalancing increases as the system becomes more complicated and less controllable. Since balancing errors cannot be eliminated even with careful handling, independent control measures have to be taken. Principally, residual volumes of infusion bottles should be weighed with spring balances and an exact log should be kept of used infusion volume (see Fig. 6).

The filtrate can be collected and kept in large measuring containers so that it can be measured again separately for intermittent or total balancing.

Finally, it has to be remembered that central venous pressure, blood pressure, pulse rate, and in special cases, pulmonary artery pressure and certainly skin turgor are of greater concern for the good clinician when deciding on more or less fluid removal from a patient.

References

1. Jeanneret P, Essellier AF, Völlm B, Schneider E (1956) Ein Nomogramm für Dauertropfinfusionen. Schweiz Med Wochenschr 49:1390
2. Kapadia CR, Bigun JEJ, Hall P, Fielding LP (1981) Improved flow control in parenteral nutrition. Br J Intravenous Ther 1:8

A New Mechanical Device for Automatic Fluid Balancing in Continuous Arteriovenous Hemofiltration

H. J. Schurek and D. Biela

One of the disadvantages of continuous arteriovenous hemofiltration (CAVH) is that a daily fluid balance of 12–20 l has to be handled manually. To overcome this laborsome and potentially inaccurate handling, we developed a simple mechanical system which enables an automatic exchange of 4.5 l substitution fluid and an adjustable volume of filtrate (between 4.5 and 6.5 l) during one nursing shift [1].

Figure 1 is a schematic drawing of the system, which consists of a vertical stand with two mechanically coupled horizontal cross beams mounted on roller bearings (Gambro, Lund, Sweden). A fluid bag of 4.5 l substitution fluid hanging at

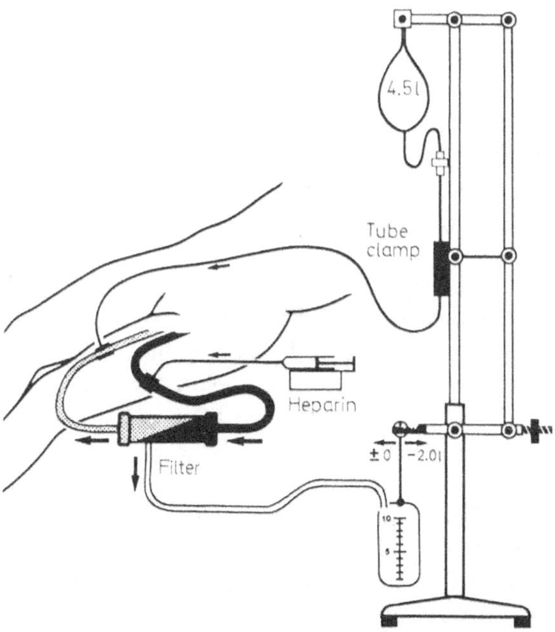

Fig. 1. Schematic presentation of the mechanical balancing system in clinical use. The position of the hanging point of the filtrate container is used to preselect negative balance at defined points giving a negative balance of ± 0, -0.5, -1.0, -1.5, -2.0 l/4.5 l substitution fluid

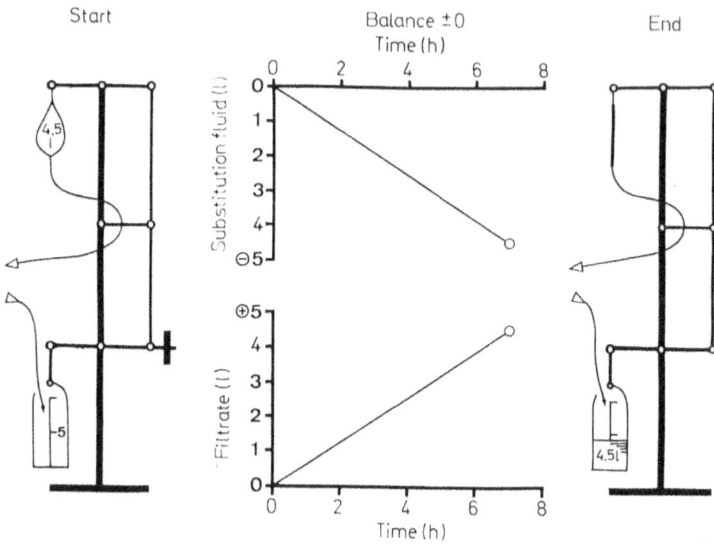

Fig. 2. Schematic presentation of an in vitro test of the system. No negative balance was intended. The signal of balance was recorded from an electronic scale bearing a fluid container (to simulate the patient's weight). A peristaltic pump was used to simulate filtration out of the fluid container into the filtrate container [1]

the upper beam is counterbalanced by a weight on the opposite side. The exact set point of the balance can be adjusted by an additional weight mobile on a screw in prolongation of the lower beam. This permits exact adjustment of the system to differences in weight of the substitution bags delivered by different suppliers. When hemofiltrate is dripping into the graduated container (10-l capacity) hanging below the substitution fluid at the lower beam, the growing imbalance opens a tube clamp mechanically setting the fluid substitution to the rate of filtration with a high accuracy.

If a negative balance was wanted, we originally [1] filled a 2-l container on the opposite side by a dripping infusion which determined the amount of the negative balance. Recently we improved the system further by modifying the hanging point of the filtrate container to preselected positions to enable an exact negative balance in steps of 0.5 l between ±0 up to 2 l per cycle. The different hanging positions have been calculated by the law of leverage. It can be shown by in vitro test as described elsewhere [1], that the accuracy of a cycle is ±10 ml/4.5 l and using a negative balance of 2 l it is better than ±20 ml/cycle. Figures 2 and 3 demonstrate two examples of an in vitro test. The balance was recorded as a total balance between filtrate and substitute on an electronic scale, the signal of which has been recorded.

This system can be handled by the staff of a general intensive care unit after a short training period. To prevent damage of the clamped silastic tube, integrated within the infusion line, the force of the tube clamp is reduced to an uncritical amount by a spring steel torque.

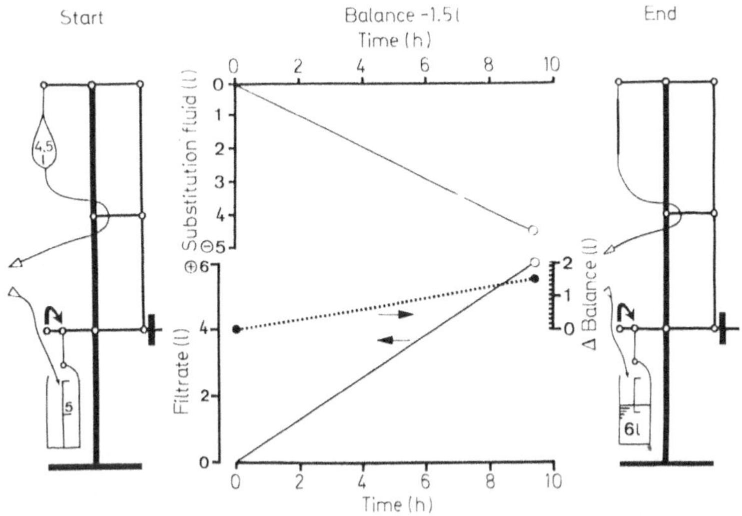

Fig. 3. Schematic presentation of an vitro test of the system as in Fig. 2 including a negative balance of −1.5 l/4.5 l substitution fluid. The accuracy of the system was better than ±20 ml/6 l filtrate volume as it was reached in this cycle

To enable a measurement of the filtration rate per minute, filtrate is dripping into a graduated plastic tube (syringe cylinder) the outlet of which can be blocked for a defined time period.

The height of the end of the filtrate tube connecting hemofilter and filtrate container is variable in order to alter the filtration rate by changes of negative pressure.

Clinical Experience

After 2 years' practice with manual handling of fluid balance, we started to use the newly developed mechanical balance system, as of April 1982, as an aid in CAVH.

In the meantime (30 months) the staff of six different intensive care units, each with a different frequency of acute renal failure, was trained in using this aid of fluid handling (first clinical prototype). From July 1984 on we got clinical experience with the newly developed negative balance design.

For the introduction of the system to the staff we used colored graphic representations of the system and of some of the systematic steps to start a balancing cycle [1].

References

1. Schurek HJ, Biela D (1983) Continuous arterio-venous hemofiltration: Improvement in the handling of fluid balance and heparinization. Blood Purification 1:186–196

A Computer Monitor to Simplify the Management of Fluid Balance During Continuous Arteriovenous Hemofiltration

J.C. Mason, R.D. Bradley, T.K. Cowell, P.J. Hilton and A.J. Wing

Introduction

Continuous arteriovenous hemofiltration (CAVH), through its cardinal virtues of maintenance of haemodynamic stability and ease of fluid removal, has already made an important contribution to the management of certain patients with acute renal failure (ARF) [3, 5]. These patients are not only severely oliguric but require cardiovascular, respiratory and nutritional support, and CAVH offers almost unlimited potential for correction of fluid overload and infusion of therapeutic solutions. For example, in our own series of 31 patients treated from 1981–1983, the average daily volume of haemofiltrate was 13.1 l which was replaced by 9.9 l of a standard substitution solution in addition to parenteral nutrition (1.5 l/day), blood products (0.8 l/day), drugs and other crystalloids (1.3 l/day). The regulation of these large volume exchanges continuously for periods up to several weeks presents difficulties for the attending staff on a scale not previously experienced. Indeed, it has been suggested [2] that arithmetic and other errors may place the patient at risk, and restriction of the filtrate flow to 5–6 l/day (slow continuous ultrafiltration, SCUF) has been recommended. In most cases this provides adequate treatment of volume overload but requires additional intermittent haemodialysis for metabolic control. Such an approach erodes the essential simplicity of CAVH and reduces its haemodynamic advantages.

Several devices to assist fluid regulation have been suggested. An attempt using weight-driven substitution fluid replacement adjusted automatically to the filtrate flow has not been widely adopted [4]. The filtration rate may be measured gravimetrically and appropriate substitution achieved by a microprocessor servo pump (Sartorius), but this means a major increase in technical sophistication and a requirement for safety monitors. In widespread practice, the filtrate is measured and the substitution fluid delivered hourly using devices varying considerably in complexity. Burettes and measuring cylinders are laborious and while volumetric pumps (I-Vac, IMED) and electronic "urinometers" (Vitalmetric) simplify this, they are expensive and still need arithmetic manipulation and charting. Furthermore, this approach does not conveniently relate haemofiltration to all the other quantitatively significant flows to and from the patient, requiring further computation.

The computer system developed at St. Thomas' Hospital provides entirely automatic monitoring of the haemofiltrate and substitution flows and additionally encompasses the total fluid balance of the patient by incorporating all other fluid exchanges. Manual record keeping has been superseded. We were anxious not to diminish the simplicity of CAVH and emphasis was placed on provision of a system which could be operated by general intensive therapy units (ITU), rather than specialist renal nurses. A microcomputer is ideally suited to the solution of repetitive numerical problems and forms the core of this unit.

Methods

Principles

Figure 1 shows the system in outline. The receptacle for haemofiltrate and the bag of substitution fluid are each suspended from electronic force gauges. Their analogue signals are fed through an interface unit and digital converter into a microcomputer which derives measurements of the container weights. Average values are used to provide a continuous display on the visual display unit (VDU) of the prevailing flow rates and cumulative volumes transferred. The display is updated every 5 s. All other fluid inputs and outputs are entered hourly through the computer keyboard by the attending nurse and the net balance is continuously displayed. The screen display can be "dumped" to the printer whenever desired and this also occurs automatically at the end of each day, providing the permanent record.

Hardware

A photograph of the system is shown in Figure 2. The apparatus is housed on two trolleys. The "master" trolley carries the microcomputer, disc drive, interface unit, VDU and printer. A 4-m cable connects it to the hemofiltration tower and permits free positioning of the units. To avoid the complexity of servo-controlled

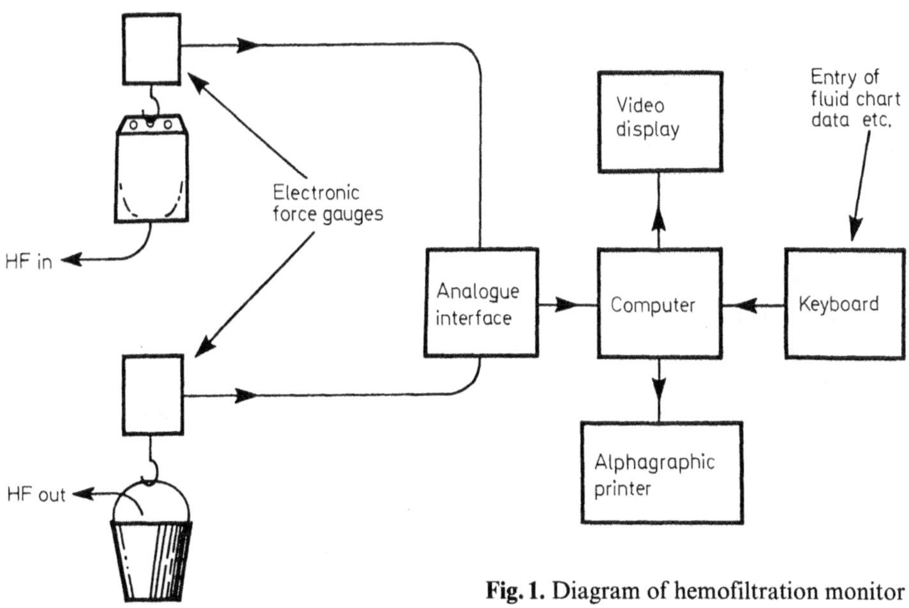

Fig. 1. Diagram of hemofiltration monitor

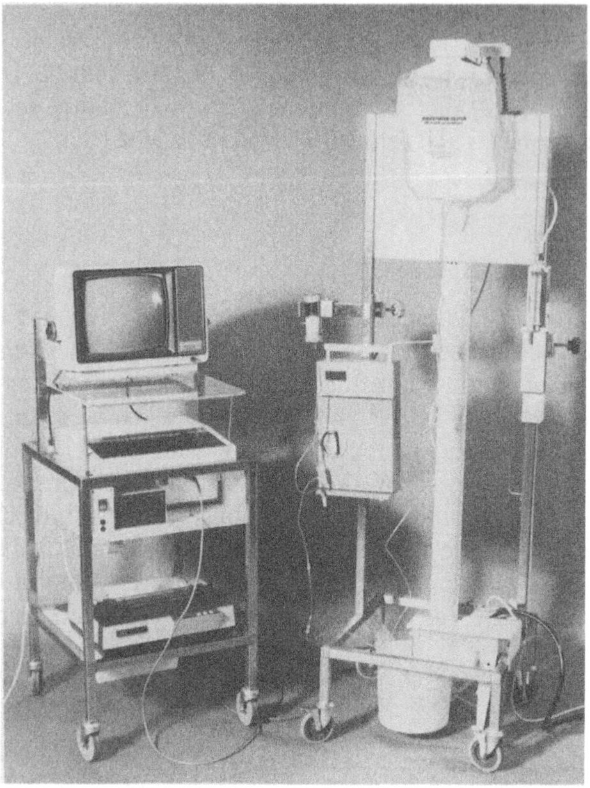

Fig. 2. Photograph of computer trolley and hemofiltration tower (full description in text)

pumps, hydrostatic pressures have been used to maintain fluid flows. The force gauge carrying the filtrate bucket is positioned close to the floor to maximise the negative pressure applied to the membrane. The second gauge is mounted on the top of a vertical piston and cylinder assembly through which compressed air or a manual ratchet permit easy elevation of the heavy (4.5 kg) bags of substitution fluid from 1.5 m (bag change position) up to 3 m above the floor. A controlled air leak regulates the descent of the unit and prevents sudden impacts. Advantage is taken of the full 10 kg range of the force gauges (Salter Abbey 100N) by using a 2:1 lever and frictionless pivot assembly. Minor nonlinearities are corrected in software for individual gauges to $<0.5\%$ full scale. Overall error is $<1\%$ and after initial equilibration for 15 min, stability over several weeks has been demonstrated. The filtration tower also carries a power supply and mountings for the hemofilter, dry warmer unit for the substitution fluid and heparin syringe pump.

Microcomputer and Software

The microcomputer [1] (Acorn BBC Model B 32K) provides a 12-bit Analogue-Digital converter with 4-channel multiplexer and 10 ms sampling time, which permits inputs from each force gauge at 50/s. A real time clock ("ticking" at 100/s) is integral and can be set and read from BASIC. The intermediate resolution monochrome graphics mode provides a 256 × 320 pixel display which with disc-filing leaves 16 kb of RAM for program and variable storage. The graphics capability is flexible and permits definition of separate text and graphics windows and simplifies screen "dumps" to printer. The program is written in BASIC with machine code additions, and stored on 5¼″ disc which also carries a calibration checking program. For safety, certain keyboard controls are inactivated during use to prevent accidental contact terminating operation. The matrix printer (NEC PC 8023) will reproduce the graphics display and print up to 136 characters per line allowing the generation of a 23-column fluid balance chart.

Operation

Emphasis has been placed on "user friendliness". By pressing two keys, the program is loaded and operation automatically commences. A short question and answer sequence follows and information concerning the patient is entered to provide labelling of subsequent printed records. The entry continues with the current time and existing state of fluid balance. The operator is reminded to check certain aspects of the apparatus and installation of the fluid containers, the weights of which are measured and operation permitted only if they fall within previously defined limits. Continuous monitoring of haemofiltration then follows.

The screen display is shown in Fig. 3. The figures at the lower left illustrate the contents of the containers while above them, the pair of opposed scales (0–1 200 ml/h) with moving printers indicate the prevailing flow rate of haemofiltrate

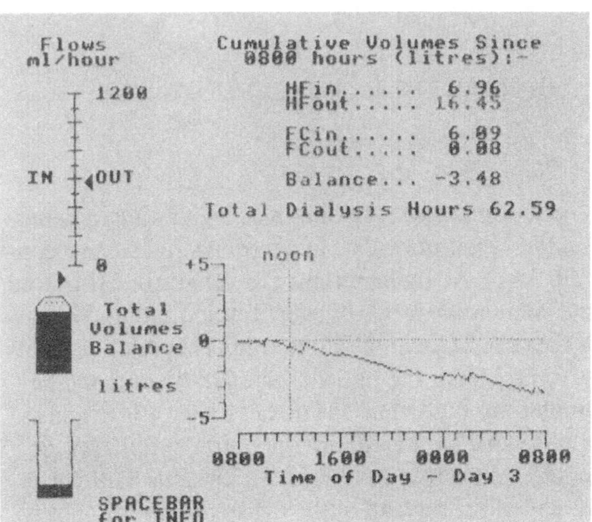

Fig. 3. VDU screen display at the end of a complete day of treatment by CAVH (details in text)

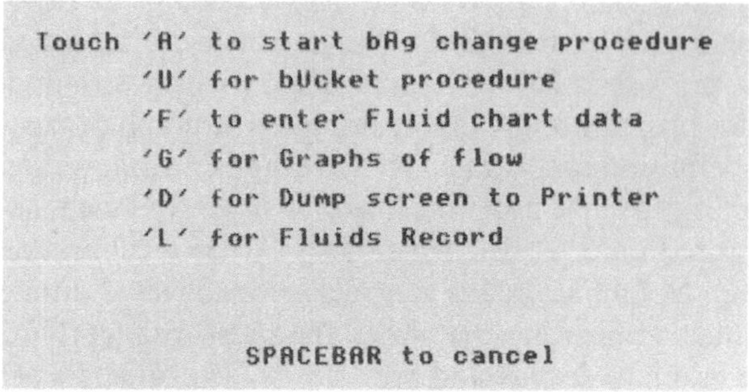

Fig. 4. VDU screen display. Menu of subroutines required during operation of CAVH computer monitor

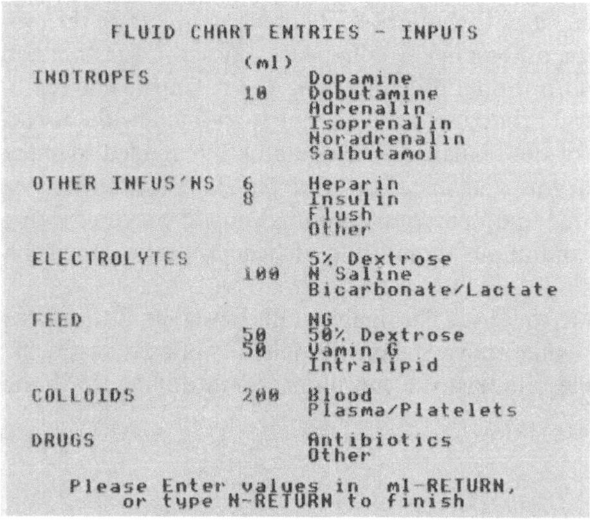

Fig. 5. VDU screen display. Example of entry of fluid input (FC) data. This is performed each hour through the keyboard

OUT and substitution fluid IN. Our practice is to obtain as high a rate of hemofiltration as possible, and to set the substitution rate appropriate to it using a constant flow device (Isoflux, Van Leer). At the top right the values for HFin and HFout refer respectively to the cumulative totals of substitution fluid and hemofiltrate from the beginning of the day. FCin and FCout are the cumulative totals of all the other volume flows to and from the patient, entered through the keyboard and conventionally handled by fluid charts. The net balance is displayed below these and every 15 min this value is entered into the central graph, progressively depicting the overall trend as the day continues. After the automatic printing of the screen display at the end of the day, all of the registers are reset to zero, the graph is cleared and the whole process starts again, without intervention.

By pressing the keyboard space bar, a menu of subroutines is displayed (Fig. 4) and after selecting the appropriate key the operator is guided through procedures such as changing the substitution bag or filtrate bucket. The nurse is not required to manipulate numbers to achieve this. Approximately hourly, "fluid chart" (FC) data is entered by selection of the relevant routine ("F", Fig. 4). A list of possible fluid entries (with two open options to allow flexibility) appears on the screen (Fig. 5) and their values are typed in. When the completion of the entry is signalled, the display reduces to show only those items with positive entries. This facilitates accurate checking and after any necessary correction, fluid outputs are handled similarly. The entire entry, with its time, is then automatically printed in conventional chart-column form, with a second row of print showing the cumulative totals of the individual items.

Audible chimes from the computer's loudspeaker, together with appropriate messages on the screen, provide prompts concerning the timing of container changes and entry of fluid data. A more forceful display signals warning if the container changes have not been properly initiated through the computer. A restart routine is available if the instrument is accidentally disconnected, permitting entry of the current numeric data.

Discussion

This computer monitor has provided the basis for CAVH in our unit for over 1 year, and has performed for several thousand hours without significant problem. It has been readily assimilated into the nursing process and fulfilled our expectations of operation by nonspecialist nurses, typically after only a few minutes of tuition. This stands in contrast to our earlier experience with CAVH in rudimentary form, when laborious fluid monitoring threatened to impose an unacceptable burden on staff who were already heavily committed in the intensive care of patients needing multisystem support. As the latter had an inevitably poor prognosis, there were adverse effects on nursing morale. The present system offers management at least as simple as peritoneal dialysis.

We have deliberately not "closed the loop" to provide automatic substitution with respect to measured filtration, although this was included in our original plans. The relationship between these flows often requires revision with respect to concurrent events such as feeding, transfusions, or unforeseen fluid losses, and the displayed graph of fluid balance against time provides a simple guide to adjust the substitution rate, setting it in the context of the overall fluid state. In certain patients, CAVH is capable of delivering filtrate volumes approaching 25 l/day, which can now be managed without difficulty and with the benefit of improved metabolic control.

The cost of this system is small in comparison with conventional dialysis equipment. Since its operation is defined in software, modification to meet newly recognised needs is comparatively simple. It is perhaps of interest to note that our "master unit" (computer, VDU and printer) when supplied with alternative inputs and programs, routinely serves several other purposes on the ICU. These include measurement of cardiac output by thermodilution, multichannel pressure recording, respiratory gas analysis by mass spectrometry and semiautomatic charting of routine observations of pulse, blood pressure etc. With respect to CAVH it allows full and easy application of this extremely useful technique.

References

1. Cowell TK (1983) The BBC Model B microcomputer in clinical instrumentation. J Med Eng Tech 7:79
2. Dodd NJ, O'Donovan RM, Bennett-Jones DN, Rylance PB, Bewick M, Parsons V, Weston MJ (1983) Arteriovenous haemofiltration: a recent advance in the management of renal failure. Br Med J 287:999
3. Kramer P, Wigger W, Rieger J, Matthaei D, Scheler F (1977) Arteriovenous haemofiltration: a new and simple method for treatment of over-hydrated patients resistant to diuretics. Klin Wochenschr 55:1121
4. Kramer P, Seegers A, De Vivie R, Matthaei D, Trautmann M, Scheler F (1979) Therapeutic potential of haemofiltration. Clin Nephrology 11:145
5. Kramer P, Bohler J, Kehr A, Grone HJ, Schrader J, Matthaei D, Scheler F (1982) Intensive care potential of continuous arteriovenous haemofiltration. Trans Am Soc Artif Intern Organs 18:28

Blood Volume and Blood Flow

Continuous Noninvasive Monitoring of Blood Volume During Arteriovenous Hemofiltration

H. Mann, S. Stiller, P. Eberle, and N. Maurin

Extracorporeal filtration of plasma water of a patient is possible without decrease in blood pressure as long as the blood volume is not critically reduced. In clinical practice blood pressure and central venous pressure are simple clinical measurements to monitor the circulation, and yet it often happens that the blood pressure suddenly drops to very low values within a few minutes after exceeding the permissible filtrate volume. Therefore filtration rates in relation to circulatory parameters have to be observed closely and interpreted with great clinical experience. It would be desirable, therefore, to measure blood volume during extracorporeal filtration in a simple way but with sufficient accuracy and if possible continuously, in order to get information about the "refilling rate."

This contribution deals with a method for continuous evaluation of the hematocrit in the extracorporeal circulation which reflects actual changes in the relative blood volume. The method is based on the simultaneous measurement of electric conductivity of the blood and the filtrate. The conductivity of the filtrate and blood depends (as well as on temperature) mainly on the electrolyte composition, but the difference of conductivity between whole blood and filtrate depends entirely on the hematocrit. If the volume of erythrocytes is constant, as in hemodialysis and hemofiltration, short-term changes of the hematocrit during blood filtration reflect changes in the relative blood volume.

Since whole blood as well as filtrate are continuously transported through the extracorporeal circulation during spontaneous filtration, conventional hemofiltration, and plasmafiltration, this method may be classified as noninvasive and comfortable for the patient.

Method

Three small refined-steel tubes are worked into the arterial tubing system which are, like the tubing, disposable (Fig. 1). Their inner diameter is the same as that for the blood tubing. At these points blood conductivity is measured with 400 cycles per second of alternating current and the temperature, as interference factor, is observed. A similar measuring mechanism is attached to the filtrate-conducting tubing (Fig. 2). From the simultaneously registered values, after eliminating the effect of temperature, the hematocrit is determined and continuously displayed as difference between whole blood and filtrate conductivity.

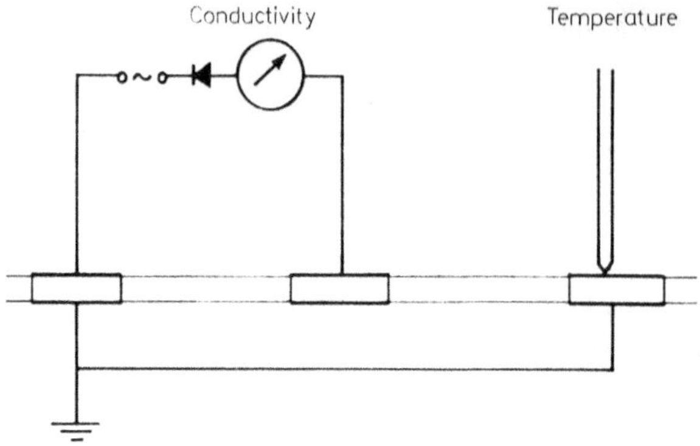

Fig. 1. Arrangement of electrodes in the blood or filtrate tubing system. The tubing electrodes are disposable

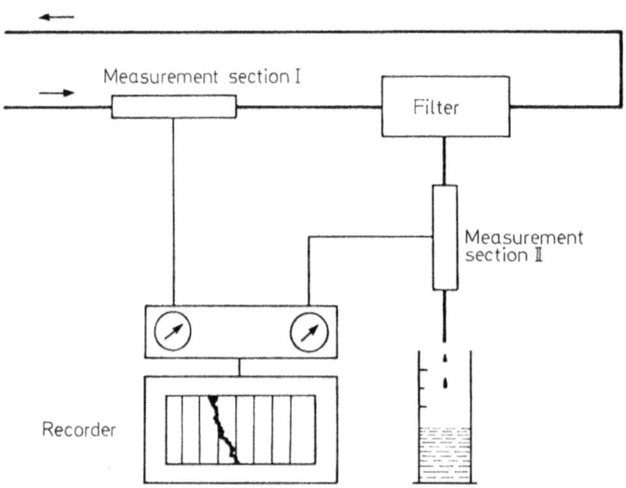

Fig. 2. Measuring setup for arteriovenous hemofiltration. Measuring point in the arterial and filtrate tubing. Continuous registration of the differential value

Figure 3 gives an example of the sensitivity of the method: the graphs show the values of the hematocrit ($V_{b/Vb}$) and the mean arterial pressure (*RR*) in relationship to a specific filtration rate of 1300 ml/h and then 300 ml/h during 4 h. After a reduction of the plasma volume and blood pressure drop, 500 ml fructose (5 g/dl) are infused. This leads to an immediate increase in the plasma volume and blood pressure which only lasts for the duration of the infusion. Then, blood pressure and plasma volume falls again because of the fluid diffused into the extracellular and intracellular space.

Next, an infusion of 1000 ml normal saline (0.9 g/dl) is administered with similar results, but only now the systolic blood pressure reaches the desired value.

Figure 4 shows the results of a patient who was severely hydropic due to renal failure; 22 l plasma water were filtered off by spontaneous ultrafiltration within 4 days. During the first treatment (11-15-80) a total of 12 l were ultrafiltered in 15 h at a filtration rate of 800 ml/h without measurable change of plasma volume or blood pressure. During the second treatment (11-17-80), at a filtration rate of 1000 ml/h the plasma volume decreased gradually but without change of blood

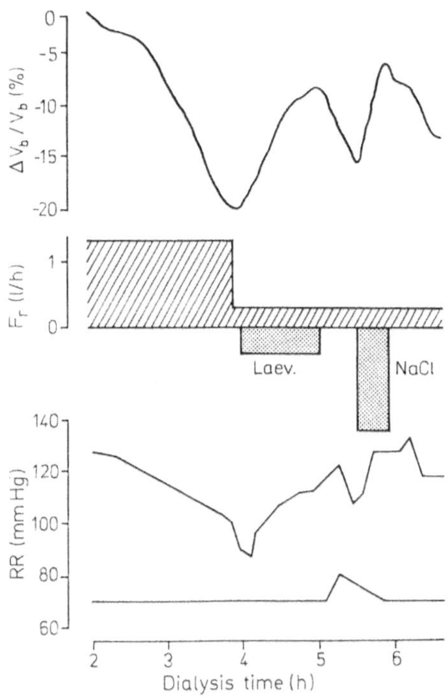

Fig. 3. Sensitivity of the measuring system: Change of hematocrit after ultrafiltration and substitution with 5% fructose and 0.9% NaCl

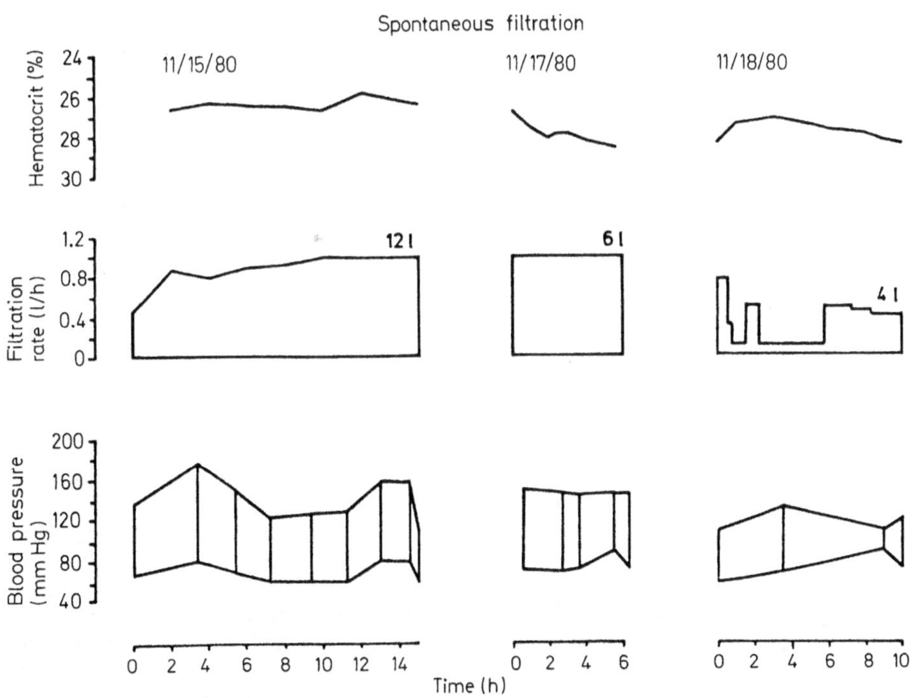

Fig. 4. Arteriovenous hemofiltration of a hydropic patient on three of four consecutive days

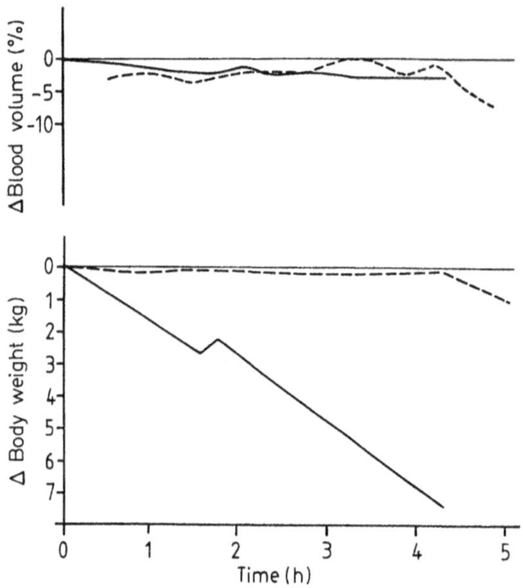

Fig. 5. Changes of blood volume in one patient at different degrees of fluid overload. *Straight lines:* hydropic state with 15 l of fluid overload. *Dotted lines:* nonhydropic state of the patient

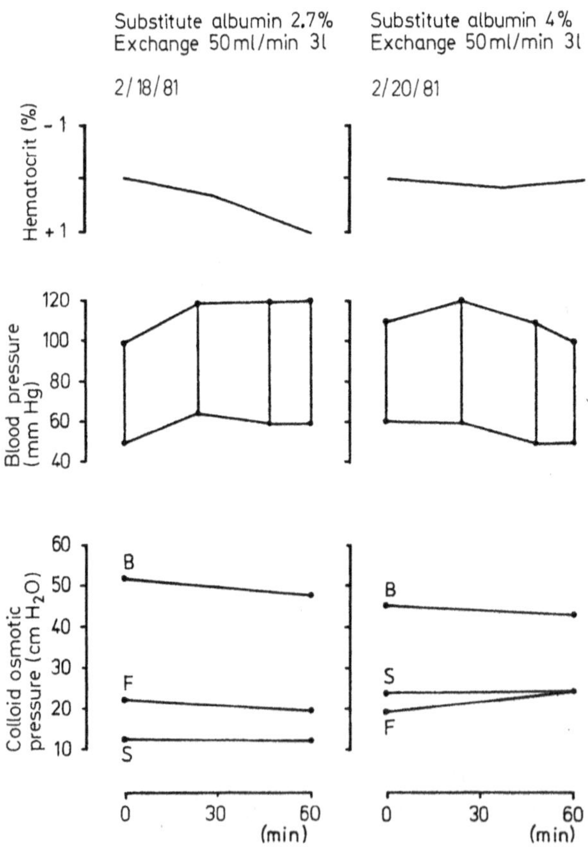

Fig. 6. Membrane plasmapheresis with substitution of albumin solutions (2.7 and 4.0 g/dl) with different concentrations. Hematocrit, colloid-osmotic pressure, and blood pressure are shown. *B*, blood; *F*, filtrate; *S*, substitution fluid

pressure. During the third treatment the filtration rate had to be reduced to avoid further increase of the hematocrit. Filtration was only adjusted to the fluid flow from the extracellular space.

In the same patient during ultrafiltration, change of blood volume was very much dependent on the degree of overhydration. This is illustrated in Fig. 5: With the first slope (straight lines) the patient was hydropic with 15 l overload. Ultrafiltration of 1700 ml/h for 4 h induced no change in blood volume. One month later the patient was no more hydropic (dotted lines). There was a decrease of 7% blood volume analogous to ultrafiltration rate during the 5th h of treatment.

During membrane plasma separation, plasma volume can decrease as a result of substituting an albumin solution with low colloid-osmotic pressure. In Fig. 6 the same patient received a 2.7% albumin solution at one time, and a 4.0% albumin solution as substitute at another time.

It can be clearly seen that the lesser concentrated albumin solution with lower colloid-osmotic pressure caused a reduction of plasma volume (elevation of hematocrit).

Discussion

The method described here [6, 7], permits the continuous registration of the hematocrit as indicator of the blood volume. The procedure is accurate and without discomfort for the patient during hemofiltration [2], plasma separation [4], and also during hemodialysis [3]. A method with a similar goal but different principle has been described elsewhere [1]. During the extracorporeal blood cleaning procedures, ultrafiltration can change the colloid-osmotic pressure, and the osmotic pressure gradient between the extra- and intracellular space, especially through changes of the extracellular sodium concentration [5], which may cause a change of the blood volume independent of extracorporeal fluid loss. It is usually difficult, under clinical conditions, to control each single factor especially when infusion therapy is administered simultaneously.

By continuous monitoring of the hematocrit as marker for blood volume, critical conditions that can occur during excessive filtration, can be recognized in time.

In this way ultrafiltration can be adjusted to the so-called "refilling rate" of the blood volume and can be continued at a clinically optimum rate until the desired volume is filtered off.

The apparatus for continuous hematocrit measuring is easily integrated into the treatment device and optimizes therapy using alarm limits for blood volume change.

Summary

Through excessive ultrafiltration and change in osmotic pressure, undesired reduction of the blood volume can occur during arteriovenous hemofiltration, conventional hemofiltration, hemodialysis, and membrane plasma separation. For continuous extracorporeal noninvasive monitoring of the hematocrit, a technically simple but sensitive method was developed which is based on simultaneous measurements of electric conductivity of whole blood and ultrafiltrate. Changes in the hematocrit during filtration reflect changes in the relative blood volume.

By using this procedure, filtration can be regulated without risking critical reduction of the blood volume.

References

1. Kenner T, Hinghofer-Szalaky H, Leopold H, Pogglitsch H (1977) Das Verhalten der Blutdichte in Relation zum Blutdruck im Tierversuch und bei Hämodialyse von Patienten. Z Kardiol 66:399
2. Mann H, Schultheis R, Homburg A, Raguse T, Rautenbach R (1978) Hämofiltration in der Intensivmedizin. Diagnostik Intensivtherapie 3:15
3. Rouby J, Rottenbourg J, Durande JP, Basset JY, Legrain M (1979) Plasma volume changes induced by regular hemodialysis and controlled sequential ultrafiltration hemodialysis. Dialysis Transpl 8:237
4. Sieberth HG (1980) Plasma exchange. Schattauer, Stuttgart
5. Stiller S, Mann H, Gürich W (1978) Theoretical aspects of various ultrafiltration methods in artificial kidney therapy. Artif Organs 2:137
6. Stiller S, Mann H (1980) Automatische Kontrolle des Blutvolumens bei extrakorporaler Dialyse und Filtration. Biomed Tech 25:286
7. Stiller S, Mann H (1980) Continuous monitoring of blood volume during hemodialysis. Proc Eur Dial Transplant Assoc 7:167

Doppler Sonographic Measurement of the Blood-Flow Rate in the Extracorporeal Tubing System During Arteriovenous Hemofiltration *

T. Eisenhauer, H. Kaiser, J. Schrader, G. Sold, P. Kramer,
U. Hüttig, F. Scheler, and H. Kreuzer

Since Doppler ultrasound flow measurement was introduced to medicine [9] and was found to be practical for measuring flow rate [3], different modifications were quickly developed so that this method of transcutaneous arterial and venous measurement of blood flow could, in practice, be increasingly used in patients [11, 12].

The method was first used on a large scale by clinical angiologists to evaluate vascular diseases, but was soon utilized in the area of nephrology, where function and hemodynamic effect of arteriovenous fistulas were of particular interest [8].

During spontaneous arteriovenous hemofiltration [6], blood-flow rate can neither be estimated by the speed of roller pumps nor by the drop rate of blood into the air bubble catcher. Therefore, a practical technique needed to be found promptly whereby blood flow through the hemofilter, besides the filtration rate, could be measured as indicator, i.e., of the dose of heparin necessary for anticoagulation of the extracorporeal blood circuit [10].

* Supported by SFB 89 Cardiology, Göttingen, Federal Republic of Germany

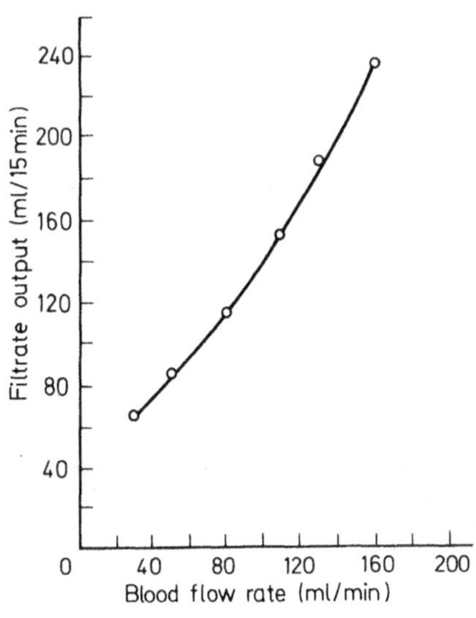

Fig. 1. Relationship between blood-flow rate and 15-min filtrate output

Although filtrate volume decreases almost linearly with gradually reduced blood flow by clamping the arterial tubing of individual patients, as seen in Fig. 1, in clinical practice situations arose where it seemed advantageous to measure blood-flow rate separately, such as in the case of (a) determination of filtration fraction during arteriovenous hemofiltration, (b) determination of blood-flow rate when the filtrate tubing is clamped off, (c) optimum heparinization of the extracorporeal system depending on blood-flow rate in bleeding-endangered patients, (d) early detection of hemofilter clotting.

Method

For blood-flow measurement, electromagnetic flowmeters [13] were found to be quite accurate. However, the disadvantage of this method is that the extracorporeal tubing system has to be opened up for the insertion of the cannulating measuring probe, risking invasion of bacteria into the blood stream and loss of blood.

It therefore seemed to make sense to use a noninvasive method such as Doppler sonography for the measurement of blood-flow rate in the extracorporeal tubing system during arteriovenous hemofiltration. Doppler sonography is based on the following principle: If a sound wave of particular frequency hits a moving object, the frequency of the reflected sound wave changes proportionally to the speed of the object, in this case the red blood cells. The mean flow (Q) is given here as function of the tubing diameter (A) and speed of sound in the blood medium (c).

$$\bar{Q} = A \times \bar{V} \tag{1}$$

The mean flow, on the other hand, is dependent on emission frequency (f_o), on reflected Doppler frequency (f_D), on the angle of incidence (α) of the ultrasound as well as on the speed of sound in the blood medium (c).

$$\tilde{V} = 1/2 f_D/f_o \times c \times 1/\cos\alpha\,, \tag{2}$$

Equation (3) follows from Eqs. 1 and 2:

$$Q = (A \times 1/2 f_D/f_o \times c \times 1/\cos\alpha\,. \tag{3}$$

In the extracorporeal tubing system, tubing diameter, angle of incidence (alpha), and propagation of sound in the blood are constant. The only variable remaining, therefore, is Doppler frequency relative to flow rate.

Figure 2 shows the measuring device.

The supporting fixture for the Doppler transducer was attached to the arterial tubing of the extracorporeal system, approximately 50 cm from the proximal tubing end. A flat probe with a 45° angle (from Meda Sonics) was securely fixed into a homemade plexiglas case. A 10-cm long groove, corresponding in size to that of the outer tubing diameter, was drilled into the bottom half of the housing. The arterial tubing was placed in such a way that, without deforming the tubing, the entire inner tubing diameter was in direct contact with the flat probe. At the distal

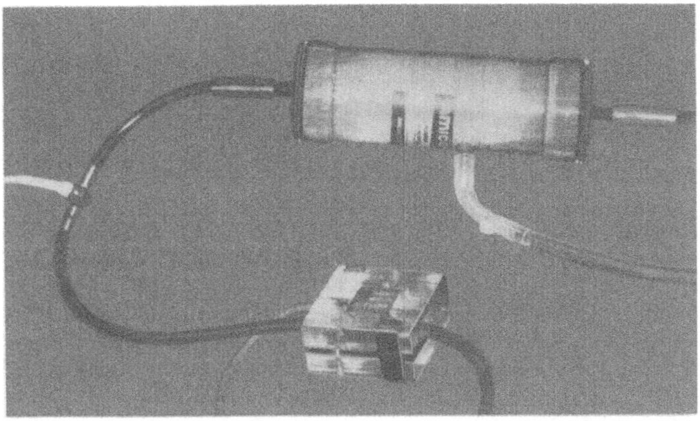

Fig. 2. Hemofilter with extracorporeal arterial and venous tubing. Electromagnetic flowmeter and Doppler flat probe are attached to the arterial line. The flat probe is fixed into a plexiglas housing in constant position to the tubing system

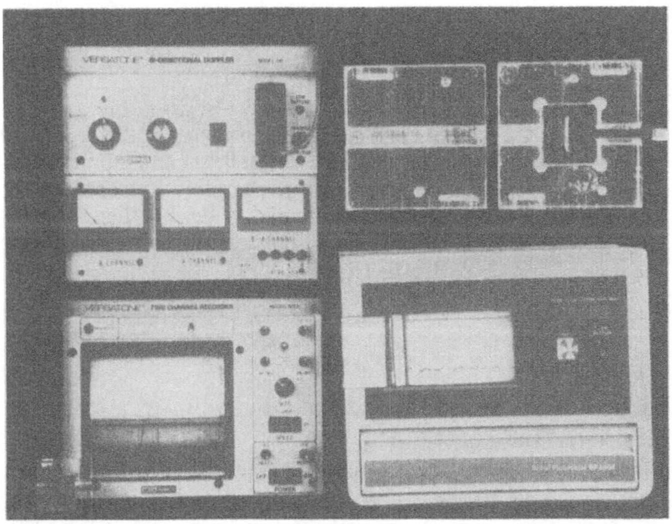

Fig. 3. Doppler instrument with flat probe in the plexiglas housing on the *upper right* and electromagnetic flowmeter on the *lower right*. (The Doppler instrument was on loan from the routine diagnostic department, angiology ambulance of the cardiology department)

end of the arterial line, approximately 20 cm before entering the hemofilter, the line was opened up and the previously sterilized and calibrated electromagnetic measuring probe inserted.

Both types of measuring devices used for the experiment are shown in Fig. 3. On the left side a bidirectional Doppler instrument with recorder (from Meda Sonics, Mountain View, USA) can be seen, and on the right side is an electromagnetic blood flowmeter (from Gould Statham, P 2204). Both instruments were used in parallel for two patients during spontaneous arteriovenous hemofiltra-

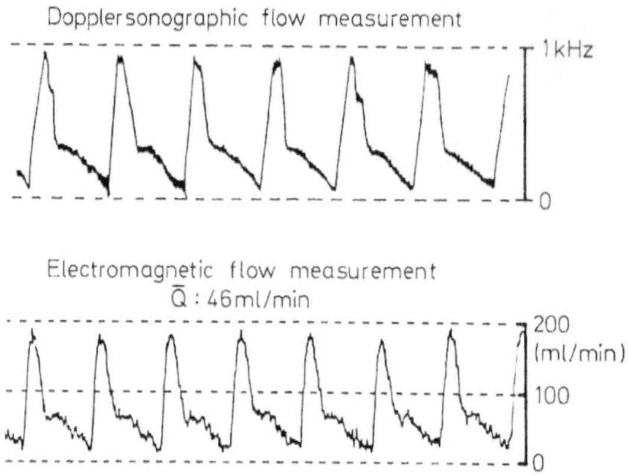

Fig. 4. Pulsatile flow curves; *top:* Doppler sonographically registered curve with standard peak corresponding to 1 kHz; *bottom:* electromagnetically measured curve

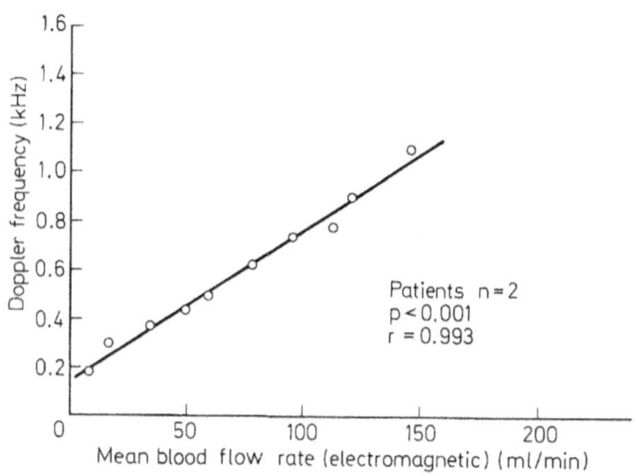

Fig. 5. Relationship between electromagnetically registered mean flow and Doppler sonographically measured maximum rate in the extracorporeal arterial line during CAVH

tion. For gradual reduction of the arterial blood flow, a clamp was attached at the proximal end of the arterial tubing.

Altogether 10 double measurements were performed, each at different bloodflow rates. Since it was not possible to obtain mean values from the Doppler instrument available to us, the Doppler frequency values are given in relationship to the values of the electromagnetic flowmeter. Postulating that the curve remains the same the maximum flow values from the Doppler signal were compared with the mean values of the electromagnetic flowmeter. Maximum flow rate was determined from 10 Doppler sonographically registered flow profiles and the mean flow rate could be read directly from the digital readouts of the electromagnetic flowmeter.

Results

Figure 4 shows a typical recording of blood flow measurements with Doppler sonography standardized to 1 kHz (1000 cycles/s). The shape of the curve was nearly identical for both patients and was in good agreement with the electromagnetically registered blood-flow curve. By graded clamping of the arterial line, mean flow rates of a minimum of 9 ml/min to a maximum of 148 ml/min were achieved. The relationship between the electromagnetically measured mean blood-flow rate and the Doppler sonographically measured maximum flow rate is presented in Fig. 5. There was a linear relationship between both types of measurements (2 patients, $n=10$ pairs of values) with a correlation of $r=0.993$ ($p<0.001$).

Discussion

Filtration rate and anticoagulation of the extracorporeal system do not solely depend on the blood-flow rate [1, 2, 7]. Filtrate output can be affected by deposits of blood factors on the membrane surface. Filtration raction can change with increased resistance caused by partial thrombosing of the capillaries, or with elevation of the hematocrit and albumin concentration. Therefore separate measurement of the filtration and blood-flow rate might occasionally be desirable.

The development of the easily performable continuous arteriovenous hemofiltration [4, 5] presented the opportunity to utilize Doppler sonography, which is available almost anywhere, for the determination of the mean blood-flow rate in the extracorporeal system.

The advantage of this noninvasive method is, specifically, the indirect blood measurement without risk of bacterial invasion or loss of blood. Also, the Doppler instrument is generally easy to handle and less expensive than an electromagnetic flowmeter.

The goal of this experiment was to demonstrate that Doppler sonographic flow measurement in the extracorporeal system is technically possible, and that reproducible values can be obtained which are sufficient for practical purposes. The immediate disadvantage of the sonographic flow measurement lies in only being able to measure indirectly. However, by installing a mean value computer into the ultrasound device it is possible, at known tubing diameter, to register the mean blood-flow rate directly.

References

1. Blanke H, Kreuzer H, Wigger W, Scheler F (1977) Die Behandlung der akuten Linksherzinsuffizienz anurischer Patienten mit der Hämofiltration. Dtsch Med Wochenschr 102:1804
2. Blanke H, Karsch KR, Kreuzer H, Wigger W, Scheler F (1978) Treatment of acute left heart failure in anuric patients by haemofiltration. VIII. World congress of cardiology 17th.–23rd Sept., Tokyo
3. Franklin DL, Schlegel WA, Rushner RF (1961) Blood flow measured by Doppler frequency shift of backscattered ultrasound. Science 132:564
4. Kaiser H, Rumpf KW, Schrader J, Sold G, Kramer P, Kreuzer H (1981) Serum myoglobin (SMb) in acute renal failure due to rhabdomyolysis treated with arteriovenous hemofiltration. XVIII. Congress of the European dialysis and transplant association, Paris
5. Kramer P, Wigger W, Rieger J, Matthaei D, Scheler F (1977) Arteriovenous hemofiltration: a new and simple method for treatment of over-hydrated patients resistent to diuretics. Klin Wochenschr 55:1021

6. Kramer P, Kaufhold G, Gröne HJ, Wigger W, Rieger J, Matthaei D, Stokke T, Burchardi H, Scheler F (1980) Management of anuric intensive-care patients with arteriovenous hemofiltration. Int J Artfic Organs 3:225
7. Kramer P, Schrader J, Bohnsack W, Grieben G, Gröne HJ, Scheler F (1981) Continuous arteriovenous hemofiltration (CAVH). A new kidney replacement therapy. Proc Eur Dial Transplant Assoc 18:743
8. Rumpf KW, Biastoch J, Kaiser H, Hölscher M, Hildebrandt HH, Lowitz HD, Kreuzer H, Scheler F (1980) „Steal"-Phänomene bei Patienten mit arterio-venösen Fisteln: Diagnostik mittels Messung von Perfusionsdruck und Fingerplethysmographie. Symposion: arterio-venöse Fisteln zur Hämodialyse, Münster
9. Satomura S (1957) Study of flow patterns in peripheral arteries by ultrasonics. J Acoust Soc Jpn 15:151
10. Schrader J, Köstering H, Kaiser H, Kramer P, Scheler F (1981) Thrombophilia in patients with acute renal failure. XVIII. Congress of the European dialysis and transplant association, Paris
11. Strandness DE Jr, McCutcheon EP, Rushner RF (1966) Application of a transcutaneous Doppler flowmeter in evaluation of occlusive arterial disease. Surg Gynecol Obset 22:1039
12. Strandness DE Jr, Schultz RD, Sumner DS, Rushner RF (1967) Ultrasonic flow detection: a useful technique in the evaluation of peripheral vascular disease. Am J Surg 113:311
13. Wyatt DG (1977) Theory, design and use of electromagnetic flowmeters. In: Hwang NHC, Normann NA (eds) Cardiovascular flow dynamics and measurement. University Park Press, Baltimore, Chapter 2

Bedside Estimation of Blood-Flow Rate

P. Kramer and W. Rosenkranz

There are two clinical situations which require a rough estimation of the blood-flow rate during continuous arteriovenous hemofiltration (CAVH):

1. Differentiation between various causes of low filtration rate: Capillary thrombosis, partial occlusion of the vascular access, low blood pressure, high colloid-osmotic pressure, high hematocrit, low blood-flow rate due to inappropriate components of the set and unknown changes of membrane permeability.
2. Suction-assisted CAVH [3] requires blood-flow rates > 100 ml/min for the use of the Diafilter-20 (Amicon), otherwise the negative pressure will result in a blocking of capillaries by red cell puree with consequent clotting of the extracorporeal circuit. For the clinically experienced it may be sufficient to fill the arterial tubing with saline after occlusion of the arterial three-way valve and to observe the blood-flow velocity through the tubing to the hemofilter. With an internal diameter of the tubing of 4 mm the front of the blood column should move at least 5 cm/s through the tubing after opening the stop cock.

In hemofilters with a filtration fraction of more than 20% the measurement of inlet/outlet hematocrit (HCT vol%) or albumin concentration (ALB g/dl) may be used for calculation of the blood-flow rate by means of a formula, which is derived from the Fick principle [2]. The Fick principle is based on the conservation of material in a three-port system and is the basis for blood-flow measurements in many organs. The filtration rate is equivalent to the extraction rate of an indicator and the change of hematocrit or albumin concentration is indirectly equivalent to concentration change of the indicator ($1 - C_{inlet}/C_{outlet}$ is equivalent to the inlet/outlet concentration difference in the Fick formula).

$$\text{Blood-flow rate (ml/min)} = \frac{\text{Filtration rate (ml/min)}}{1 - HCT_{inlet}/HCT_{outlet}} \tag{1}$$

$$\text{Blood-flow rate (ml/min)} = \frac{\text{Filtration rate (ml/min)}}{1 - ALB_{inlet}/ALB_{outlet}}. \tag{2}$$

The great disadvantage of this method is the small difference between inlet and outlet hematocrit or albumin concentration. In our experience the differences in hematocrit range between 2 and 5 vol%, whereby the accuracy of hematocrit determination is only ± 1 vol%.

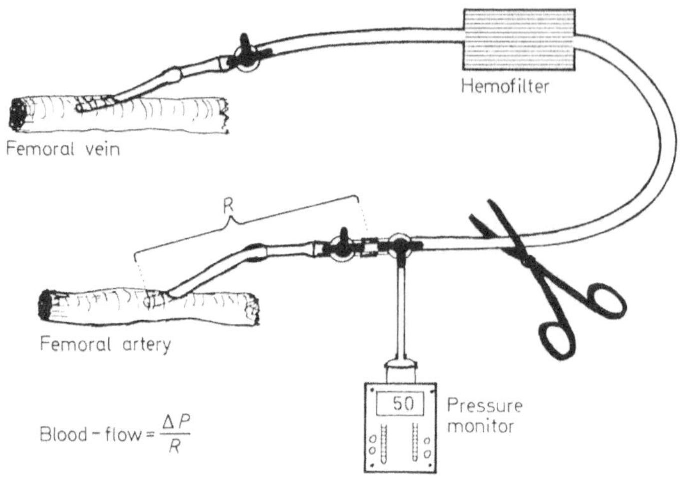

Fig. 1. Schematic illustration of the bedside method for estimation of blood-flow rate

Therefore, we should like to introduce a simple bedside estimation of blood-flow rate, which is derived from Ohm's law or the Hagen-Poiseulle's equation [1] and based on pressure measurements.

The blood flow in a tubing system is proportional to the pressure drop along a stenosis. The blood flow may be calculated if the resistance of the stenosis and the viscosity of the blood are known. Practically, the cannula (8-Charr-Vygon-CAVH-catheter) and the first arterial three-way valve are the defined stenosis, and the pressure line is connected to the second arterial three-way valve as shown in Fig. 1. The pressure drop along the "stenosis" is determined by measuring first under free-flow conditions and then after occlusion of the arterial tubing. The difference between the two valves represents more or less the pressure drop or pressure gradient. Most of our patients have, for the purpose of intensive supervision, an arterial pressure transducer connected to the femoral cannula. In these cases it is very simple to estimate the blood-flow rate: The mean arterial pressure is taken from the digital display, then the arterial blood line is occluded for more than 5 s using thumb and index finger. The pressure increase shown on the display is comparable with the pressure drop along the "stenosis."

In order to simplify the blood-flow estimation, the relationship between pressure increase (or pressure drop) along the "stenosis" in relation to blood-flow rate and hematocrit was investigated. Figure 2 demonstrates results of studies on the blood flow studied under in vivo conditions (37 °C; oxygen and glucose substituted blood; pulsatile blood flow with Harvard-pump-driven membrane heart) in relation to pressure drop along the "stenosis" and hematocrit [4]. The Amicon-CAVH set (1983) including Diafilter-20 (0.2 m^2) and the 8 Charr-Vygon vascular catheters were used for the artificial circulation. Systolic, diastolic, and venous backflow pressure as well as the flow and pressure profiles were comparable with in vivo conditions.

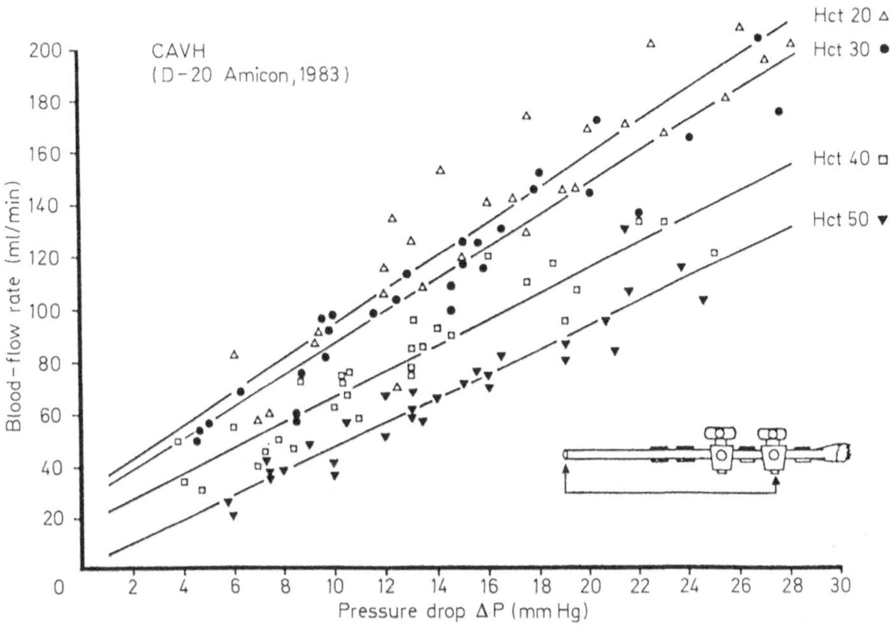

Fig. 2. Relationship between blood-flow rate and pressure drop along the arterial cannula and the first three-way valve

Figure 2 displays the results. If the patient has a hematocrit of 30 vol% and a pressure drop of 15 mmHg, the estimated blood flow would be clearly over 100 ml/min. Unfortunately, this "nomogram" has to be renewed, whenever another arterial cannula or three-way valve is used. Also, the estimations of blood-flow rate are not valid, if the patient has a severe stenosis proximal to the tip of the cannula. Nevertheless, in daily intensive care practice this rough estimation of blood-flow rate has proven useful. If the pressure drop is over 15 mmHg, a low filtration rate cannot be due to low blood-flow rate and suction may be applied. Before suction-assisted CAVH is started one should, however, exclude a stenosis of the iliac artery (good peripheral pulses?) and a partial blocking of the cannula (rapid filling of a 20 cc syringe?).

References

1. Feigl EO (1974) Physics of the cardiovascular system. In: Ruch TC, Patton HD (eds) Physiology and biophysics, vol II. Saunders, Philadelphia, p 10
2. Feigl EO (1974) Measurement of blood pressure and blood flow. In: Ruch TC, Patton HD (eds) Physiology and biophysics, vol II. Saunders, Philadelphia, p 23
3. Kaplan AA, Longnecker RE, Folkert VW (1983) Suction-assisted continuous arteriovenous hemofiltration. Trans Am Soc Artif Intern Organs 29:408–412
4. Kramer P, Rösick F, Rosenkranz W, Hellige G, Scheler F (1985) Determinanten der Filtrationsfraktion bei arterio-venöser Hämofiltration. Verh Dtsch Ges Inn Med 90:983–986

Fluid and Electrolyte Substitution

Management of Electrolyte and Acid-Base Metabolism with Continuous Arteriovenous Hemofiltration

W. Wigger, K. Grieben, D. Matthaei, and P. Kramer

General Aspects

Continuous arteriovenous hemofiltration (CAVH) is intended to perform the following functions as a miniature artificial kidney in the treatment of oligoanuria: correlation of overhydration, electrolyte imbalance, metabolic acidosis, and uremia.

The loss of fluid accompanied by convective removal of electrolytes and uremic substances is usually continously replaced with potassium-free Ringers lactate solution. The ultrafiltrate concentration of nonplasma protein bound electrolytes (Na^+, Cl^-, K^+, PO_4^{--}, HCO_3^-, lactate$^-$) is similar to that of plasma [5, 8]. In Table 1 concentrations of various plasma and ultrafiltrate electrolytes of patient K.U. (Fig. 2) are compared as an example. The ultrafiltrate concentration of calcium and magnesium amounts to only 50%–70% of that of plasma. HCO_3^- determination of the ultrafiltrate is of little significance since concentration changes occur as soon as the ultrafiltrate comes into contact with air because the blood pH value is usually higher than the filtrate pH (Fig. 1) which may be explained by absence of buffering proteins in the ultrafiltrate and by loss of CO_2.

For the purpose of balancing acid-base metabolism, it can be postulated that the bicarbonate loss during CAVH corresponds to the product of the standard bicarbonate of blood × ultrafiltrate volume. Concentration changes in plasma are caused by plasma water exchange and can be regulated specifically with vari-

Table 1. Electrolyte concentration in plasma and ultrafiltrate with CAVH and pump-driven hemofiltration (20 l in 4 h) of patient K. U. (Fig. 2)

	Electrolyte concentration (meq/l)			
	CAVH		Pump-driven hemofiltration	
	Plasma	Ultrafiltrate	Plasma	Ultrafiltrate
Na^+	149	147	144	144
K^+	6.6	6.5	4.8	4.9
Ca^{++}	3.8	2.2	4.2	3.0
Cl^-	99	101	105	105
HCO_3^-	23		24	
Lactate$^-$	3.0	3.1	3.2	3.1

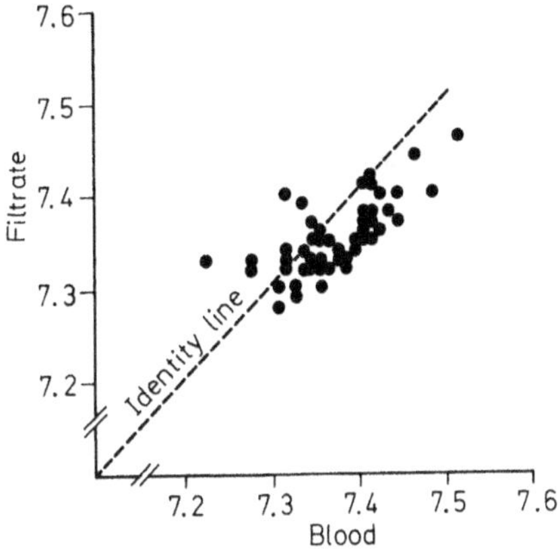

Fig. 1. Comparison between ultrafiltrate and plasma pH values during hemofiltration

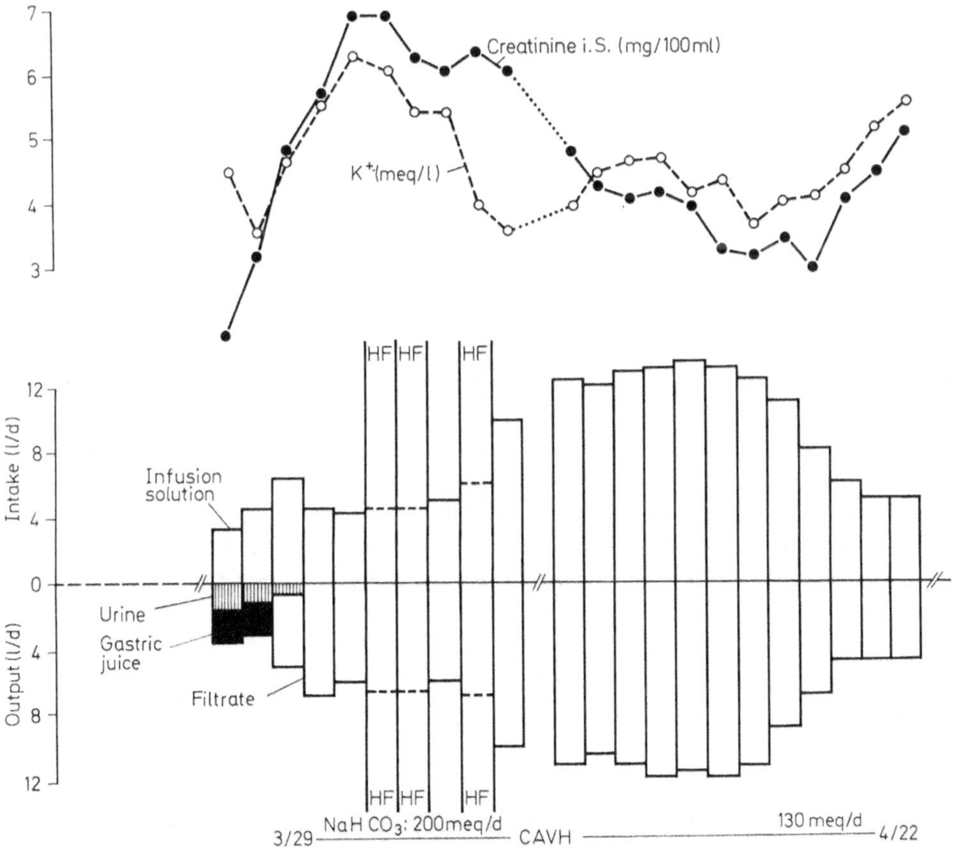

Fig. 2. Changes of plasma potassium and plasma creatinine in relation to the substitution volume for ultrafiltrate during CAVH and pump-driven hemofiltration (HF) of patient K.U. (53 y) with posttraumatic acute renal failure

Table 2. Composition of different infusion solutions for CAVH, pump-driven hemofiltration, and for performing forced diuresis. Electrolyte concentrations are given in meq/l

	Standard infusion solution[a]	Infusion solution for forced diuresis [2]	Substitution solution for CAVH[b]	Substitution solution for pump-driven hemofiltration[c]
Na^+	140	80	142	142
K^+	4	15	–	2
Ca^{++}	5	–	4	4
Mg^{++}	2	–	1.5	1.5
Cl^-	106	75	103	105
$Lactate^-$	45	–	44.5	44.5
HCO_3^-	–	20 (in 5% glucose solution)	–	–

[a] Sterofundin Braun-Melsungen
[b] SH 05 Schi-Wa
[c] HF 24 (ESH 142) Fresenius

ous compositions of substitution solutions (Table 2). In contrast to forced diuresis [2], the infusion solution used for CAVH has to contain electrolyte concentrations very similar to those of plasma water [4].

Overhydration (but neither uremia nor hyperkalemia) can be prevented with a 24-h filtrate volume of 3 l including the volume intake for enteral and parenteral high caloric nutrition and intake of medications. This allows for administration of suitable infusion solutions which have to be given to the patient for "conservative" correction of electrolyte imbalances [1].

Metabolic Acidosis

Sodium bicarbonate ($NaHCO_3$ in meq = base deficit × kg body weight × 0.3).

Hyperkalemia

Sodium, calcium, glucose, insulin (i.e., 200 meq of NaCl, 300 ml 40% glucose +50 IU insulin, 20 ml 20% calcium-gluconate [3, 6], with simultaneous metabolic acidosis $NaCHO_3$ has to be added separately instead of NaCl [7].

Hyponatremia

Sodium (concentrated solution with Cl^- or HCO_3^- taking into account an extracellular space of 20% the body weight for calculation of dose).

Hypochloremia

Arginine or lysine-hydrochloride (is dosed as sodium salt concentrate in hyponatremia).

These conservative measures, however, have only a short delaying effect. If it is not possible to increase the exchange volume, pump-driven hemofiltration or hemodialysis have to be used.

Control of Hyperkalemia with CAVH

At pure fluid removal in renal failure, plasma concentrations do not change and dangerous elevation of plasma potassium has to be expected. A replacement for 3 l filtrate with potassium-free solution removes, according to Fig. 3, only 15–20 meq/day of potassium and is therefore inadequate.

Figure 2 shows the protocol for treatment of an anuric patient with acute renal failure, particularly with respect to the relationship between ultrafiltrate substitution volume and change of concentration of uremic parameters. At low volume exchange, creatinine and potassium increased and sodium bicarbonate had to be administered because of metabolic acidosis. Intervention with pump-driven hemofiltration at 10 l/4 h was only effective after repeated treatment. With CAVH, at 10 l/day, the plasma potassium and creatinine levels could then be maintained at approximately 4 meq/l respectively, mg/dl, for more than a week.

Larger ultrafiltrate substitution volumes are necessary when the acute renal failure is the result of a hypercatabolic illness that leads to hyperkalemia, a most dangerous early complication of low-flow CAVH. At a plasma potassium concentration of 6 meq/1,10 l ultrafiltrate have to be replaced with a potassium-free solution in order to remove the relatively small amount of 60 meq/day potassium, as seen in the nomogram in Fig. 3. For these patients, therefore, a high filtration rate has to be achieved right from the beginning, and all parenterals as well as tube feedings have to be potassium free.

Accompanying measures are corrections of acidosis (Table 3) possibly through gastric juice drainage or administration of ion-exchange resins through a gastric tube or as an enema.

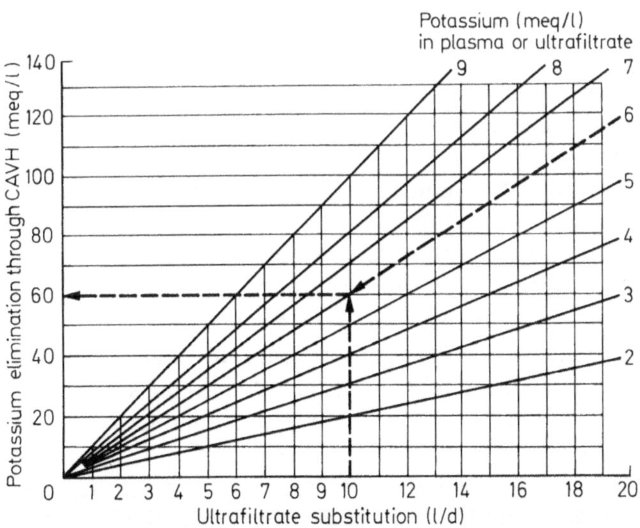

Fig. 3. Nomogram for estimating potassium elimination through CAVH with known plasma concentrations and known volume of potassium-free substitution solution (i.e., with plasma potassium of 6 meq/l and exchange volume of 10 l per day, 60 meq per day are eliminated)

Table 3. Rules of thumb for potassium metabolism management

1. Total potassium, 4000 meq (70 kg body weight)
2. Extracellular potassium, 65 meq (70 kg body weight)
3. Potassium turnover, normal, 60–100 meq/day (predominantly through urine)
4. Potassium turnover, renal insufficiency (diet), 30–60 meq/day
5. Potassium elimination through CAVH (see Fig. 3)
6. With hyperkalemia less deviation of intracellular K^+ from the normal value than with hypokalemia
7. Acidosis effects increase in plasma potassium: reduction of pH by 0.1 = increase in potassium of ~ 0.6 meq/l
8. Catabolic cell destruction causes plasma potassium increase: 200 g tissue = increase of plasma potassium of ~ 0.4 meq/l

In addition, catabolism has to be kept as low as possible by nutrition because cell destruction leads to increased plasma potassium in anuric patients (Table 3). With extensive traumatic, toxic, or hypoxic cell destruction, CAVH is generally overtaxed (destruction of 2 kg tissue results in anuria in a doubling of the plasma potassium). In this case, hemodialysis has to be used early unless the fluid turnover exceeds 20 l/day.

It should be mentioned, however, that with this high fluid turnover and optimal nutrition, hypokalemia and hypophosphatemia are more frequently encountered and require appropriate substitution.

Control of Metabolic Acidosis by CAVH

For balancing metabolic acidosis, the exchange solution has to be alkalizing. For this purpose, lactate with a concentration of 45 meq/l is commonly used. Even considering the loss of a total of 150 meq bicarbonate through 12 l ultrafiltrate per day (standard bicarbonate 12.5 meq/l) the amount of lactate in the substitution solution is sufficient for balancing the base defict of 14 meq/l (i.e., body weight of 70 kg: 14 meq/l × 21 l = 294 meq base deficit; substitution volume of 10 l: 45 meq/l × 10 = 450 meq lactate minus 150 meq loss of HCO_3^- = 300 meq buffering capacity).

It is our experience that buffering with lactate, which is entirely degraded to bicarbonate, is adequate for large ultrafiltrate substitution volumes (> 10 l/day) because of slow and continuous administration. However, for low volume replacement, as is the case in Fig. 2, sodium bicarbonate has to be added via separate infusion because of its limited solubility in calcium-containing standard solutions. During the course of acute renal failure, $NaHCO_3$ should be substituted for protection of the proximal tubule, whereby plasma sodium is kept between 145 and 150 meq/l and base excess at +5 meq/l. This in connection with relative hydration of the patients is important for protection of the proximal tubule of the anuric kidney (see pitfalls of CAVH).

According to our data, plasma lactate concentration increases during CAVH (12 l/day) are hardly ever seen even in patients with manifested lactate acidosis. For patients with manifested lactate acidosis, lactate therefore does not have to

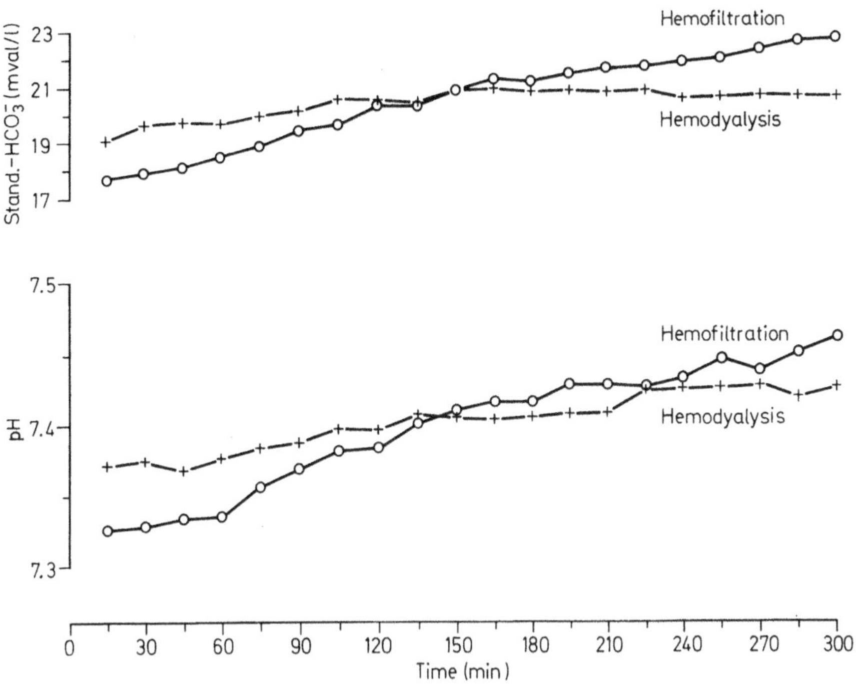

Fig. 4. Standard bicarbonate and pH values of blood during pump-driven hemofiltration (lactate 45 meq/l) and conventional hemodialysis (acetate 34 meq/l) of nine patients who were treated alternately 3 × with both methods. Each point represents the mean value of 27 individual measurements

be replaced with bicarbonate until the clinical situation improves. It can be generally stated that with continuous ultrafiltrate substitution of more than 10 l/day (45 meq lactate per liter), patients usually end up with an excess of base and that lactate input of only 34 meq/l is sufficient for longer-term use of CAVH; the degradation of lactate to bicarbonate is hardly even disturbed.

We also did not observe an increase in plasma lactate with pump-driven hemofiltration (10 l per 3 h) with 45 meq/l lactate concentration in the substitution solution.

In Fig. 4 the changes of standard bicarbonate during pump-driven hemofiltration (lactate 45 meq/l) are compared with to those of conventional hemodialysis (acetate 34 meq/l). Only for fast exchange (20 l in 4 h) with pump-driven hemofiltration an average increase of 6 meq/l of lactate was noted for eight other patients at the end of treatment but which already normalized during the next 2 h.

Control of Hypernatremia by CAVH

Besides the already described CAVH indications typical for uremia, hypernatremia, which can be well controlled with minimum volume exchange, should be mentioned. The liquor-sodium concentration decrease, contrary to that of the plasma concentration, is delayed with forced correction of hypernatremia [1, 6]

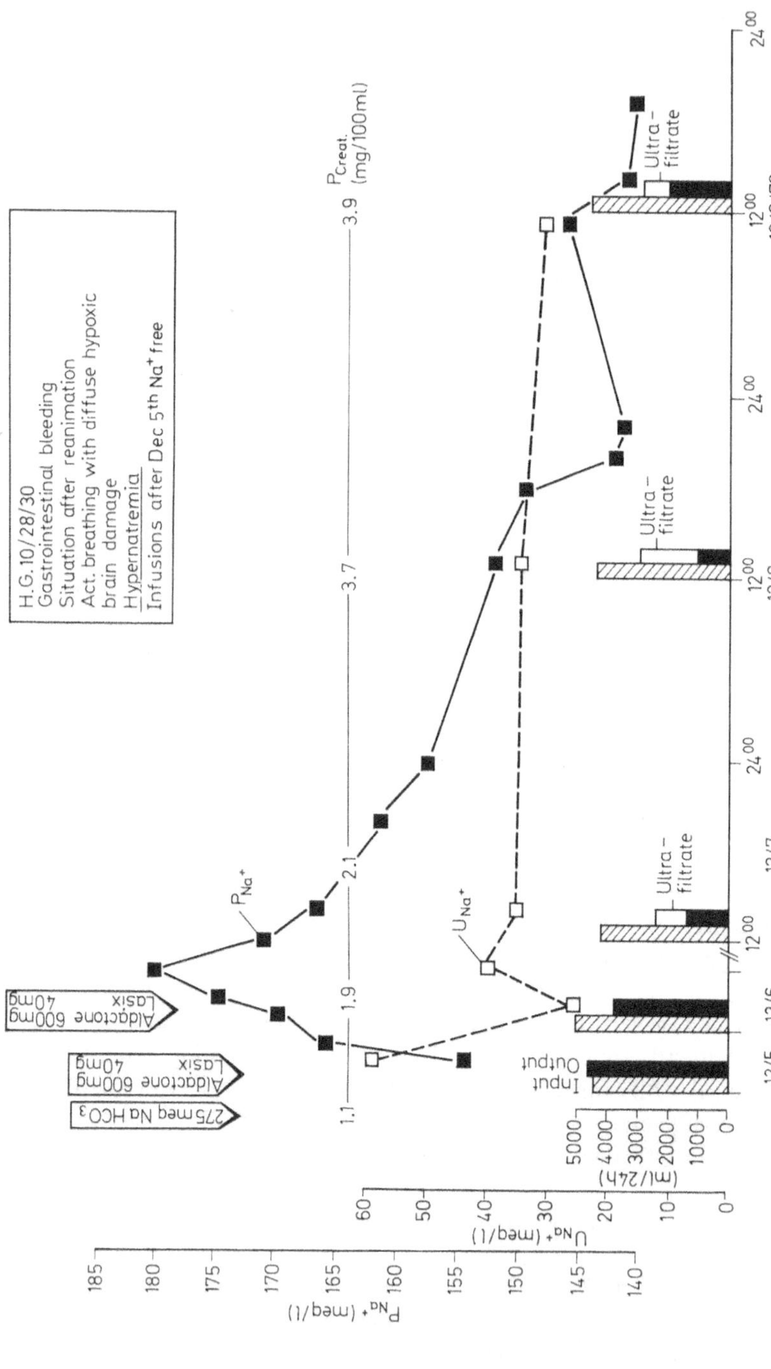

Fig. 5. Treatment of a case of hypernatremia with arteriovenous hemofiltration and ultrafiltrate substitution with 5% glucose solution

and poses a specific risk. Despite normalizing of the plasma sodium concentration, worsening of the symptoms can therefore occur due to a cerebral edema.

For that reason, administration of sodium-free solutions is often not possible since patients need to be kept rather dry to avoid brain edema. A therapy-resistant increase in plasma sodium with overhydration is occasionally observed after hypoxic brain damage. Characteristically, sodium concentrations in the urine are low (30–40 meq/l) as recorded in the example in Fig. 5 despite the increase in plasma sodium up to 180 meq/l. With the "central nervous" hypernatremia even the aldosterone antagonist and the loop diuretic were ineffective. But with 1 l ultrafiltrate substituted with 5% glucose solution, we were able to remove as much sodium from the patient as he eliminated in 4 l urine. This way we were able to reduce the plasma sodium, continuously in the course of 48 h until it was at normal.

Other Electrolyte Losses

Phosphate is eliminated with the ultrafiltrate in plasma-equivalent concentrations. Therefore in anuric patients, 10 l plasma water exchange are sufficient to eliminate the necessary amount of phosphate. If a patient can be brought to an anabolic state through optimal parenteral nutrition while CAVH is performed with a volume exchange far above 10 l per day, it may become necessary to substitute phosphate and sometimes even potassium. It generally holds true that with large volume exchange the danger of overdosage is relatively small since elimination increases parallel with increases in plasma concentration.

Conclusions

Based on our experiences we can summarize that independent of the specific situation of anuric patients, the control of fluid and electrolyte balancing is more manageable with CAVH and less dangerous than with diuretic therapy or forced diuresis in beginning renal insufficiency. With diuretics, urine volume and urine electrolyte concentrations can only be regulated very coarsely. With CAVH, the electrolyte concentrations of the ultrafiltrate are known because they correspond to the plasma concentrations, which are determined routinely, and filtration rate can be regulated exactly. Finally, straight fluid removal is still possible at a blood pressure where, as a rule, urine elimination ceases.

References

1. Bauer H (1982) Der Wasser- und Elektrolythaushalt des Kranken. In: Frey R, Kern F, Mayrhofer D, Halmagyi M (eds) Anästhesiologie und Wiederbelebung, Vol 65. Springer, Berlin Heidelberg New York
2. Frotscher U (1973) Forcierte Diurese. Fresenius Wissenschaftl Inform 4:78–93
3. Halhuber MJ, Kirchmair H (1962) Notfälle in der inneren Medizin. Urban und Schwarzenberg, München p 152
4. Kramer P, Kaufhold G, Gröne HJ, Wigger W, Rieger J, Matthaei D, Stokke T, Burchardi H, Scheler F (1980) Management of anuric intensive-care patients with arteriovenous hemofiltration. Int J Artif Organs 3:225

5. Matthaei D, Kramer F, Grieben K, Schrader J, Ansorg R, Scheler F (1982) Advantages of continuous arteriovenous hemofiltration in the management of acute renal failure. Contrib Nephrol 32:175–180
6. Scheler F, Wigger W, Quellhorst E, Willms B (1966) Zur Klinik des Hypernaträmiesyndroms. Verh Dtsch Ges Inn Med 640–645
7. Seybold D (1977) Elektrolyt- und Wasserhaushalt bei Niereninsuffizienz. In: Gessler U (Hrsg) Urämie. Äsopus, München, S 116
8. Thieler H, Baufeld A (1979) Brauchbarkeit des Dialysats für Laboratorien zur Kontrolle der kontinuierlichen Peritonealdialyse (CAPD). Dt Gesundh Wesen 34:713

Potential Risks of Large-Volume Intravenous Fluid Therapy by Bacteria, Endotoxins, Trace Elements, and Particulate Matter

F.K. Port

Continuous arteriovenous hemofiltration (CAVH) has become a well-established alternative to dialysis therapy for acute renal failure (ARF) due to the multiple major advantages related to CAVH as discussed elsewhere in this book. The continued poor patient survival despite better alimentation, cardiovascular stability, and other advantages is an unresolved problem with CAVH. Late unexpected fatal complications despite successful maintenance by CAVH occur frequently at a time when the patient appears to recover from multiple organ failure. This puzzling observation was shared by all members of an international panel at a symposium on CAVH for ARF at the University of Michigan in March 1984. In search for possible explanations for these late complications this chapter will review potential problems related to large-volume i.v. fluid administration.

Filtrate replacement solutions are generally available commercially as 4.5-l substitution fluids in Europe or as commercial saline and glucose solutions in 1-l bags to which calcium, magnesium, and bicarbonate is added to make up a similar physiologic solution as is the case in the United States. Our current formulation includes the simultaneous infusion of 1-l normal saline with 10 mEq calcium chloride, 1-l normal saline with 6 mEq magnesium chloride, 1-l normal saline without additive or with KCl as needed and 1-l of 5% glucose in water with 150 mEq sodium bicarbonate. The latter additive may be increased or decreased according to the patient's special need. Preparation of i.v. substitution fluids from tap water has been successfully employed in intermittent hemofiltration [1, 2]; however, this approach does not appear economical for CAVH because of the smaller number of patients treated simultaneously and the lower infusion rates.

While clinical problems related to large-volume infusates can be due to factors such as faulty electrolyte composition or errors in fluid balance, the following will address those potential problems that relate to various contaminants in parenteral fluids.

Bacteria

Bacterial contamination of i.v. fluid bags has been studied extensively during multiple outbreaks of bacteremia that were due to infected i.v. fluids, particularly when glass bottles were used [3, 4]. With intermittent hemofiltration using replacement volumes of 18–27 l during 4–5 h treatments, there have been episodes of septic shock and death that were traced to infected infusate solutions in 4.5-l bags. In a survey of 135000 such treatments, septic shock was observed in 0.018% leading to death in half of the affected patients [5]. Infusate cultures were positive in 87% of these patients. The presence of high levels of endotoxin is likely to have occurred with bacterial growth in infusate, particularly for solutions containing glucose as a nutrient. We have shown that pseudomonas bacteria inoculated in spent dialysate would have a high growth rate and an increase in endotoxin concentrations 10^1–10^4 ng/ml while the growth of the same bacteria in water was associated with no increase in the endotoxin concentration [6]. Contamination of commercially prepared solutions may occur during manufacturing and should be noted by quality control sampling [7]. Contamination may occur later due to microscopic defects in fluid containers [5]. Bacteria may be introduced during the injection of additives to i.v. solutions [8]. Our current practice of using 3 or 4 additives for each 4-l infusate, therefore, adds a significant risk. To minimize this risk, additives should be injected by the pharmacy personnel using aseptic technique under laminar flow and after such preparation or after connection to infusion lines the solutions should not be left at room temperature for more than 12–24 h [4]. Potential contamination at the bedside during connection or manipulation of the infusion set becomes clinically important when the infusion sets are left in place for prolonged periods of time [8] as may occur after clotting of the hemofilter or with vascular access problems.

Endotoxin

Endotoxic shock may develop even in the absence of bacteria. The heparin infusion required for CAVH is a potential source for high levels of endotoxin as demonstrated in an outbreak of pyrogenic reactions in a hemodialysis center [9]. Solutions sterilized by bacterial filters with pore sizes as low as 0.04 μm may contain high levels of endotoxin since this polysaccharide is not limited by such a filter. Therefore, a sensitive limulus lysate assay should be employed since sterile cultures do not rule out endotoxin as a cause for infusion-related fevers.

Trace Elements

During manufacturing of parenteral fluids, unwanted trace elements may remain in the solution. Commercial substitution fluids for hemofiltration in 4.5-l bags have been analyzed by von Herrath et al. [10]. Their findings include aluminum at 30 μg/kg which accounts for a daily parenteral dose of 300 μg aluminum for 10-l replacement fluids. This is somewhat greater than the normal intestinal absorption from an oral dose of 2.2 gm aluminum hydroxide [11], but a clinical significance for this dose in CAVH is doubtful. Other trace elements found in these commercial solutions include (in μg/kg) silicium 140, strontium 30, sulfur 977, and zinc 153, as well as several other elements [10]. A toxic role for these agents is still to be determined.

Particulate Matter

The following is a list of the variety of agents which may be infused with parenteral fluids:

Spallation of silicone particles from infusion tubing
Polyvinylchloride globules
Diethylhexolphthalate
Rubber particles
Asbestos
Cellulose and other fibers
Precipitates of salts or medications
Miscellaneous or unidentified particles

Precipitates in parenteral fluids are primarily due to additives or poor solubility of drugs. We searched for precipitates due to the simultaneous infusion of bicarbonate-containing glucose solution with calcium and magnesium salts in normal saline solution, but found no traces when forcing the solution through bacterial filters. Furthermore, our measurements of ionized calcium indicated no precipitation of calcium carbonate.

The finding of plasticizers being leached from i.v. bags and tubings by blood products and hyperalimentation solutions [12, 13] should be a concern because patients on CAVH frequently receive such infusions. Concentrations of plasticizers in electrolyte solutions have been much lower, but the large volumes used in CAVH may add an important burden. Accumulation of plasticizers in tissues, particularly in liver, has been reported but its clinical significance is as yet uncertain [12, 13].

The United States Pharmacopeia has standards for particulate matter permitting fewer than 5 particles of more than 25 μm size and fewer than 50 particles of more than 10 μm size per ml sterile solution [14]. The British Pharmacopeia considers smaller particles and allows up to 100 particles >5 μm in size and up to $1000>2$ μm in size, per ml [15]. The list of particles reported in parenteral fluids has been shortened over the last one or two decades; however, recent reports still include rubber particles, polyvinylchloride globules, asbestos, diethylhexolphthalate, fibers including cellulose, and as yet unidentified materials [16]. Testing for particulate matter requires the use of in-line filters of certain pore sizes and analysis of the filter surfaces [17].

An additional source for microparticles may be the blood tubing. The release of large numbers of silicone particles from the inner surface of the tubing of blood pump segments has been observed in hemodialysis patients [18, 19]. These observations may be significant for CAVH since substitution fluid is usually administered via pumps attached to the infusion tubing. The possible spallation of particles from the inner surface of the tubing has not been studied rigorously for i.v. infusion sets.

Clinical Problems Related to Particulate Matter

The suspected clinical importance of particulate matter has been difficult to prove. Several studies using 0.45 and 5.0 μm in-line filters showed a markedly reduced incidence of infusion phlebitis suggesting a relationship to particulate matter [20, 21]; however, other unrelated causes for this complication clearly exist. Arterial fiber emboli have been documented in multiple organs of patients following cardiac catheterization or heart surgery [22]. Studies in rats using various sizes of inert polystyrene spheres showed that particles of 10 μm size primarily affected the lungs, while smaller particles of 4 μm size were found also in liver and spleen [23]. In these rat experiments labored respirations were observed following exposure to microspheres even though these microspheres were inert and produced no tissue reaction.

Spallated particles from pump segments could be observed at autopsy of hemodialysis patients in multiple organs, particularly in liver but also in spleen, lung, and other organs [18, 19]. It is important to note that spallation of particles remained undetected even though retrospective analysis of autopsy material indicates that this problem had existed for many years [24]. The very recent observation of these particles in liver and other organs had not been considered significant in the initial autopsy reports. One can therefore speculate that patients who have multiple organ failures and require CAVH may also have abnormalities at autopsy that may be misinterpreted as being insignificant or secondary to the multiple primary conditions.

Preventative Measures

For trace elements and dissolved chemicals, no preventative measures are available and stricter guidelines for the manufacturing of parenteral fluids may have to be considered.

Regarding bacterial contamination, maintenance of sterile techniques and inspection of i.v. fluid bags for defects or tears, as well as for clarity of the fluid remains an important issue. The 0.2 μm in-line filter is effective for essentially all bacteria and fungi from contaminated solutions while the 0.45 μm filter is only effective for the majority of bacteria [25]. Bacterial products such as endotoxin, however, penetrate this standard filter freely so that endotoxic shock may occur even though no bacteria entered the patient. A newly developed in-line filter with a high positive charge is capable of absorbing endotoxin from i.v. fluids. This membrane is probably effective in withholding endotoxin that may be present in large-volume parenterals without exceeding the manufacturer's minimum detectable endotoxin concentration by limulus lysate assay; however, its capacity for heavily contaminated fluids requires further study. Filters of 0.04 μm pore size are available but offer no advantage over the 0.2 μm filters because these tighter filters are still highly permeable to endotoxin and also to viruses [26]. The optimal approach to fluid purification is the use of an additional hemofilter. These hemofilters have proven effective in withholding both endotoxin and bacteria [1, 2]; their relatively high cost, however, is expected to limit widespread application.

There is a need for detailed studies to consider the potential risk of particulate matter in patients with multiple organ failure receiving large-volume parenteral fluids. Until studies are available to prove or disprove the risks associated with contaminants in large-volume parenteral fluids, the in-line use of the 0.2 μm filter with or without the positive charge is capable of retaining particulate matter below the controlled size of United States and British standards. For hyperalimentation solutions, the use of bacterial filters has been strongly recommended and this practice should clearly be continued.

It is hoped that future investigation will clarify whether or not the proposed precaution of using the in-line filter for bacteria and particulate matter is advisable. The widespread observation of late unexpected deaths and continued high mortality in patients treated with CAVH prompted this recommendation according to our current knowledge even though a cause and effect relationship has not been established.

References

1. Henderson LW, Beans E (1978) Successful production of sterile pyrogen free electrolyte solution by ultrafiltration. Kidney Int 14:522–525
2. Shaldon S, Beau MC, Deschodt G, Flavier JL, Nilsson L, Ramperez P, Mion C (1983) Three years of experience with on-line preparation of sterile pyrogen free infusate for hemofiltration. Int J Artif Organs 6:25–26
3. Felts SK, Schaffner W, Melly MA, Koenig MG (1972) Sepsis caused by contaminated intravenous fluids. Ann Intern Med 77:881–890
4. Maki DG, Rhame FS, Mackel DC, Bennett JV (1976) Nationwide epidemic of septicemia caused by contaminated intravenous products. I. Epidemiologic and clinical features. Am J Med 60:471–485
5. Frei U, Koch KM (1983) Fever and shock during haemofiltration. Contrib Nephrol 36:107–114
6. Port FK, Bernick JJ (1983) Pyrogen and endotoxin reactions during hemodialysis. Contrib Nephrol 36:100–106
7. Duma RJ, Latta T (1976) What have we done – the hazards of intravenous therapy. N Engl J Med 294:1178–1180
8. D'Arcy PF, Woodside W (1973) Drug additives: a potential source of bacterial contamination of infusion fluids. Lancet 2:96
9. Kantor RJ, Carson LA, Graham DR, Petersen NJ, Favero MS (1983) Outbreak of pyrogenic reactions at a dialysis center. Am J Med 74:449–456
10. von Herrath D, Schaefer K, Hufler M, Pauls A, Koch KM, Gohl H, Ljunggren L, Gardiner P (1983) Complications of hemofiltration. Int J Artif Organs 6:49–52
11. Kaehny WD, Hegg AP, Alfrey AC (1977) Gastrointestinal absorption of aluminum from aluminum-coating antacids. N Engl J Med 296:1389–1390
12. Kevy S, Jacobson M (1983) Hepatic effects of the leaching of phthalate ester plasticizer and silicon. Contrib Nephrol 36:82–89
13. Neergaard J, Nielsen B, Faubry V, Christensen DH, Nielson OF (1971) Plasticizers in PVC and the occurrence of hepatitis in a haemodialysis unit. Scand J Urol Nephrol 5:141–145
14. United States Pharmacopeia, 20th revision (1980) p 863
15. British Pharmacopeia (1980) Cambridge University Press, Cambridge, p 578
16. Turco SJ (1981) Hazards associated with parenteral therapy. Am J Therap Clin Nutr 8:9–50
17. Blanchard J, Thompson CM, Schwartz JA (1976) Comparison of methods for detection of particulate matter in large-volume parenterals. Am J Hosp Pharm 33:144–150
18. Bommer J, Waldherr R, Gastner M, Lemmes R, Ritz E (1981) Iatrogenic multiorgan silicone inclusions in dialysis patients. Klin Wochenschr 59:1149–1157
19. Leong ASA, Disney APS, Gove DW (1982) Spallation and migration of silicone from blood-pump tubing in patients on hemodialysis. N Engl J Med 306:135–136
20. DeLuca PP, Rapp RP, Bivins B, McKean HE, Griffen WO (1975) Filtration and infusion phlebitis: a double-blind prospective clinical study. Am J Hosp Pharm 32:1001–1007
21. Evans WE, Barker LF, Simone JV (1976) Double-blind evaluation of 5 μm final filtration to reduce postinfusion phlebitis. Am J Hosp Pharm 33:1160–1163
22. Dimmick JE, Bove KE, McAdams AJ, Benzing G III (1975) Fiber embolization – a hazard of cardiac surgery and catheterization. N Engl J Med 292:685–687

23. Gesler RM, Garvin PJ, Klamer B, Robinson RU, Thompson CR, Gibson WR, Wheeler FC, Carlson RG (1973) The biological effects of polystyrene latex particles administered intravenously to rats, a collaborative study. Bull Parenter Drug Assoc 27:101–113
24. Brommer J, Waldherr R, Ritz E (1983) Silicone storage disease in long-term hemodialysis patients. Contrib Nephrol 36:115–126
25. Anonymus (1975) I.V. filters. Medical Letter 17:35–36
26. Port FK, Bernstein IA (1981) Hepatitis risk from hemodialysis pressure monitors. An in vitro investigation. Artif Organs 5:638–641

Parenteral Nutrition

Parenteral Nutrition in Patients with Acute Renal Failure Treated by Continuous Arteriovenous Hemofiltration

V. E. Trapp, A. Kehr, P. Striebel, and P. Kramer

Enteral Versus Parenteral Nutrition

Only few patients with complicated acute renal failure (ARF) can be sufficiently and safely fed enterally. The main problems of enteral feeding are compiled in Table 1. Especially in cases with shock, unconsciousness, stomach or intestinal bleeding, diarrhea, large fluid losses, or metabolic disorders, enteral nutrition is problematic for various reasons [23, 33].

Furthermore, it has to be considered that in more than one-third of patients fed through a gastric tube, small amounts of feeding may reflux into the trachea in spite of intubation [63]. The advantages of enteral nutrition, namely, binding of gastric acid and administration of large quantities of calories with little fluid, are of minor importance since the introduction of potent acid release inhibitors and because of unlimited parenteral fluid administration available with continuous arteriovenous hemofiltration (CAVH).

During treatment with CAVH, administration of fluid is almost unlimited, to the extent that the following warning mentioned in most textbooks is not true anymore: "The greatest danger exists in the excessive fluid and electrolyte (sodium !) intake that can be particulary deleterious for patients with cardiac and renal insufficiency" [60]. For most patients who develop ARF (particularly in "multiple organ failure") parenteral nutrition is indicated. It is considered the primary treatment particularly for ARF with gastrointestinal bleeding, hepatorenal syndrome, metabolic imbalances, or elevated catabolism, as well as for renal failure caused by cardiac insufficiency [15].

Table 1. Problems of enteral nutrition

1. Anorexia, nausea, emesis
2. Enteral tubing not placeable
3. Pressure lesions or probe ulcers
4. Aspiration hazard
5. Digestive insufficiency (i.e. pancreatic insufficiency)
6. Resorption disorder (i.e. congestive heart failure)
7. Osmotic overcharge with diarrhoea by hypercaloric nutrition
8. Perforation hazard after gastrointestinal surgery or injury
9. Contraindication in patients with ileus

Table 2. Advantages of partenteral nutrition

1.	Relief of stomach, pancreas, small and large bowls
2.	Defined administration of calories, substrates, electrolytes, vitamins and trace elements
3.	Easy adjustment of nutrition to individual expenditure
4.	Hyperalimentation always possible during CAVH

Advantages of CAVH for Parenteral Nutrition (Table 2)

Early use of CAVH has to be considered when central venous access is necessary for administration of hyperosmolar fluids (> 800 mosmol/l) especially in oliguric patients. CAVH offers, in addition to practically unlimited infusion volume, the possibility for administration of hyperosmolar solutions under optimal conditions. Usually the femoral artery and vein are cannulated [38, 39] for CAVH and the parenterals are given through the venous return line. (Note: If the parenterals are infused into the arterial line, more of the administered substance is lost into the filtrate.) Mostly a mixture of 1500 ml 40% glucose solution and 1000 ml 10% amino acid solution is infused into the venous return line at infusion rates of 1.5–2.5 ml/min.

This solution with an osmolality of 1734 mosmol/l is diluted in the extracorporeal system with 10 ml substitution fluid and at least 50 ml heparinized blood. By mixing the parenteral solution with 60 ml blood isotonic fluid, its osmolality is reduced to 345 mosmol/l before entering the iliac vein. Thus, by lowering osmolality close to blood isotonic values, vessel damage and thrombosis can be avoided.

In addition, the development of thrombi is prevented by constant infusion of heparin. As this is given into the extracorporeal circuit, the heparin concentration of the blood flowing into the iliac vein is the highest in the circulation. This corresponds with the clinical experience that occluding thrombi of the femoral vein occur only seldom even after the catheter has been in place for several weeks.

Amino Acid Loss by CAVH

The values of serum and ultrafiltrate concentrations of 20 different amino acids (essential and nonessential) including the metabolic product 3-methyl-histidine are compared in Fig. 1. The points in the graph are predominantly grouped around the identity line. Only glutamic acid and tryptophane concentrations are significantly lower in filtrate than in serum. Based on these results it can be postulated that the loss of most of the amino acids correlates directly with the serum concentration and the filtration rate.

Serum concentrations and loss of different amino acids with the filtrate are compiled in Table 3. The patients received 100 g amino acids per day as constant infusion. The total loss of free amino acids was about 2 g per day. It is estimated that an additional 2 g amino acids are lost in a conjugated form or as peptides [37]. Compared with the administered amount, the total loss is negligible. With increased parenteral amino acid administration the serum concentrations of most

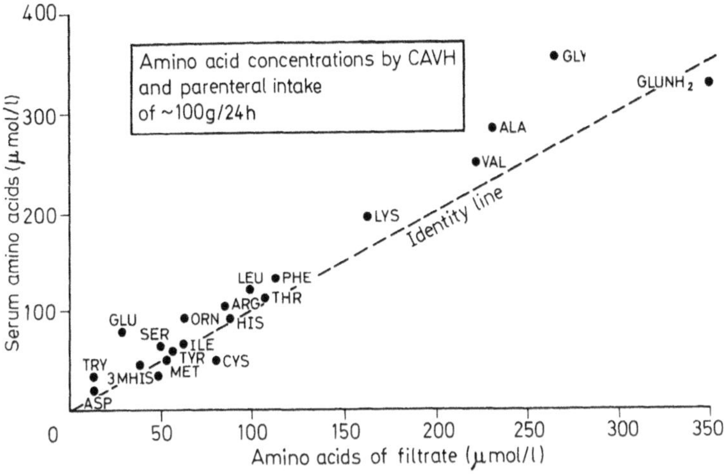

Fig. 1. Comparison of serum and filtrate concentrations of 20 different amino acids and the metabolic product 3-methylhistidine. Each point represents two mean values of 12 single measurements

amino acids were elevated proportionally. This is demonstrated in Fig. 2 with alanine, threonine, methionine, and glutamine. The administered amino acid solution contained neither glycine, serine, asparagine, glutamine, nor glutamatic acid, and yet the concentration of these amino acids did not fall. The sharp increase in glycine may be due to the large amount of alanine given with the amino acid solution.

Amino Acid Loss by Hemodialysis and Pump-Driven Hemofiltration

Under conditions of intermittent hemodialysis, several authors noted losses of amino acids of 2–40 g during 6–12 h [25–27, 36]. Detailed examination of the amino acid loss during hemodialysis showed that 3.8 g free essential, 0.9 g conjugated essential, 8.7 g free nonessential, and 6.9 g conjugated nonessential amino acids were lost [25].

Correspondingly, a fall of serum amino acid concentrations was noted during hemodialysis [58]. Serum amino acid concentration also decreased by pump-driven hemofiltration in dogs [50].

Hemodialysis is more effective for removing small molecules like amino acids (mol. wt. 75–240 daltons) than is hemofiltration. Elimination of amino acids increases as in CAVH proportionally to serum in the concentration [36]. In chronic hemodialysis patients, the total loss of amino acids was estimated to be 3%–4% of the intake [61].

Amino Acid Metabolism in ARF

In ARF different and partly contradicting changes of amino acid metabolism were observed. On the one hand, amino acid mobilization from the muscle tissue

Table 3. Mean plasma concentration and elimination of essential (EAA) and non-essential (NEAA) amino acids by CAVH (24 h-filtrate volume of 5–8 l) in patients with acute renal failure (n = 7) during administration of 100 g amino acids (EAA 41%), Aminosteril R (Fresenius)

	Initial value µmol/l	After 24 h µmol/l	µmol/24 h	Elimination mg/24 h
EAA				
Isoleucine	64.8 ± 23.8	65.0 ± 26.9	457 ± 356	60.0 ± 43.3
Leucine	120.7 ± 25.5	118.4 ± 48.2	752 ± 575	98.6 ± 75.4
Lysine	180.6 ± 19.6	194.0 ± 33.7	1249 ± 860	182.6 ± 125.7
Methionine	39.1 ± 10.9	48.4 ± 36.2	476 ± 566	71.0 ± 84.4
Phenylalanine	127.1 ± 30.3	131.6 ± 41.1	– –	– –
Threonine	99.6 ± 21.2	114.0 ± 31.2	692 ± 514	82.5 ± 61.2
Tryptophan	29.8 ± 17.4	32.9 ± 18.4	81 ± 81	16.5 ± 16.2
Valine	230.0 ± 34.0	242.1 ± 87.1	1680 ± 1311	196.8 ± 153.6
"Semi-essential amino acids"				
Arginine	91.4 ± 39.8	94.9 ± 29.4	463 ± 339	80.7 ± 59.0
Histidine	83.0 ± 13.9	88.4 ± 26.7	593 ± 417	92.1 ± 64.7
NEAA				
Alanine	241.4 ± 39.4	258.4 ± 78.8	1570 ± 1278	139.8 ± 113.9
Asparagine	18.3 ± 6.5	22.6 ± 15.9	133 ± 86	17.6 ± 11.3
Citrulline	26.1 ± 13.9	34.6 + 20.3	162 ± 80	28.4 ± 14.0
Cystine	44.1 ± 44.6	36.1 ± 40.7	592 ± 491	143.0 ± 118.1
Glutamine	294.0 ± 60.4	340.0 ± 92.4	2577 ± 1838	376.6 ± 268.6
Glutamic acid	74.6 ± 41.9	79.3 ± 51.3	155 ± 154	22.8 ± 22.6
Glycine	343.6 ± 303.3	284.9 ± 73.9	1510 ± 1149	113.3 ± 86.2
Ornithine	127.1 ± 30.3	93.9 ± 37.5	381 ± 261	50.3 ± 34.5
Serine	61.9 ± 14.7	60.6 ± 7.3	357 ± 243	37.5 ± 25.5
Tyrosine	68.4 ± 19.7	60.0 ± 10.7	445 ± 333	80.6 ± 60.4
EAA (free) total elimination				639*
NEAA (free) total elimination				1043

* Without phenylalanine

is enhanced [29], on the other hand, insulin-mediated amino acid uptake is reduced [5]. Increase of hepatic gluconeogenesis was reported [22]. Furthermore, an elevation of the serum concentrations of phenylalanine, cystine, methionine, and a moderate decrease of histidine was observed [16]. Elimination was prolonged for glutamic acid, proline, phenylalanine, and ornithine, and was shortened for histidine. The turnover rate was lower for asparaginic acid, glutamic acid, proline, and branched-chain amino acids, but higher for glycine, methionine, and lysine [17]. However, there are authors who believe that no characteristic amino acid pattern occurs in ARF [3].

Fig. 2. Serum concentrations of five different amino acids before and behind the hemofilter and in the filtrate of a patient during CAVH and an increasing amino acid infusion rate

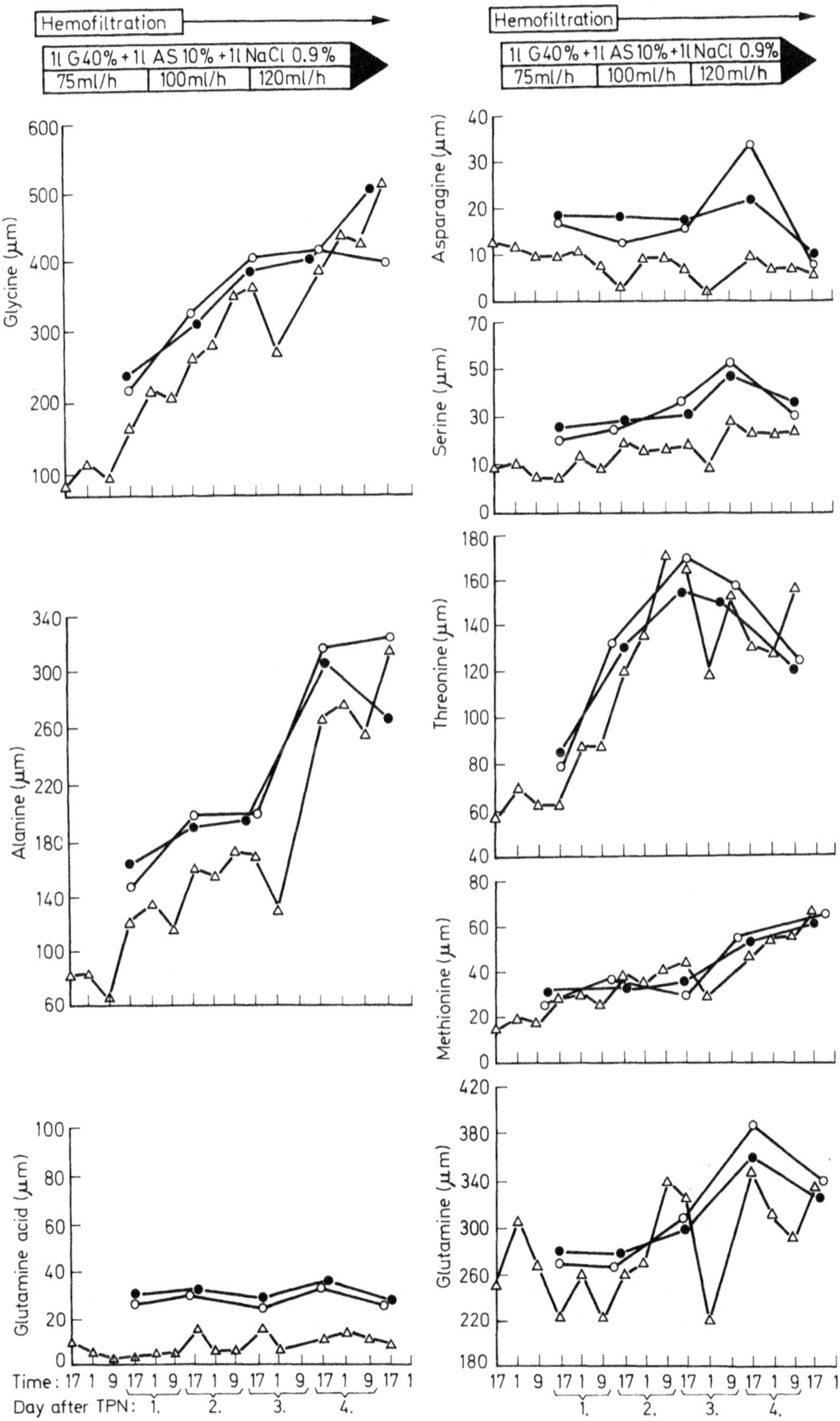
Hemofiltration
1l G40% + 1l AS 10% + 1l NaCl 0.9%
75ml/h
100ml/h
120ml/h
Glycine (µm)
Alanine (µm)
Glutamine acid (µm)
Asparagine (µm)
Serine (µm)
Threonine (µm)
Methionine (µm)
Glutamine (µm)
Time: 17 1 9 17 1 9 17 1 9 17 1 9 17 1 9 17 1
Day after TPN: 1. 2. 3. 4.

Amino Acid Requirements in ARF

Contrary to the formerly usual protein or amino acid restriction for patients with ARF [31, 33, 40], we now tend to give generous amounts of high grade nitrogen substrates preferably as mixed amino acid solutions. With a large supply of all amino acids, the body should have sufficient substrate for protein synthesis. It can be assumed that at most 5% of the infused amino acids were lost with the ultrafiltrate during CAVH. Thereby the amino acids which are retained in ARF have the highest elimination rates. Since amino acid filtration increases proportionally with serum concentration, the possibility of metabolic disturbances by retention of certain amino acids is minimal under CAVH.

There are further reasons to disregard the danger attributable to particular amino acids. Even in healthy individuals considerable fluctuations of the amino acid concentrations can be observed depending on age, sex, time of day, and food intake. Occasionally, side effects were noticed with administration of incomplete amino acid solutions. In children with ARF, hyperalimentation with exclusive infusion of essential amino acids caused hyperchloremic acidosis with high blood ammonia values.

These changes were improved using complete amino acid solutions [52]. An increase in blood ammonia was also noted in adults if the amino acid solution did not contain L-arginine [19].

Various authors have proposed complete amino acid solutions for ARF patients treated with other renal replacement therapy [30, 35, 45, 46]. For this treatment, a ratio of essential to nonessential amino acids of 2:1 to 3:1 is recommended because a better nitrogen balance can be achieved with this mixture [30, 46, 56].

Since the intermediate amino acid metabolism is disturbed in ARF, the synthesis of nonessential amino acids from essential amino acids may be limited. Nonessential amino acids, however, are necessary for synthesis of high grade proteins; for healing processes and for optimal resistance against infection, a high amino acid intake of 1.3–2.1 g/kg body weight per day is required [10, 41]. Nutrition with sufficient high-grade nitrogen substrates resulted in a higher rate of survival and earlier recovery of kidney function [1, 2, 9].

Nitrogen Elimination and Amino Acid Administration

With high nitrogen turnover, 90% of the eliminated nitrogen is urea nitrogen. This proportion may fall to 50% with low protein nutrition [18]. Urea can be regarded as a relatively nontoxic degradation product of the protein metabolism. Patients with ARF show the same improvement of uremic symptoms irrespective of whether they were treated with urea-containing or urea-free dialysate [51].

Chronic uremic patients improved with hemodialysis even when the blood urea concentration was maintained at 200–300 mg/dl. When the urea concentration exceeded 200–300 mg/dl these patients tended to feel ill, exhausted, and itchy, had headaches, suffered from vomiting, and exhibited a tendency to bleeding [28, 31].

Generally, urea can be considered a mild uremic toxin especially when high amino acid intake causes the high plasma concentration of urea. In ARF blood

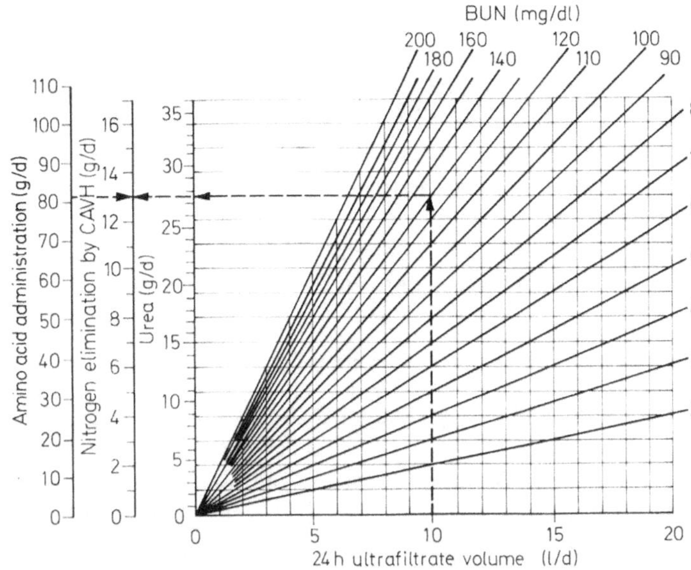

Fig. 3. Nomogram for the determination of nitrogen elimination as urea derived from BUN and 24-h ultrafiltrate volume. By means of the nomogram one is able to read the amino acids equivalent for the eliminated amount of nitrogen. An example is drawn where the 24-h ultrafiltrate volume is 10 l and the BUN is 130 mg/dl. Under these conditions the patient would have eliminated 27.5 g urea or 13 g nitrogen. For compensation of this nitrogen loss 81 g amino acids should be infused. (For total nitrogen loss, see details in text)

urea nitrogen (BUN) should be kept below 150 mg/dl (during CAVH). However, if this is achieved through restriction of amino acid intake it is predominantly a cosmetic intervention because the proportion of other uremic substances like guanidines, amines, indoles, and phenols will not decrease with the inevitably increasing catabolism.

It is generally true that the ratio of urea to pure aromatic amines, phenols, and monosubstituted guanidines is significantly higher for ARF than for chronic uremia [42]. Concentration of these substances can only be lowered through effective hemofiltration but not through reduced amino acid administration. In case of doubt it is better to accept a higher BUN rather than insufficient amino acid administration. Nitrogen elimination by CAVH corresponds approximately with the product of BUN and ultrafiltrate volume.

The nomogram in Fig. 3 permits an estimation of the daily output of urea and urea-nitrogen as well as the lowest amount of amino acids, which should be administered for compensation of nitrogen loss.

To the nitrogen, which is eliminated as urea with the ultrafiltrate, about 2 g have to be added, which are eliminated with the filtrate in the form of other nitrogen-containing substances like amino acids, peptides, amines, creatinine, etc. [37]. Besides that, the loss of nitrogen through feces (about 2 g) and through perspiration (about 1 g) has to be taken into account.

Assuming a filtrate volume of 10 l/day and an average BUN of 150 mg/dl a patient would eliminate a total of 13 g urea-nitrogen (Fig. 3). For compensation of the other nitrogen losses this patient should receive 30 g amino acids (5 g nitrogen) in addition to the 80 g shown on the scale. (Clinical practice has shown that the analysis of ultrafiltrate and all other drainage fluid for nitrogen by means of Kjeldahl's method is a more accurate method for determination of the nitrogen balance. Only with CAVH – and not with other intermittent treatments – reliable data for a controlled parenteral nutrition can be obtained.)

With the high amino acid intake (as recommended above), the ratio between BUN and plasma creatinine exceeds 15, but this must not be interpreted as an expression of severe catabolism. With chronic uremic patients this value increases from 3.4 to 8.6 if protein intake is improved from 20 to 60 g/day [65].

Energy Requirement for Anabolic Amino Acid Utilization

To prevent the infused amino acids being used more than normally as fuel, other energy carriers, preferably in the form of glucose, have to be given in large amounts. For anabolic utilization of amino acids most authors recommend a caloric intake of 125–200 kcal/g nitrogen [20, 21, 24, 54]. The weight ratio of carbohydrates to amino acids should be between 5:1 and 8:1 (1 g glucose = 4.1 kcal, 1 g amino acids = 0.16 g nitrogen).

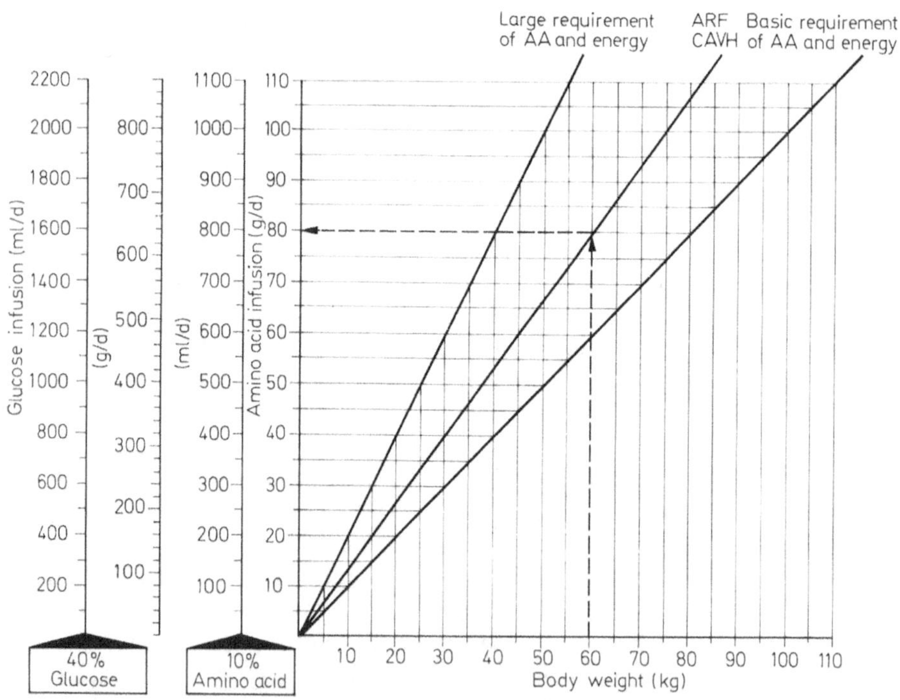

Fig. 4. Nomogram for quick determination of the necessary infusion of amino acid solution (10%) and glucose solution (40%) based on an energy intake of 50 kcal/kg of body weight/day for intensive-care patients with acute renal failure (ARF) treated by continous arterio-venous hemofiltration (CAVH). The values for basic and high energy requirement are 37 or 74 kcal/kg of body weight/day, respectively. (For further details, see text)

The protein or amino acid requirements can amount to twofold the daily energy expenditure in patients after trauma or surgery. The maximum turnover of essential amino acids is reported to be 2.1 g/kg body weight/day [15]. In order to achieve a positive nitrogen balance in hypercatabolic patients without ARF, 2 g amino acids/kg body weight/day are given together with sufficient energy [48].

In Fig. 4 (nomogram) the high ratio of 1:8 of amino acids to glucose was chosen to keep the amino acids oxidation as low as possible. In reference to Lee [46], our nomogram depicts three different degrees of energy supply recommended for nutrition of ARF patients:

1. Basic energy requirement of 37 kcal/kg body weight/day with a nitrogen turnover of 5–10 g/day (i.e., ARF by cardiac circulatory failure or acute pancreatitis)
2. Average energy requirement of 50 kcal/kg body weight/day with a nitrogen turnover of 10–15 g/day in patients treated with CAVH (i.e., ARF after medium-severe surgery, trauma, intoxication, and on ventilation therapy)
3. High energy requirement of 74 kcal/kg body weight/day represents a nitrogen turnover of more than 15 g/day (i.e., ARF as complication of polytrauma, sepsis, burns, cerebral trauma)

After grouping the patients, the necessary amino acid and glucose requirement can be determined from the nomogram in the relation to body weight. Usually, a mixture of 600 g glucose (1500 ml 40% glucose) and 100 g amino acids (1000 ml 10% amino acid) is infused during the first 24 h at a lower rate. In addition, fat emulsions may be given for reduction of nitrogen loss [6].

Infusion of Various Energy Carriers

Because of some particularities of carbohydrate metabolism in uremia, exclusively glucose is recommended as carbohydrate-fuel in ARF [43]. Glucose substitutes, such as fructose, xylose, and sorbite, should not be used since metabolism disturbance (i.e., lactacidemia) may occur. Furthermore, the metabolic pathways of glucose are known better and the cellular uptake as well as the oxidation can be influenced by insulin. In addition, glucose can easily be measured in blood and urine. Since glucose tolerance is often reduced in patients with ARF, and large amounts of glucose have to be administered, it is sometimes necessary to give more than 300 IU of insulin/day (12 IU/h) using an accurate syringe pump [4]. The insulin infusion rate is adjusted so that blood glucose does not exceed 250 mg/dl. Because of very low serum concentration (10–30 μU/ml) and because of albumin binding, insulin loss with the filtrate (maximal 1 IU/day) is minimal [37].

The loss of glucose with the filtrate is relatively small. According to Fig. 5 only 19 g glucose were lost during infusion of 600 g per day. Since the glucose concentrations are identical in plasma and filtrate, elimination rate varies with blood glucose values. Even with a rather high volume exchange (i.e., 15 l/day) and a high blood glucose (i.e., 400 mg/dl) only 60 g or 10% of the infused amount are lost.

Some authors found fatty changes of the liver after 8–14 days of hypercaloric carbohydrate-rich nutrition [11, 12, 49]. Otherwise it could be demonstrated that by infusing fat in the order of 5% of the total caloric requirements, carbohydrate-

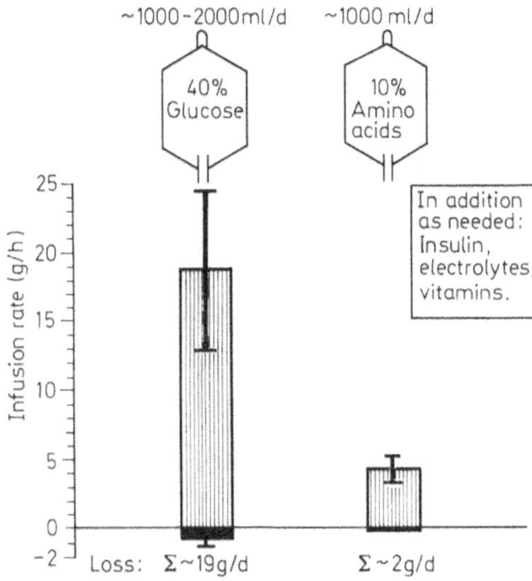

Fig. 5. Comparison between glucose and amino acid infusion and loss through filtrate

induced fatty changes of the liver could largely be avoided [7, 62]. With an energy requirement of 3000 kcal/day, 150 kcal as fat (1 g fat = 9.3 kcal) corresponding to 150 ml of a 10% fat emulsion, would cover the minimum need. We recommend giving 250 ml of a 10% fat emulsion continuously during 24 h.

This quantity contains the daily requirements of 8 g essential fatty acids necessary for reparative processes, especially for formation of biological membranes [8, 57, 64]. Together with this lipid emulsion, fat-soluble vitamins can be infused.

Endogenic lipolysis and fat oxydation [55] as well as protein degradation are inhibited by high plasma levels of insulin [65]; both effects are desirable.

Substitution of Electrolytes, Vitamins, and Trace Elements

Calcium and magnesium are contained in the usual substitution solution (calcium 2.0, magnesium 0.75 meq/l) and should replace the expected losses. (For substitution of potassium see the article by Wigger et al., this volume.)

Phosphate

Since the substitution fluid does not contain phosphate it has to be substituted occasionally. With CAVH 200–800 g phosphate are eliminated per day. Renal failure usually results in an increase of plasma phosphate but with continuous elimination by CAVH concentration of inorganic phosphate may drop considerably [8] particularly if patients are brought to a state of anabolic metabolism.

In cachectic patients, severe hypophosphatemia often occurs especially when hyperalimentation is accomplished with amino acids and glucose [14]. Carbohydrate-induced elevation of phosphorylation and increased formation of inorganic phosphorus compounds are believed to be the cause [17]. Severe hypophos-

Table 4. Practical suggestions for the parenteral nutrition in ARF treated by CAVH. Substitution of the ultrafiltrate with potassium-free Ringer lactate solution (Na^+ 142, Ca^{++} 2, Mg^{++} 0.75, Cl^- 103, lactate$^-$ 44.5 mg/l)

Energy requirement	Low	Medium	Significantly elevated
kcal/24 h	2584	3140	4360
kcal/kg body weight/24 h	39	48	67
Amino acids [g/kg body weight/24 h]	1.2	1.5	2.3
Glucose 40% [a] [ml]	1250	1500	2000
Amino acids (AA) 10% [b] [ml]	850	1000	1500
with EAA:NEAA ≧ 1:1 without electrolytes, without carbohydrates			
Fat emulsion 10% [c] [ml]	200	300	500
Fat soluble vitamins [e]	1 Amp.	1 Amp.	1 Amp.
Water soluble vitamins [e]	1 Amp.	1 Amp.	1–2 Amp.
Trace element mixture [f]	1 Amp.	1 Amp.	1 Amp.
Potassium-malate (or poss. KCL, KPO_4)	according to serum level		
Glucose 1-Phosphate (or Na-Phosphate)	according to serum level		
Insulin [g]	separate with pump according to blood glucose		
Glucose [g/24 h]	500	600	800
Fat [g/24 h]	20	30	50
Amino acids [g/24 h]	85	100	150
AS/total calories	1:7.9	1:7.7	1:7.1
Total volume [ml/24 h]	2330	2830	4040
Infusion rate [ml/h]	87.5	104.2	145.8

[a] No fructose, no glucose substitutes
[b] EAA Braun, EAA Pfrimmer, KE Nephro, Fresenius (EAA 92%), Aminomel L 10 without carbohydrates, Salvia Boehringer Mannheim (EAA 44.6%), Aminosteril KE 10% Fresenius Homburg (EAA 41%), Aminoplasma L 10%, B. Braun Melsungen (EAA 39.2%)
[c] Intralipid 10% Vitrium, Deutsche Kabi München, Lipofundin S 10%, B. Braun Melsungen
[d] Vitintra Adult, Deutsche Kabi Vitrum GmbH München or Vitalipid
[e] Soluvit, Deutsche Kabi Vitrum GmbH München
[f] Addamel
[g] Soluble insulin, i.e., Actrapid Novo, Altinsulin Hoechst

phatemia, however, may cause fungal and bacterial infections [14]. Quaddok et al. demonstrated a 50% reduction of chemotactic, phagocytic, and bactericidal activity of the leukocytes by reduced ATP concentration [14]. Besides that, at low phosphate levels, the survival time of thrombocytes is reduced to 25% and peripheral O_2 release is reduced through decreased erythrocytic 2,3-diphosphoglycerate and ATP concentration [34, 47]. Lowered ATP concentration may lead to a decrease in cardiac output through impaired energy supply. This can be particularly disadvantageous in patients with ARF because of cardiac insufficiency. For these reasons it is necessary to monitor plasma or ultrafiltrate values of inorganic phosphate regularly in patients on CAVH. Substitution of glucose-1-phosphate should be preferred, as the carrier glucose needs not to be taken into account.

Vitamins (Table 4)

The exact daily vitamin requirement for ARF patients is not known [24] and therefore different doses of the various vitamins are used [20, 21, 24, 53, 54].

It is recommended that the same dose of vitamins should be administered as is administered to patients with other diseases who are on parenteral nutrition: 1 amp. of water-soluble and 1 amp. of fat-soluble vitamins per day. The loss of vitamins through CAVH can be considered negligible. On the other hand, it can be assumed that with increased retention of a certain vitamin, elimination through CAVH increases proportionally.

Trace Elements

In patients with ARF, essential trace elements are certainly iron, iodine, cobalt, zinc, copper, and probably also chromium, manganese, and fluoride [24]. Since trace elements are predominantly found protein bound and in low plasma concentrations, only a small quantity is lost during CAVH. The usual amount of a trace elements mixture is adequate and should be given in patients on prolonged total parenteral nutrition.

Practical suggestions for performing total parenteral nutrition in patients with ARF on CAVH are compiled in Table 4.

References

1. Abel RM (1978) Total parenteral nutrition of acute renal failure. Compr Ther 3:16
2. Abel RM, Beck CH, Abbott WM, Ryan JA, Barnett GO, Fischer JE (1973) Improved survival from acute renal failure after treatment with intravenous essential L-amino acids and glucose. Results of a prospective, double-blind study. N Engl J Med 288:659
3. Abel RM, Shih UE, Abbott WM, Beck CH, Fischer JE (1974) Amino acid metabolism in acute renal failure. Influence of intravenous essential L-amino acid hyperalimentation therapy. Ann Surg 180:350
4. Allison SP (1973) Medicine 11, 730 (1973). Carbohydrate and fluid metabolism in trauma. Proc R Soc Med 66:484
5. Arnold WC, Holliday MA (1978) Effects of uremia on insulin-mediated amino acid transport. Clin Res 26:838
6. Bark S, Holm L, Håkansson I, Wretlind A (1976) Nitrogen-sparing effect of fat emulsion compared with glucose in the postoperative period. Acta Chir Scand 142:423
7. Beck CJ, Mellati AM, Dupre J, Rubenstein D (1970) Conversion of glucose to lipid by human adipose tissue. Metabolism 19:988
8. Becker H, Schuring R, Schilling R (1980) Praktische Durchführung der parenteralen Ernährung bei Oligo-Anurie. In: Ibe K (Hrsg) Klin Ernährung 2, Krankheitsadaptierte Ernährungstherapie. Zugschwerdt, München, S 146
9. Bevilacqua RG, Neto ED, Margarido NF, Osaka JT, Lima-Gonçalves EE (1981) Effects of nutrition on the experimental ischemic renal failure. Eur Soc Parent Ent Nutr [Abstract], p 45
10. Bistian BR, Blackburn GL, Scrinshaw NS, Flatt JP (1975) Cellular immunity in semistarved states in hospitalized adults. Am J Clin Nutr 28:1148
11. Burke JF, Wolfe RR, Mullany CJ, Mathews DE, Bier DM (1979) Parameters of optimal glucose infusion and possible hepatic and respiratory abnormalities following excessive glucose intake. Glucose requirements following burn injury. Ann Surg 190:274

12. Chang S (1974) Fatty liver produced by hyperalimentation of rats. Am J Gastroenterol 62:410
13. Cohen RD, Woods HF (1976) Clinical and biochemical aspects of lactic acidosis. Blackwell, Oxford
14. Craddock PR, Yawata Y, van Santen L, Gilbenstadt S, Silvis S, Jacobs HS (1974) Aquired phagocyte dysfunction. A complication of the hypophosphatemia of parenteral nutrition. N Engl J Med 290:1403
15. Druml W (1980) Parenterale Ernährung bei Niereninsuffizienz. In: Eckart J, Kleinberger G, Lochs HW (Hrsg) Klin Ernährung 3, Grundlagen und Praxis der Ernährungstherapie. Zugschwerdt, München
16. Druml W (1981) Parenterale Ernährung beim akuten Nierenversagen: Verwertung parenteral verabfolgter Nahrungsbestandteil. In: Lochs H, Grünert A, Druml W (Hrsg) Klin Ernährung 5, Aktuelle Probleme der klinischen Ernährung. Zugschwerdt, München
17. Druml W, Bürger U, Kleinberger G, Lenz K (1981) Utilisation of amino acids in acute renal failure. 3rd Eur Congr Parent Ent Nutr (Espen) Abstract, Maastricht
18. Eastham RD (1979) Chemical values. In: Clin Med Vol 4, Wright, Bristol, p 106
19. Fahey JL (1957) Toxicity and blood ammonia rise resulting from intravenous amino acid administration in man: the protective effect of L-argenin. J Clin Invest 36:1647
20. Fischer JF (1974) Hyperalimentation. Med Clin North Am 63:973
21. Fleming CR, Beart RW jr, Berkner S, McGill DB, Gaffron R (1980) Home parenteral nutrition for management of the severely malnourished adult patient. Gastroenterology 79:11
22. Fröhlich J, Schölmerich H, Hoppe-Seyler G, Maier KP, Talke H, Schollmeyer P, Gerok W (1974) The effect of acute uremia on gluconeogenesis in isolated perfused rat livers. Eur J Clin Invest 4:453
23. Göschke H, Buess H, Gyr K, Leutenegger A, Ott S, Stadler GA, Thölen H, Fahrländer H (1977) Elementare Diät als Alternative zur intravenösen Ernährung bei schweren gastrointestinalen Krankheiten. Schw Med Wochenschr 107:43
24. Nutrition Advisory Group (1979) Guidelines for essential trace element preparation for parenteral use. J Ent Parent Nutr 3:263
25. Hecking E, Miladinovic Z, Dörr M, Port FK (1976) Aminosäurenverlust im Dialysat. Nieren Hochdruckkrankheiten 2:95
26. Hecking E, Dörr M, Mader H, Miladinovic Z, Port FK, Schicketanz K, Zobel R (1977) Der Ersatz dialysebedingter Verluste von Aminosäuren: Fortschritte in der parenteralen Ernährung. Klin Anästhesiol Intensivther 13:140
27. Hecking E, Dörr M, Mader H, Zobel R (1978) Dialysatverlust und Substitution von Aminosäuren bei Hämodialysepatienten. In: Grundlagen und neue Aspekte der parenteralen und Sondenernährung. INA 13:283
28. Hegstrom RM, Morrai JS, Pendras JP, Burnell JM, Scribner BH (1962) Two years experience with periodic hemodialysis in the treatment of chronic uremia. Trans Am Soc Artif Intern Org 8:266
29. Hörl WH, Heidland A (1979) Aminosäuretherapie bei akutem Nierenversagen – Untersuchungen an der binephrektomierten Ratte. In: Siebert (Hrsg) Akutes Nierenversagen. Thieme, Stuttgart
30. Holliday MA, Wassner S, Ramirez I (1978) Intravenous nutrition in uremic children with protein energy malnutrition. Am J Clin Nutr 31:1854
31. Johnson WJ, Hagge WW, DiNapoli RP, Rosevear JW (1972) Effects of urea loading in patients with far-advanced renal failure. Mayo Clin Proc 47:21
32. Kleinberger G, Gabl F, Gassner A, Lochs H, Pall H, Pichler M (1978) Hypophosphatämie bei parenteraler Ernährung niereninsuffizienter Patienten. Wien Klin Wochenschr 90:169
33. Kluthe R (1978) Probleme der parenteralen Ernährung und Sondenernährung bei Nierenkrankheiten. Internist 18:79
34. Knochel JP (1977) The pathophysiology and clinical characteristics of severe hypophosphatemia. Arch Intern Med 137:203

35. Kopple JD (1979) Nutrition and the kidney. In: Hodges (ed) Human nutrition – a comprehensive treatise. Metabolic and clinical application, vol 4
36. Kopple JD, Swendseid ME, Shinaberger JH, Umezawa CY (1973) The free and bound amino acids removed by hemodialysis. Trans Am Soc Artif Intern Organs 19:309
37. Kramer P, Matthaei D, Arnold R, Ebert R, Köbberling J, McIntosh C, Schwinn E, Scheler F, Ludwig H, Reichel J, Spitella G (1977) Changes of plasma concentration and elimination of various hormones by hemofiltration. Proc Eur Dial Transplant Assoc 14:144
38. Kramer P, Wigger W, Rieger J, Matthaei D, Scheler F (1977) Arteriovenous hemofiltration: A new and simple method for treatment of over-hydrated patients resistent to diuretics. Klin Wochenschr 55:1121
39. Kramer P, Kaufhold G, Gröne HJ, Wigger W, Rieger J, Matthaei D, Stokke T, Burchardi H, Scheler F (1980) Management of anuric intensive-care patients with arteriovenous hemofiltration. Int J Artif Organs 3:225
40. Kult J, Heidland A (1975) Dosierungs- und Anwendungslinien für die intravenöse Zufuhr von Nährstoffen bei Patienten mit Niereninsuffizienz. Klin Anästesiol Intensivther 7:175
41. Law DK, Dudrick SJ, Abdou RL (1973) Immunocompentence of patients with protein-caloric malnutrition. Ann Int Med 79:545
42. Leber HW, Ampt D, Schütterle G (1973) Monosubstituierte Guanidine, Phenole und aromatische Amine im Serum von Patienten mit akuter und chronischer Niereninsuffizienz. In: Dittrich VP, Skrabal F (Hrsg) Aktuelle Probleme der Dialyseverfahren und der Niereninsuffizienz. Bindernagel, Friedberg, S 436
43. Lee HA (1976) The role of intravenous nutrition in the management of acute renal failure. S Afr Med J 50:1703
44. Lee HA (1977) The management of acute renal failure following trauma. Br J Anaesth 49:697
45. Lee H (1978) The nutritional management of renal diseases. In: Dickerson JWT, Lee HA (eds) Nutrition in the clinical management of disease. Arnold London, p 210
46. Lee HA, Jackson MA (1978) Parenteral nutrition in acute renal failure. In: Zöllner N, Karger S (ed) Parenterale Ernährung. Karger, Basel, p 153
47. Lee HA, Sharpstone P, Ames AC (1967) Parenteral nutrition in renal failure. Postgrad Med J 43:81
48. Liljedahl SO (1980) Die Behandlung von Verbrennungen. In: Ahnefeld FW (Hrsg) Klin. Ernährung 1, Parenterale Ernährung. Zugschwerdt, München, S 124
49. Lindor KD, Chem B, Fleming CR, Abrams A, Hirschkorn MA (1979) Liver function values in adults receiving total parenteral nutrition. JAMA 241:2398
50. Mann H (1977) Amino acid loss during hemofiltration. J Dialysis 1:697
51. Merrill JP, Legrain M, Höigne R (1953) Observation on the role of urea in uremia. Am J Med 14:519
52. Motil KJ, Harmon WE, Grupe WE (1980) Complications of essential amino acid hyperalimentation in children with acute renal failure. J Parent Ent Nutr 4:32
53. Müller J, Stock W, Schindler L, Hübner W, Pichelmaier H (1980) Ambulante parenterale Ernährung. Infusionstherapie 1:13
54. Myers RM, Smink RD, Goldstein F (1974) Parenteral hyperalimentation. Five years clinical experience. Am J Gastroenterol 62:313
55. Owen OE, Trapp VE, Reichard A Jr, Azzoli MA, Smith R, Boden G (1980) Effects of therapy on the nature and quantity of fuels oxidized during diabetic ketoacidosis. Diabetes 29:365
56. Pelosi G, Proietti R, Arcangeli A, Magalini SL, Bondoli A (1981) Total parenteral nutrition infusate. An approach to its optimal composition in post-trauma acute renal failure. Resuscitation 9:45
57. Riella MC, Broviac JW, Wells M, Scribner BH (1975) Essential fatty acid deficiency in human adults during total parenteral nutrition. Ann Int Med 83:786
58. Rosen H, Meroney WH, Levenson SM (1958) Plasma amino acid in patients with renal failure. Effect of extracorporeal hemodialysis. Clin Sci 17:653

59. Sandstead HH (1980) Trace elements in uremia and hemodialysis. Am J Clin Nutr 33:1501
60. Strohmeyer G (1974) Diätetik und künstliche Ernährung. In: Buchborn E (Hrsg) Therapie innerer Krankheiten. Springer, Heidelberg, S 578
61. Tepper T, van der Hem K, Tuma GJ, Arisz L, Donker AJM (1978) Loss of amino acids during hemodialysis: quantitative and qualitative investigation. Clin Nephrol 10:16–20
62. Thaler H (1978) Fettleber. In: Hornbostle, Kaufmann, Siegenthaler (Hrsg) 2nd edn, vol 6. Innere Med. in Praxis und Klinik. Thieme, Stuttgart, S 231
63. Winterbauer RH, Durning RB Jr, Barron E, McFadden MC (1981) Aspirated nasogastric feeding solution detected by glucose strip. Ann Int Med 95:67
64. Wolfram G, Zumtobel V, Zöllner N (1977) Die Bedeutung der essentiellen Fettsäuren für Patienten mit einer akuten Krankheit. In: Wretlina A, Frey R, Eyrich K, Makowski H (Hrsg) Fettemulsionen in der parenteralen Ernährung. Reihe Anästhesiologie u. Wiederbelebung, Bd. 103. Springer, Berlin Heidelberg New York
65. Woolfson AM, Heatley RW, Allison SP (1979) Insulin to inhibit protein catabolism after injury. N Engl J Med 300:14

Energy Balance and Survival in Patients with Acute Renal Failure

J. R. Mault and R. H. Bartlett

Introduction

The metabolic management of acute renal failure (ARF) is an ongoing battle of medical economics. While the nutritional demands of ARF patients are typically elevated with multisystem failure and hemodialysis, fluid restrictions and the stress of frequent dialysis preclude administration of adequate nutrition. Confronted with a dwindling supply and increased demands, these patients utilize body stores to pay the balance. However, as carbohydrate reserves are depleted, more and more endogenous protein must be catabolized to supply the energy requirements. Urea is now generated at a faster rate, requiring more frequent hemodialysis. Administration of nutrition, especially protein, is even further restricted in hopes of minimizing urea generation. It is obvious that this scenario leads down a dark path.

With the advent of continuous arteriovenous hemofiltration (CAVH), the above-described situation may be avoided. Studies conducted by Kramer et al. [1–3], and others [4–6], have shown that CAVH is a safe and effective means of managing uremia and fluid balance, continuously, without hemodynamic instability and fluid restriction. ARF patients can now receive an unlimited amount of nutrition when treated with CAVH. However, it should be kept in mind that too much nutrition may also cause problems [7]. Assessment of nutritional requirements is therefore necessary to determine an "optimal" amount.

In this chapter, we will discuss various clinical methods of determining energy and protein requirements. The results of studies of energy and protein balance in ARF will also be reveiwed.

Assessment of Metabolic Demands

The amount of energy required to maintain basic bodily functions is known as the basal metabolic rate (BMR) and is expressed in joules or kilocalories per day. The BMR has a precise relationship with age, body size, and gender, and can be estimated from nomograms based upon these parameters [8]. While such nomograms may accurately predict the energy requirements of healthy, normal subjects, the metabolic rate of any given patient may significantly differ according to clinical circumstances. Because the metabolic rate has been shown to increase with sepsis, operation, and hemodialysis, in addition to the type and severity of disease, actual measurement of some metabolic parameter will enhance clinical judgement. A parameter which takes these changes into account is called the resting energy expenditure (REE) and is expressed as kilocalories per day.

Clinical measurement of REE is accomplished primarily through indirect calorimetry. Indirect calorimetry is based upon direct measurement of oxygen consumption (VO2) and the stoichiometry of basic catabolic pathways to determine the actual energy expenditure. Having measured VO2, the metabolic rate is derived using the formula:

$$\mathrm{REE} = \mathrm{VO2}\ (\mathrm{l/min}) \times 5\ \mathrm{kcal/l\ O2\ consumed} \times 1440\ \mathrm{min/day}.$$

The respiratory quotient may be determined by taking the measurement of carbon dioxide production (VCO2) and dividing that by the oxygen consumption. Each energy substrate produces a different respiratory quotient according to the stoichiometry.

In the clinical setting, oxygen consumption can be determined by closed-circuit rebreathing spirometry, mixed-exhaled gas analysis, or it can be calculated through the Fick equation.

Closed-circuit rebreathing spirometry is based upon circulation of oxygen from a reservoir to the subject, then through a carbon dioxide absorber and back to the reservoir. Assuming no leaks within the closed rebreathing circuit, the net volume loss over time equals the oxygen consumption. Exhaled VCO2 is also measured in-line before absorption by the calcium hydroxide scrub. This system permits accurate and continuous measurement of gas exchange on spontaneously breathing or mechanically ventilated patients at any inspired oxygen concentration and is the method of choice. A closed-circuit rebreathing device of this type has recently been described [9]; see Fig. 1.

Mixed-exhaled gas analysis allows measurement of oxygen consumption by subtracting expired volume and oxygen concentration from inspired oxygen concentration and volume. Carbon dioxide production can also be determined by this method. While mixed-exhaled gas analysis is simple and accurate for study of normal subjects, it is unsuitable for patients on supplemental oxygen or mechanical ventilators. This is due to variation of the inspired oxygen concentration and compression of gases from breath to breath.

Finally, oxygen consumption may be calculated through the Fick equation by measuring arterial and mixed-venous oxygen content and cardiac output using the formula:

$$\mathrm{VO2} = \mathrm{A-VDO2} \times \mathrm{CO}.$$

The oxygen consumption values obtained through this equation are only approximations, at best. The numerous assumptions inherent to thermal dilution and dye cardiac outputs and calculation of oxygen content result in a large standard error in the final value. In addition, this technique does not measure VCO2. On the other hand, a Fick-calculated oxygen consumption will allow the practitioner to distinguish between specific ranges of energy requirement and is considered a more accurate means of assessment than is the use of nomograms for critically ill patients.

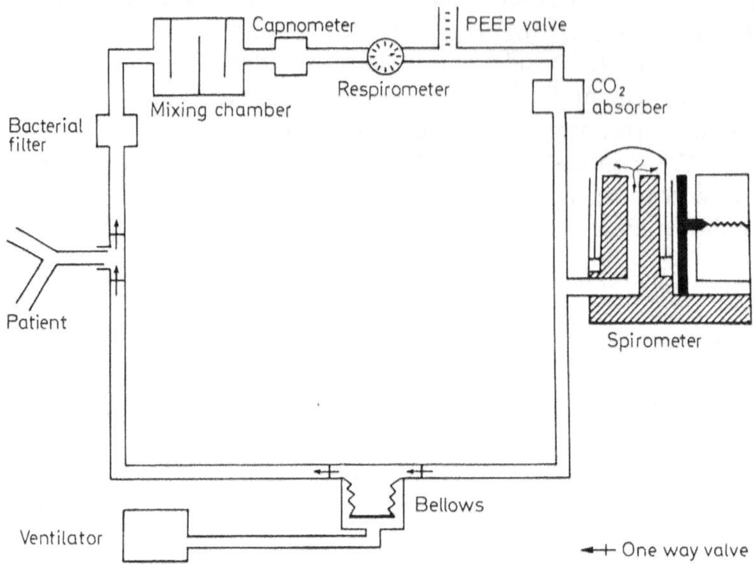

Fig. 1. Schematic diagram of a closed-circuit rebreathing spirometer. A ventilator-activated pneumatic expiratory value (not shown) is included in the *PEEP valve*. From Bartlett et al. [9], by permission, C. F. Mosby Company

With the introduction of CAVH, quantitative measurement of protein catabolism in ARF has been simplified. In patients treated with CAVH, calculation of the urea generation rate (G) is done by measuring the nitrogen content in 24-h collections of ultrafiltrate, nasogastric suction, wound drainage, urine, etc., while accounting for changes in blood urea nitrogen and fluid balance. The protein catabolic rate (PCR) is then calculated using the formula:

$$PCR = (9.35 \times G) + 11.$$

The units for PCR are grams of protein (or amino acids) catabolized over the period of measurements [10].

Once the energy and protein requirements have been determined, the final task in sound nutritional management is to maintain a balance ledger. Daily caloric and protein balances should be tabulated by subtracting the amount catabolized from the amount administered. Cumulative energy and protein balances are calculated by adding consecutive daily balances. (Note: The objective of nutritional therapy is to prevent breakdown of endogenous protein and promote protein anabolism; therefore, protein should *not* be considered an energy substrate when tabulating the caloric balance.)

Studies of Nutritional Balance in ARF

Previous investigators have concluded that much of the morbidity and mortality of ARF patients may result from inadequate metabolic care and poor nutrition

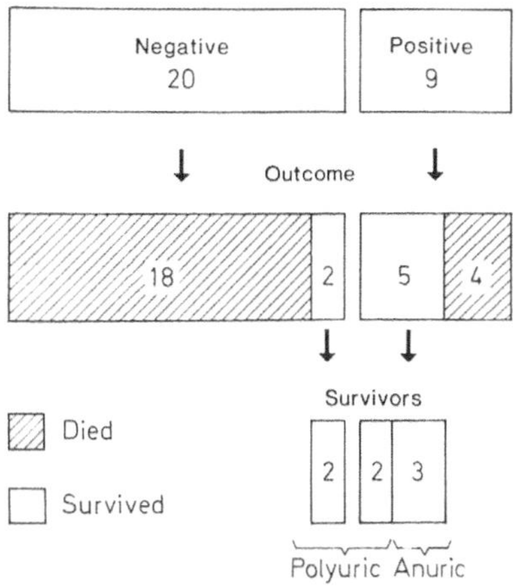

Fig. 2. The relationship between cumulative caloric balance (CCB) and outcome. Survival of acute renal failure patients in negative CCB was 10% while 56% of patients in positive CCB survived the acute episode. Of the seven survivors, four were polyuric and three were anuric. From Mault et al. [13], with permission

in their management. Asbach [11] studied nutritional support for ARF by administering carbohydrates and protein with frequent dialysis. Although caloric balance was not measured, the degree of protein catabolism in the study patients could be distinctly reduced by increasing caloric support.

In a controlled double-blind study, Feinstein [12] provided 1300–3500 kcal/day to ARF patients in comparing different glucose and amino acid solutions. Although energy balance was not measured, several important relationships between energy intake, catabolism, and final outcome were defined in this study. Energy intake (in kcal/kg) was significantly higher in those patients whose ARF resolved. Also, most patients were severely catabolic and required large amounts of calories and protein to counteract or reduce the catabolic effects of the disease and enhance protein anabolism.

Using a closed-circuit rebreathing apparatus, we have conducted a study relating energy balance to outcome in ARF [13]. In the 2-year course of this study, 67 patients were treated for ARF in the surgical ICU. Thirty-seven of these patients survived the acute episode (were discharged from the SICU) resulting in a 55% rate of survival; 29 of these 67 patients were selected for detailed metabolic studies. This study population was characterized by multiple organ failure and extended mechanical ventilation with or without sepsis. When indicated, uremia was treated by hemodialysis in this study. The results of this investigation identified a strong correlation between cumulative caloric balance (CCB) and survival of the acute episode. Of the 29 patients studied, 20 completed the study in negative CCB and two of these patients survived (10%); whereas, nine patients ended the study in positive cumulative caloric balance and five of these nine survived (56%). The difference in survival between the two groups was statistically significant using Chi-square analysis ($P < 0.01$); see Fig. 2. Also, CCB of survivors was significantly higher than of patients who died ($P < 0.05$). The mean CCB of survivors

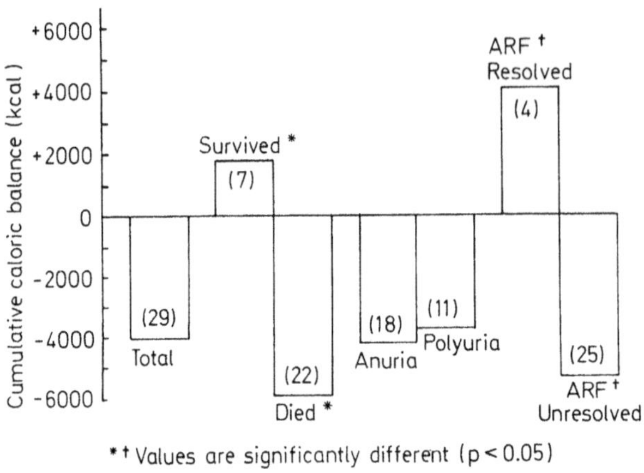

Fig. 3. Cumulative caloric balance (CCB) according to various categories. CCB of patients who survived was significantly higher than in those who died ($P<0.05$). CCB for patients whose renal failure resolved (all of whom survived) was significantly higher than in patients with unresolving renal failure. From Mault et al. [13], with permission

was positive, averaging +1800 kcal, while mean cumulative caloric balance of patients who died was negative, averaging −6000 kcal (see Fig. 3). No difference existed in the amount of calories and protein given to either group. In this study, it was also observed that the metabolic rate of these ARF patients was elevated 35%–40% above the normal range, thus making it even more difficult to maintain these patients in positive energy balance. Protein balance was not measured in this study.

The timing of nutritional support may be equally important. In a study of general critical illness, including ARF, patients were matched according to diagnosis and divided into positive ($n = 27$) and negative ($n = 35$) balance groups based on their cumulative caloric balance on day 7 (Kresowik T. F. and Bartlett R. H. unpublished findings). The overall survival of the positive balance group was 74%, while the negative balance group was 46% ($P = 0.025$, Chi-Square).

CAVH and Nutritional Balance

CAVH appears to be the treatment of choice for providing optimal nutrition to ARF patients. While the hemodynamic instability and hypermetabolism associated with hemodialysis often preclude aggressive nutritional therapy, CAVH offers several advantages which facilitate effective nutritional management. Unlike the hypermetabolism induced by hemodialysis [14], we have seen no increase in oxygen consumption directly attributable to CAVH. Others [1–6] have also reported an absence of hemodynamic instability as a direct result of CAVH (neglecting errors in managing fluid balance). Amino acid losses through CAVH [15] are insignificant compared with what is commonly seen with peritoneal dialysis. These considerations, in addition to continuous control of fluid balance without fluid restrictions demonstrate that CAVH is a powerful tool for providing nutrition to ARF patients.

In the first seven patients we have treated with CAVH, all were easily maintained in positive daily and cumulative caloric balance. Interestingly, the protein catabolic rate of these patients averages 80–100 g per day, illustrating the catabolic state of these patients. Because of the versatility in managing fluid balance with CAVH, hyperconcentrated glucose and lipid "renal" formulations are no longer necessary.

Conclusion

As we search for the answer to illuminating the dark paths these ARF patients have encountered in the past, nutritional management is receiving serious attention. It is now well established that the nutritional requirements of these patients are much above normal. At the same time, there is an obvious need for accurate assessment of nutritional requirements. Of the several methods available, closed-circuit rebreathing spirometry is the most versatile and accurate. Maintenance of positive energy and nitrogen balance, which has been associated with increased survival and decreased protein catabolism, should become a primary objective in nutritional management. Energy administration is recommended at a level of REE + 200–300 kcal/day. Protein should be supplied to maintain positive nitrogen balance plus some surplus which is as yet to be determined. Early nutrition may also be crucial in the final outcome of these patients.

CAVH is a safe and effective means of accomplishing the nutritional objectives described above. Continuous control of fluid balance without fluid restrictions, hemodynamic instability, or hypermetabolism make CAVH an ideal supportive therapy for nutritional management of acute renal failure.

References

1. Kramer P, Wigger W, Rieger J, Matthaei D, Scheler F (1977) Arteriovenous hemofiltration: a new and simple method for treatment of over-hydrated patients resistent to diuretics. Klin Wochenschr 55:1121–1122
2. Kramer P, Schrader J, Bohnsack W, Grieben G, Grone HJ, Scheler F (1979) Therapeutic potential of hemofiltration. Clin Nephrol 11(3):145–149
3. Kramer P, Kaufhold G, Grone HJ, Wigger W, Rieger J, Matthaei D, Stokke T, Burchardi H, Scheler F (1980) Management of anuric intensive care patients with arteriovenous hemofiltration. Int J Artif Organs 3(4):225–230
4. Lauer A, Saccaggi A, Ronco C, Belledonne M, Glabman S, Bosch JP (1983) Continuous arteriovenous hemofiltration in the critically ill patient. Ann Intern Med 99:450–460
5. Matthaei D, Kramer P, Grieben K, Schrader J, Ansorg R, Scheler F (1982) Advantages of continuous arteriovenous hemofiltration in the management of acute renal failure. Contrib Nephrol 32:175–180
6. Kaplan AA, Longnecker RE, Folkert VW (1984) Continuous arteriovenous hemofiltration. Ann Intern Med 100:358–367
7. Askanazi J, Nordenstrom J, Rosenbaum SH, Elwyn DH, Hyman AI, Carpontier YA, Kinney JM (1981) Nutrition for the patient with respiratory failure. Glucose vs fat. Anesthesiology 54:1373–1377
8. Wilmore DW (1977) The metabolic management of the critically ill. Plenum Medical, New York
9. Bartlett RH, Dechert RE, Mault JR, Ferguson SK, Kaiser AM, Erlandson EE (1982) Measurement of metabolism in multiple organ failure. Surgery 92:771–778

10. Sargent J, Gotch F, Borah M, Piercy L, Spinozzi N, Schoenfeld P, Humphreys M (1978) Urea kinetics: a guide to nutritional management of acute renal failure. Am J Clin Nutr 31(9):1696–1702
11. Asbach HW, Stoeckel H, Schuler HW, Conradi R, Wiedmann K, Mohring K, Rohl L (1974) The treatment of hypercatabolic acute renal failure by adequate nutrition and haemodialysis. Acta Anaesthesiol Scand 18:225–260
12. Feinstein EI, Blumenkrantz MJ, Healy M, Koffler A, Silberman H, Massry SG, Kopple JD (1981) Clinical and metabolic responses to parenteral nutrition in acute renal failure. Medicine 60:124–137
13. Mault JR, Bartlett RH, Dechert RE, Clark SF, Swartz RD (1983) Starvation: a major contributor to mortality in acute renal failure? Trans Am Soc Artif Intern Organs 29:390–395
14. Mault JR, Dechert RE, Bartlett RH, Swartz RD, Ferguson SK (1982) Oxygen consumption during hemodialysis for acute renal failure. Trans Am Soc Artif Intern Organs 28:510–515
15. Paganini EP, Flaque J, Whitman G, Nakamoto S (1982) Amino acid balance in patients with oliguric acute renal failure undergoing slow continuous ultrafiltration (SCUF). Trans Am Soc Artif Intern Organs 28:615–620

Drug Dosage

Drug Dosage in Patients on Continuous arteriovenous Hemofiltration

K. W. Rumpf and P. Kramer

Introduction

Diseases of organs which play a role in the elimination of drugs may lead to major changes in normal pharmacokinetics. This is not only of theoretical but also of practical importance, since a decrease in drug elimination may cause a dramatic increase in serum and tissue concentrations resulting in a higher risk of dose-related toxic side effects. Diseases of the liver and the kidneys (the organs which are of prime importance in the elimination of drugs) may cause extreme prolongation of the biological half-life of drugs. Therefore, exact adaptation of drug doses according to the degree of functional impairment is obligatory.

Numerous papers concerning the alteration of pharmacokinetics in chronic renal failure have been published and dosing guidelines of great clinical usefulness have been compiled [1]. Nevertheless, nephrologists are often confronted with dosing problems for drugs for which sufficient data concerning their pharmacokinetics in renal failure does not exist. In this case a simple pragmatic procedure often cannot be avoided: Drugs are administered in doses used in normal persons, or in doses which elicit measurable effects, and patients are strictly controlled as to the appearance of toxic side effects.

In patients whose renal function has declined to a degree requiring dialysis treatment – hemodialysis, pump-driven hemofiltration, intermittent peritoneal dialysis, continuous ambulatory peritoneal dialysis (CAPD), continuous arteriovenous hemofiltration (CAVH) – the situation becomes even more complicated, since these methods eliminate drugs to an extent which is not clearly predictable.

In these patients, two opposing mechanisms have to be considered: The primary renal disease may cause a delayed elimination of drugs, whereas the dialysis therapy may lead to enhanced drug elimination. When using *discontinuous* dialysis procedures – hemodialysis, pump-driven hemofiltration, intermittent peritoneal dialysis – the resulting dosing problems may be overcome or at least alleviated by the administration of drugs at the end of dialysis sessions. Thus, the interfering influence of the dialysis clearance is limited to the short time period during dialysis treatment. This approach is not feasible when *continuous* dialysis procedures (CAPD, CAVH) are used.

Factors Influencing Drug Elimination by CAVH

Particularly during CAVH the hemofilter clearance may be considerable and adjustment of drug doses may be required.

Several factors influence drug elimination by hemofiltration, one factor being the molecular weight of the drug. Although many drugs have molecular weights far below the cut-off of modern hemofiltration membranes and should therefore appear in the ultrafiltrate, this is not the case for many other drugs because of plasma protein binding. The protein-bound fraction of a drug is not filterable; only the fraction not bound to protein is cleared by the hemofilter.

Thus, during CAVH, dosing of highly protein bound drugs may be done according to residual renal function only and adjustment to CAVH clearance is not necessary. One has to take into account, however, that the extent of drug protein binding may be diminished in patients with kidney failure. Therefore some drugs are better eliminated by CAVH than would be expected from data on protein binding in normal persons.

Another factor influencing the elimination of drugs during CAVH is the apparent volume of distribution. A large distribution volume reduces the amount of drug eliminated by CAVH, especially if the rate of transfer of the drug from tissue to plasma is slow.

The factor of prime importance in drug elimination during CAVH, however, is the filtration rate. As illustrated in Fig. 1 for sulfamethoxazole, ampicillin, and clofibrate the hemofilter clearance during pump-driven hemofiltration increases linearly with the filtration rate; this is true for most drugs. When using hemofilters with certain noninert membranes with ion exchange properties (i.e. polyacrylonitrile / methallylsulphonate), however, substantial amounts of certain drugs may be bound to the membrane, resulting in different elimination characteristics [3, 4]: although the clearance of the drug may appear to be low in such a case (as judged from plasma and ultrafiltrate concentration), the total amount eliminated by hemofiltration may be substantial because of drug binding to the membrane.

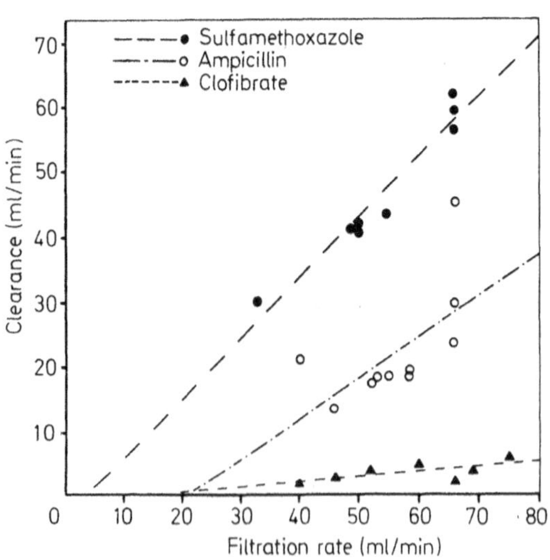

Fig. 1. Linear relationship between filtration rate and drug clearances during pump-driven hemofiltration for clofibrate, ampicillin, and sulphamethoxazole

Hemofiltration – Clearances of Drugs

Concrete data on drug elimination by hemofiltration (pump-driven as well as arteriovenous hemofiltration) is sparse. In a previous investigation [3], we demonstrated that several drugs exhibit a linear relationship between clearance value and filtration rate in pump-driven hemofiltration. This holds true for sulfamethoxazole, ampicillin, and clofibrate (Fig. 1). Clearances of ampicillin and clofibrate closely correspond to values expected from data for protein binding of these drugs, whereas the clearance of sulfamethoxazole is higher than might be expected. This may be interpreted as evidence for reduced protein binding of the drug in uremic patients. Similar results were obtained for doxycyclin [3].

Measurement of the clearances of cardiac glycosides [2] yielded values of 36.7 ± 6.6 ml/min for digoxin and 4.6 ± 2.8 ml/min for digitoxin at filtration rates of 49 ± 9 ml/min. Although these values were obtained during pump-driven hemofiltration, the clearance of these drugs during CAVH may be estimated from these data by taking into account the lower filtration rate of CAVH as compared with pump-driven hemofiltration.

A rather astonishing phenomenon was found when the drug elimination of gentamicin and doxycyclin during pump-driven hemofiltration was investigated using a dialyser-membrane (RP-6, Rhone-Poulenc) consisting of a copolymer of polyacrylonitrile and methallylsulphonate, the latter exhibiting ion exchange properties [3, 4]. The phenomenon was not found with other, electrochemically inert membranes such as cuprophane, cellulose nitrate, and cellulose acetate membranes. Theoretically it may be anticipated that polysulphone membranes have properties similar to the polyacrylonitrile/methallylsulphonate membranes. These membranes which are negatively charged at physiologic pH are able to bind positively charged drugs, as could be demonstrated in-vitro studies [4]. This membrane binding is probably responsible for the remarkable time course of drug concentrations in the filtrate during pump-driven hemofiltration which could be demonstrated for gentamicin and doxycyclin. Figure 2 shows the exponential decrease of plasma gentamicin concentration with time, whereas the drug concentration in the filtrate increases. This results in a linear increase of the filtrate/plasma

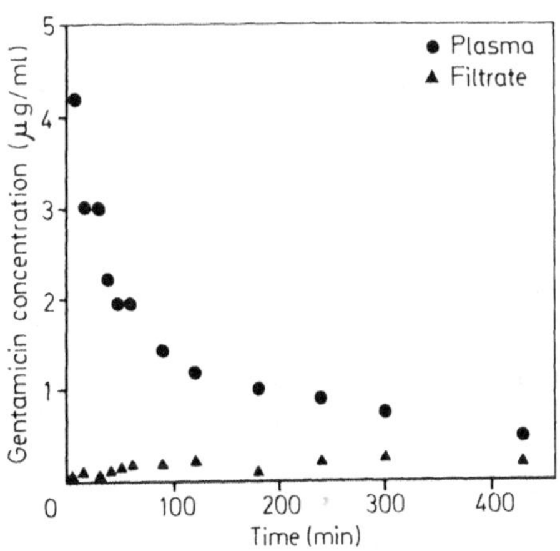

Fig. 2. Time course of gentamicin concentration in filtrate and plasma during a hemofiltration treatment. In spite of decreasing plasma concentration filtrate concentration increases with time

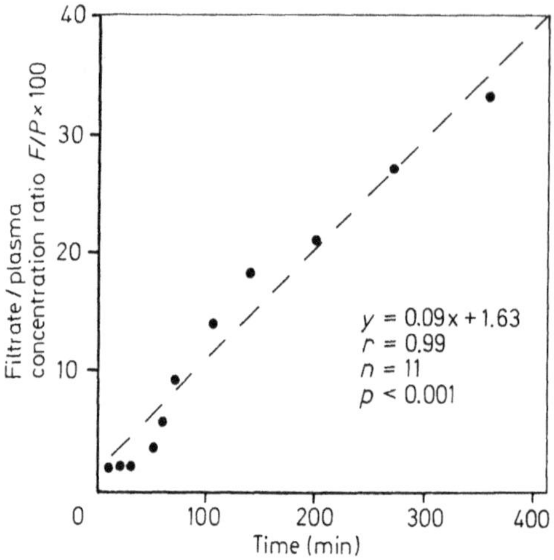

Fig. 3. Time course of the filtrate/plasma concentration ratio for gentamicin during pump-driven hemofiltration

concentration ratio (Fig. 3) and a continuous increase of the drug clearance. This paradoxical phenomenon may be explained as follows: As a consequence of the binding capacity of the hemofiltration membrane for gentamicin (as well as for doxycyclin, and presumably for other positively charged drugs) only small amounts of the drug pass the membrane with the filtrate; the drug is trapped by the methallylsulphonate moiety of the membrane. With increasing saturation of the binding sites, a higher proportion passes the membrane resulting in an apparent increase of drug clearance when calculated from the concentrations of plasma and filtrate.

Binding of drugs to certain hemofiltration membranes may be of clinical importance for those drugs administered in a single dose or if hemofilters have frequently to be changed during multiple dose therapy. This is illustrated by the fact that the binding capacity of the RP-6 dialyser for gentamicin is much higher than gentamicin doses administered to patients with renal failure [4]. However, the clinical relevance of drug binding to hemofilter membranes should be minimized if drugs are given in multiple doses and if the hemofilters are not changed frequently; in these cases early saturation of the membrane should occur. To our knowledge no work has been done with currently used hemofiltration membranes with ion exchange properties such as the polysulphone membranes which presumably should also exhibit drug-binding capacity.

Drug Dosage During CAVH

In spite of the sparsity of concrete pharmacokinetic data concerning dosage regimens during CAVH, it should be possible to establish practical guidelines for a rational drug therapy in patients on CAVH. Since glomerular filtration (usually measured as the creatinine clearance) constitutes an essential factor in the renal elimination of drugs, guidelines for drug dosage are usually given according to the values of the creatinine clearance, or alternatively, to the plasma creatinine [1]. This has proven to be a practical method, although many drugs are not solely eliminated by glomerular filtration but also by tubular secretion; apparently, glomerular lesions parallel tubular damage.

Since the permeability of currently used hemofilters is rather similar to that of the glomeruli, the concentrations of low molecular weight substances in the filtrate resemble those of glomerular filtrate. For example, the filtrate concentration of creatinine (which freely passes the hemofilter membrane) equals that of plasma. Therefore the creatinine clearance of the hemofilter is numerically identical with the filtration rate:

$$\text{Creat. Clear.}_{\text{CAVH}} = \frac{\text{Creat. Filtrate conc.}}{\text{Creat. Plasma conc.}} \times \text{Filtration rate}$$

$$= \text{Filtration rate}. \qquad (1)$$

CAVH is a continuous dialysis procedure, therefore the total creatinine clearance of a patient on CAVH is given by

$$\text{Creat. Clear.}_{\text{tot.}} = \text{Creat. Clear.}_{\text{CAVH}} + \text{Creat. Clear.}_{\text{renal}}. \qquad (2)$$

This total creatinine clearance may be used as a basis for drug dosage guidelines for patients on CAVH. Relevant data and guidelines for many drugs have been compiled and tabulated [1]. The method outlined above is suitable and correct for all drugs whose renal elimination is exclusively glomerular. However, for drugs with substantial tubular elimination this method may lead to errors in drug dosing: The currently used hemofilters simulate glomerular filtration, but not tubular secretion and metabolism.

Usually the endogenous renal creatinine clearance of patients on CAVH is negligible, so that the total creatinine clearance equals the filtration rate:

$$\text{Creat. Clear.}_{\text{tot.}} = \text{Creat. Clear.}_{\text{CAVH}} = \text{Filtration rate} \qquad (3)$$

It must be stressed, however, that in CAVH patients who still have a considerable residual renal function underdosing may occur if endogenous drug elimination is not taken into account. On the other hand, in anuric patients on CAVH drug doses are the same as in end-stage renal failure [1].

At the moment, it is not possible to establish dosage guidelines for all drugs for CAVH patients. Frequently, clinicians are forced to treat patients according to the effects or side effects observed during treatment. In view of this situation drug monitoring may be very helpful. This is particularly true for drugs used in intensive care patients, such as cardiac glycosides, antiarrhythmic drugs, and antibiotics of the aminoglycoside type.

References

1. Bennett WM, Aronoff GR, Morrison G, Golper TA, Pulljam J, Wolfson M, Singer I (1983) Drug prescribing in renal failure: dosing guidelines for adults. Am J Kidney Dis 3:155–193

2. Kramer P, Matthias C, Matthaei D, Scheler F (1977) Elimination of cardiac glycosides through hemofiltration. J Dialysis 1:689–695
3. Rumpf KW, Rieger J, Doht B, Ansorg R, Scheler F (1977) Drug elimination by hemofiltration. J Dialysis 1:677–688
4. Rumpf KW, Rieger J, Ansorg R, Doht B, Scheler F (1977) Binding of antibiotics by dialysis membranes and its clinical relevance. Proc Eur Dial Transplant Assoc 14:607–609

Importance of Continuous and Slow Fluid Withdrawal in Patients with Impending Cardiogenic Shock

H. Nordbeck, H. Blanke, H. Kaiser, and H. Kreuzer

Fluid Balance in Cardiac Failure

The prognosis of cardiac insufficiency depends primarily on the underlying disease. But it also has to be considered that in cardiac insufficient patients, often a very unstable equilibrium of the fluid balance exists, and that the prognosis is also considerably influenced by deviations of this equilibrium. The more the myocardium is limited by the underlying disease the smaller the equilibrium deviations that can lead to cardiogenic shock.

Basically cardiac insufficiency is defined as (a) reduced output with (b) diminished peripheral perfusion, (c) sufficient venous blood supply, and (d) activation of compensatory mechanisms.

As compensatory mechanism for the reduced cardiac output, elevated sympathicotonia is found, which leads among other changes to an increase in central venous pressure. But the decrease in cardiac output also leads to diminished perfusion of the kidney with increased sodium and fluid retention. With fluid retention the central venous pressure increases further and colloid-osmotic pressure decreases. The diminished colloid-osmotic pressure as well as the elevated central venous pressure lead, according to the Starling mechanism to formation of edema

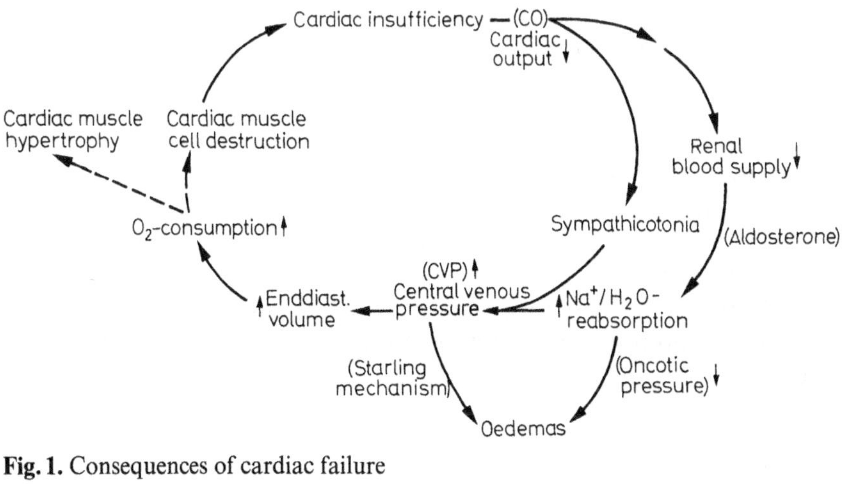

Fig. 1. Consequences of cardiac failure

in the dependant parts of the body. In addition, the antidiuretic hormone and an activation of the thirst center may cause increased fluid retention and intake.

In Fig. 1 the effects of cardiac insufficiency are depicted schematically. As a result of the elevated central venous pressure, the end-diastolic volume and the wall tension of the ventricles rises, whereby oxygen consumption of the myocardium is increased. Since in most cardiac failure patients coronary blood supply is limited and further increase of myocardial blood supply for more oxygen is not possible, additional cardiac muscle cells are destroyed. This worsens cardiac insufficiency and can lead to a "vicious circle." However, if the increased O_2-consumption is met with an adequate coronary reserve, hypertrophy of the myocardium results with decreased symptoms of cardiac insufficiency.

Compensatory Mechanisms in Cardiac Failure

Principally, the already mentioned cardiac muscle hypertrophy of the residual myocardium, elevated sympathicotonia and the Frank-Starling mechanism are regarded as compensatory mechanisms in diminished cardiac output. Through increased end-diastolic filling, the latter leads to elevated stroke volume. However, this increase of the stroke volume by means of the Frank-Starling mechanism – partly depending on the underlying myocardial disease – can only be effective up to a certain limit of ventricle preexpansion. If this limit is exceeded, the stroke volume decreases again significantly. In a case of severe initial cardiac damage, however, a change of the fluid balance of as low as 500 ml – increase or decrease in blood volume – can result in a clinically significant change in cardiac output.

As compensatory mechanism for cardiac insufficiency the elevated sympathicotonia results mostly in a rise of heart rate; the positive inotropic effect of the body's own catecholamines plays more or less a secondary role. During the adaptation phase the already mentioned hypertrophy of the myocardium is then of critical importance.

Possibilities for Treating Cardiac Failure (Fig. 2)

For the therapy of decompensated cardiac insufficiency, besides keeping the body in resting position, all measures have to be considered that can improve the fluid balance for cardiac function. First, exceeding the critical limit of the Frank-Starling mechanism can be avoided by lowering the end-diastolic volume. Second, the oxygen consumption of the residual myocardium can also be decreased so that reversibly damaged cells have a chance to recover.

In particular, the following *conservative measures* should be considered:

1. Strict body rest so that low volume load is assured through the lowest possible peripheral blood supply
2. For the increase in cardiac performance, digitalis has to be considered as one of the positive inotropic substances at chronic stages, and sympathomimetics at acute stages
3. By lowering the pre- and afterload with vasodilators, the cardiac effort is lessened and with the same O_2-consumption of the myocardium the cardiac output can be increased

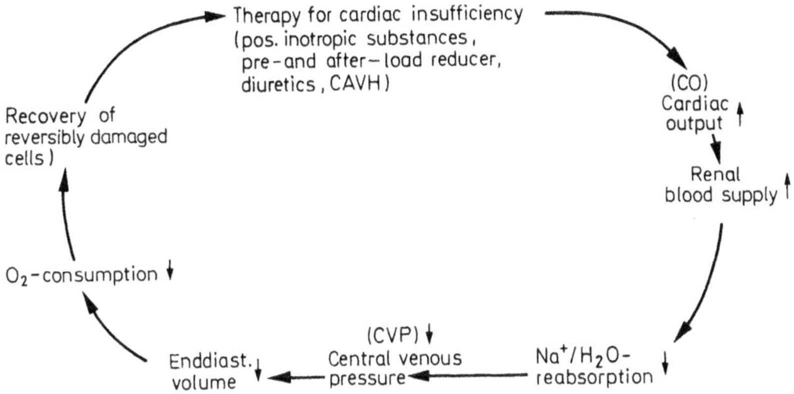

Fig. 2. Consequences of cardiac failure treatment

Table 1. Effect of diverse fluid balancing on cardiac insufficiency

Decreased volume	Normal to slightly elevated volume	Elevated volume
Reduced end-diastolic volume	Elevated end-diastolic volume	Significantly elevated end-diastolic volume
Frank-Starling mechanism not efficient	Frank-Starling mechanism positive effect	Frank-Starling mechanism negative effect
Cardiac output (CO) reduced	Normal to increased cardiac output (CO)	Diminished cardiac output (CO)
Diminished peripheral pressures	Normal peripheral pressures	Diminished peripheral pressures
Increase in the dose of sympathomimetics is necessary	Reduction of the dose of sympathomimetics is possible	Increase in the dose of sympathomimetics is necessary

The goal of these measures is to increase especially the renal blood supply through increased cardiac output to achieve increased fluid removal. For fluid removal principally drugs could be considered which increase renal blood supply selectively but which are nowadays obsolete in practice for the therapy of cardiac insufficiency, since they are not selective enough.

Most often in cardiac insufficiency fluid metabolism has to be corrected with diuretics. However, if the kidneys are resistant to diuretics, measures for increased fluid removal such as osmodiarrhea (i.e., Karion F), peritoneal dialysis, intermittent hemodialysis, mechanical hemofiltration, and continuous arteriovenous hemofiltration (CAVH) have to be considered.

The goal of those measures is to reduce the central venous pressure through fluid removal whereby the end-diastolic volume is reduced. The great importance of optimal fluid balancing in cardiac insufficiency is shown schematically in Table 1.

1. With normal to slightly elevated intravascular volume, an increase in end-diastolic volume is found which through the Frank-Starling mechanism results in a normal to slight increase of cardiac output. As a result of normal or

slightly increased cardiac output, normal peripheral pressures are obtained and the dose of the sympathomimetic drugs can be lowered.

2. Reduction of the extracellular fluid results in reduced intravascular volume and therefore also in a decrease in end-diastolic volume. Increase in cardiac output through the Frank-Starling mechanism is not possible and the peripheral pressure falls despite elevated sympathicotonia. An increase in the dose of sympathomimetic drugs is nessecary to maintain vital functions.
3. With elevated intravascular volume and significantly increased end-diastolic volume, the critical limit of the Frank-Starling mechanism is exceeded and cardiac output falls. Despite increased sympathicotonia, lower peripheral pressure results and the dosage of sympathomimetic drugs has to be increased to maintain vital functions. However, the decreased cardiac output leads to a volume increase through diminished renal perfusion and with increasing extracellular volume and decreasing cardiac output the previously mentioned "vicious circle" can occur which has to be interrupted therapeutically. With oligoanuria resistant to diuretics extrarenal fluid removal is indicated, in particular through CAVH.

Clinical Results with Hemofiltration

In the intensive care unit of internal medicine, extrarenal fluid removal was performed with CAVH in a total of 26 patients with acute cardiac insufficiency. As cause for the left heart failure, 14 patients suffered from coronary heart disease, partly after a recent myocardial infarction and partly after infarctions in the more distant past. Two patients suffered from cardiomyopathy and seven patients were decompensated as a result of valve disease. For two patients the cause of left heart failure was septicemia, one patient had left heart failure as a result of a hypertensive crisis. The ages of the patients treated with CAVH ranged from 40 to 80 years. All patients were oliguric despite massive doses of diuretics, which made them candidates for extrarenal fluid removal.

The duration of hemofiltration varied for these 26 patients from 2 to a maximum of 492 h. Total filtrate volumes of 300–200000 ml were achieved. Despite parenteral infusion of various drugs and i.v.-fluids a negative fluid balance could be achieved through arteriovenous hemofiltration in all patients. Ten patients out of the 26 were recompensated and survived for a long period of time. However, eight patients although recompensated for a short period of time by CAVH, died from secondary complications of the underlying disease.

From the results it can be concluded that CAVH therapy as "ultima ratio" is generally unsuccessful in advanced cardiogenic shock. This is especially true for patients in whom further cardiac muscle cell destruction is expected by shock or on account of the underlying disease.

The effect of fluid removal by CAVH is demonstrated in Fig. 3 in a patient with cardiogenic shock. In this 60-year-old patient, a suture rupture occurred after aortic valve replacement. CAVH was started during cardiogenic shock. At the beginning of hemofiltration, pressure in the pulmonary artery was as high as the peripheral arterial pressure which, however, dropped continuously during the course of hemofiltration while the peripheral arterial pressure increased.

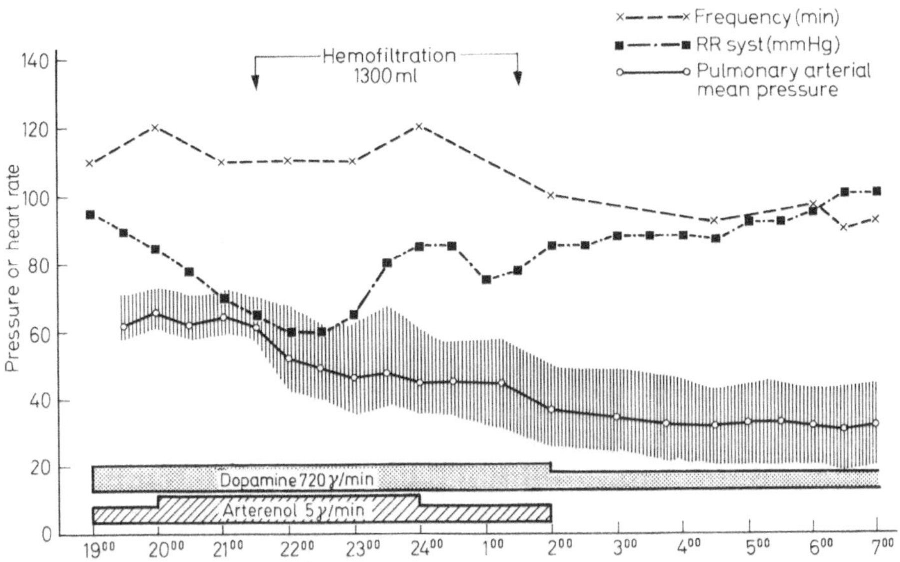

Fig. 3. Course of hemodynamic parameters of a patient with aortic insufficiency type IV, effect of fluid removal through CAVH

At the same time, heart rate went down and the catacholamine dose could be reduced. Twelve hours after finishing hemofiltration a valve revision was successfully performed in this patient.

Figure 4 displays the clinical course of a 54-year-old male after aortic valve replacement and aortocoronary bypass. He was transferred from thoracic surgery because of left heart failure with beginning renal failure and respiratory insufficiency. Acute renal failure developed as a result of cardiac insufficiency but recovered after 3 weeks of intensive care treatment. At the beginning of CAVH the central venous pressure was 15–16 mmHg. The dopamine dose was over 1000 mg/day. After a negative fluid balance of 2 l with hemofiltration, the central venous pressure normalized while the peripheral arterial pressure increased so that the dopamine dose could be reduced. With a relatively stable fluid balance over the next days and a normal central venous pressure, the patient reacted normally to dopamine increasing his cardiac output. On the 12th day of CAVH, central venous pressure rose and the dopamine dose had to be increased.

It could be shown later by recalculation of the fluid balance that the patient had received too much i.v. fluids continuously over some days.

By increasing the fluid removal, pressures normalized; thus, the dopamine dose could be reduced again. Six days later the central venous pressure dropped to 1 cm H_2O, and the peripheral arterial pressure could only be maintained by increasing the dopamine dose. The explanation was again an error of the fluid balance. Only after raising the central venous pressure through a positive fluid balance the peripheral arterial pressure values became normal despite reduction of the dopamine dose.

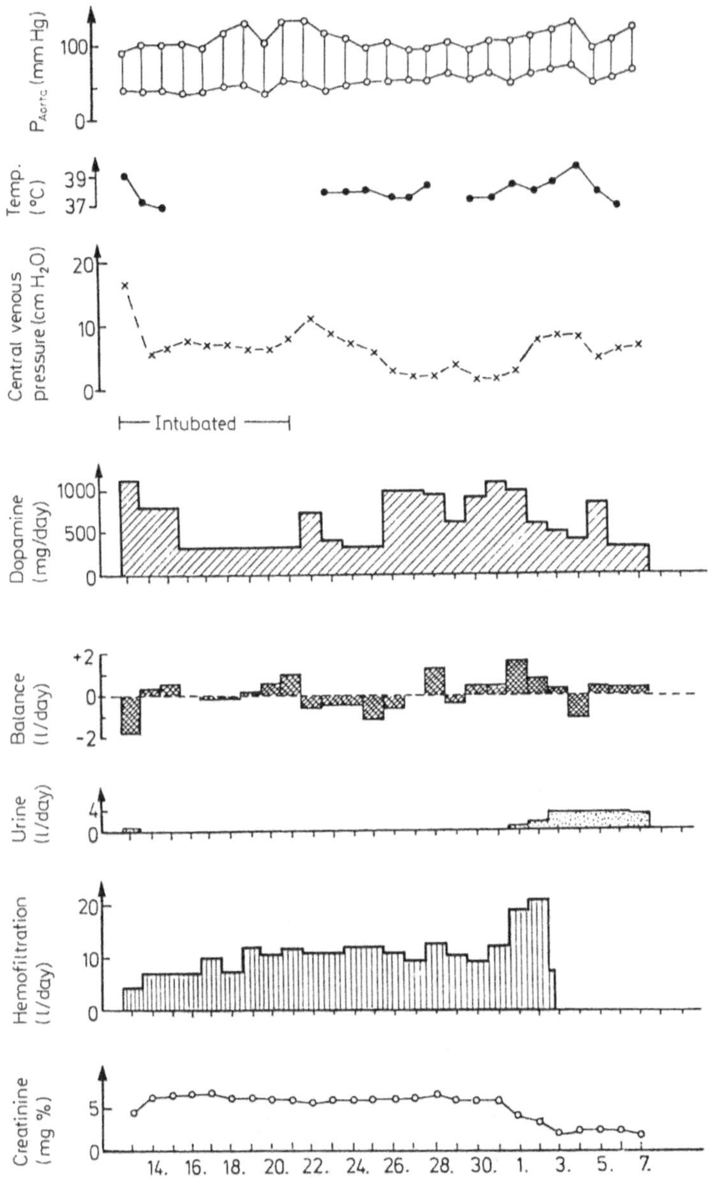

Fig. 4. Treatment of acute renal failure with CAVH of a patient after aortic valve replacement and coronary bypass operation

More than 200000 ml were filtered off this patient during 3 weeks of CAVH with filtration and substitution rates of up to 1000 ml/h. The difficulties in balancing this fluid turnover arose as a result of the pump which was used to regulate the fluid substitution, but produced an error of as much as 20%. The values entered in the curve were corrected after subsequent tests with the pump.

As can be seen from the results of the last patient, especially for patients with impending cardiogenic shock, small inaccuracies of fluid balance lead to significant circulatory changes which then require a change of the catecholamine dose. Therefore, particularly in these patients exact fluid balancing is necessary because reversibly damaged myocardium will only recover under optimum rehabilitation conditions.

Conclusions

The presented patient examples show how important well controlled fluid balance is for patients with acute cardiac failure, particularly with severely damaged myocardium. Extrarenal fluid removal is necessary in acute cardiac insufficiency when oliguria exists despite all measures for improvement of cardiac output and despite diuretics. The advantages of CAVH are obvious:

The procedure is a very simple emergency procedure which may be used in combination with all procedures for improving cardiac output including cardiac-assist systems (aortic balloon pumping). The fluid removal can be well controlled, but volumetric pumps or electronic flow balances are recommended for an accurate fluid balance. With exact monitoring of the pulmonary artery pressure, systemic blood pressure, central venous pressure, and pulse rate, the ideal point of the Frank-Starling curve for the patient's particular situation can be determined with some clinical experience and maintained without change despite continuous infusion of parenteralia and administration of medications. Since the time for preparation is short, CAVH can be started quickly and the effects of fluid removal can be seen soon. It has been our experience that the rate of side effects is minimal. In continuous peritoneal dialysis, which was used 10 years ago in these particular patients, however, fluid removal is slow and difficult to control. Furthermore diaphragmatic breathing excursions are limited so that an already critical respiratory situation generally becomes worse. With intermittent hemodialysis or mechanical hemofiltration, the rapid fluid shifting during 5 h of treatment time every day does not allow titration of the left ventricle filling pressure to the optimal cardiac output. This can only be achieved with CAVH; even small volume fluctuations and therefore deviations from the ideal point for cardiac function on the Frank-Starling curve can be avoided.

References

1. Baylen BG, Johnson G, Tsang R, Srivastava L, Kaplan S (1980) The occurrence of hyperaldesteronism in infants with congestive heart failure. Am J Cardiol 45:305
2. Blanke H, Kreuzer H, Wigger W, Scheler F (1977) Die Behandlung der akuten Linksherzinsuffizienz anurischer Patienten mit der Hämofiltration. Dtsch Med Wochenschr 102:1804
3. Davis JO (1980) The pathogenis of peripheral cardiac edema. Contrib Nephrol 21:68
4. Kramer P, Wigger W, Langescheid C, Scheler F, Matthaei D, Rieger J (1977) Arteriovenous hemofiltration: a new and simple method for treatment of overhydrated patients resistant to diuretics. Klin Wochenschr 55:1121
5. Kreuzer H, Blanke H (1979) Der Einsatz der Hämofiltration auf der Intensivstation. Mitt Klin Nephrologie 8:131
6. Siegenthaler W (1976) Klinische Pathophysiologie. Thieme, Stuttgart

Pulmonary Interstitial Edema: An Indication for Continuous Arteriovenous Hemofiltration?

T. Stokke, H. Burchardi, W. Koller, and H. Benzer

Causes and Consequences of the Pulmonary Interstitial Edema

In intensive care medicine the pulmonary interstitial edema is often an early symptom of the acute respiratory distress syndrome (ARDS), the first clinical manifestation of the beginning acute lung failure. ARDS is the pulmonary complication of severe mostly nonpulmonary injury, like polytrauma, hemorrhagic shock, sepsis, and infections (e.g., peritonitis), pancreatitis, eclampsia, or certain intoxications (such as bromcarbamides or paraquat). Thus, etiology is nonuniform, and pathophysiology, diagnosis, and therapy still present unresolved problems.

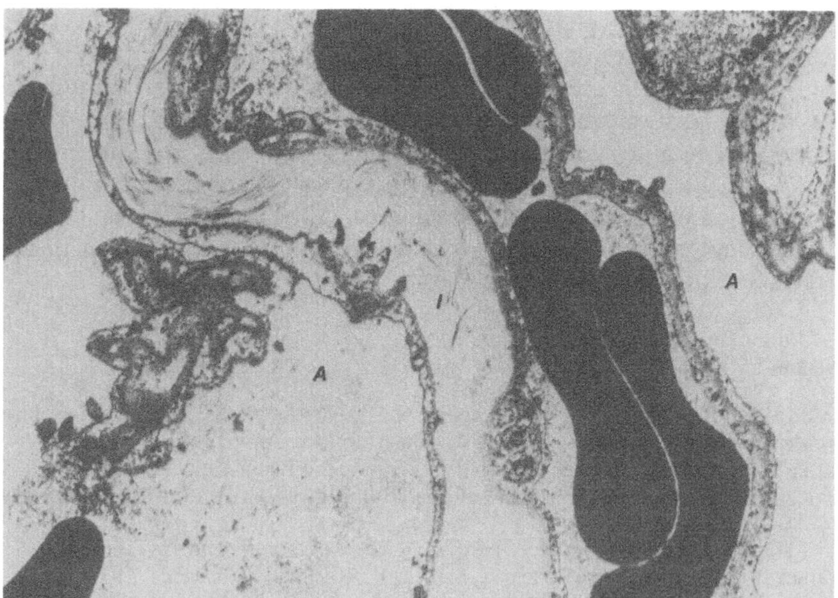

Fig. 1. Electron microscopic finding in early ARDS (percutaneous intravital lung biopsy): A marked edema in the broadened interstitial space (*I*) (including a capillary) between two alveoli (*A*). From [10]

Generally, interstitial edema develops on the basis of increased capillary membrane permeability in the lung. The hydrostatic pressure in the lung capillaries does not seem to play a causal role; however, when permeability disorders exist, any increase in hydrostatic pressure will result in severe consequences and aggravate the interstitial edema.

The participation of several complex physiologic regulatory systems are under debate: The coagulation and fibrinolytic system (including fibrin-degrading products), the protease-antiprotease system (especially elastase), the complement system (C5a), the plasmin-kallikrein system, the arachidon acid metabolism, but also released mediators from leukocytes (such as toxic oxygen radicals) selectively trapped in the lung. Figure 1 originates from a percutaneous intravital lung biopsy of a patient with ARDS [10] and shows a pronounced pulmonary interstitial edema.

Pulmonary interstitial edema considerably affects respiratory mechanics and pulmonary gas exchange and, in advanced states, constitutes an acute life-threatening situation for the patient. Primarily, the oxygenation is impaired (mainly by intrapulmonary shunt) which leads to arterial hypoxemia. But, since the reserves in pulmonary function are large, hypoxemia first will be detected clinically when the edema has already progressed considerably.

On the other hand, therapy has to be started early and consequently in order to be successful. Delayed and inconsequent therapy will endanger pulmonary function persistently.

Treatment of the Pulmonary Interstitial Edema

The most important measures for treatment of the interstitial edema are generally agreed upon as being:

1. Mechanical ventilation, especially with positive end-expiratory pressure (PEEP). The main effect of PEEP is in counteracting alveolar collapse reducing venous admixture and in raising the reduced lung volume (functional residual capacity). However, PEEP never diminishes intrapulmonary extravascular fluid accumulation.
2. Controlled fluid balance, especially avoidance of fluid overload. Generally, according to the Starling principle, elevated hydrostatic and reduced colloid-osmotic capillary pressure in the lungs raise the fluid influx into the interstitial space. Therefore, hydrostatic pressure has to be normalized, or better, reduced as much as compatible with an adequate cardiac output.

The therapeutic value of an increase of the intravascular colloid-osmotic pressure (COP) by application of albumin or colloidal solutions is still controversial. On the one hand, a large group of therapists trust in the effectiveness of the Starling principle and increase the COP in plasma by amounts of albumin and colloidal substances in order to stop or even invert the fluid influx into the interstitial space. Clinical and animal experiments like those of Lundsgaard-Hansen et al. [6] and Skillman et al. [7, 8] demonstrated good results by combining concentrated albumin infusion with diuretic medication.

On the other hand, there is now an increasing group of therapists who refuse the colloidal concept. There are indeed acceptable reasons for this. In particular the noncardiogenic pulmonary interstitial edema (especially in ARDS) is characterized by a marked increase in permeability of the capillary membrane; thus, in every case, there will be a considerable leakage of colloidal substances (especially albumins) through this membrane and COP will rapidly be adjusted also in the interstitial space. From this theoretical aspect, Staub and his group [1, 9] could not assume any positive effect of the colloid therapy in these cases. Also, the oncotic pressure gradient (COP – hydrostatic pressure) introduced by Weil [14] for diagnosis of hypooncotic states did not prove to be of clinical value [12, 13]. The significant extravasation of albumin into the interstitial space following albumin administration even seems to worsen the interstitial edema [2, 12].

Several clinical investigations support these assumptions. Comparisons between standardized colloidal and crystalloidal volume replacement in resuscitation revealed no benefit resulting from the albumin therapy [5, 13] in cases of pulmonary permeability disorders. Nevertheless, it remains extremely important to control fluid balance and to avoid fluid overload. Many try to accomplish this by administering large amounts of diuretics, which may, however, be ineffective or difficult to control. Here, continuous arteriovenous hemofiltration (CAVH) is more effective in making the management of fluid balance easily controllable.

In this context we want to point out a specific problem during respirator weaning. With PEEP ventilation, the intrathoracic, intravascular volume decreases and venous return is impeded. Therefore, often the intravascular volume has to be raised to counteract the negative circulatory effect of PEEP. But, when PEEP is reduced again or respiration is ended (once the condition has improved) central blood volume is restored and a dangerous hyperhydration may follow. A massive dehydration has to be performed to prevent a reexacerbation of the pulmonary function. For patients with increased pulmonary capillary membrane permeability, even a transitory hypervolemia can worsen the pulmonary condition considerably. Even the slightest overinfusion of a previously well-balanced patient can frequently lead to a fulminant edema if the necessary water elimination cannot be achieved immediately.

Here we see an additional indication for CAVH. By constant fluid removal we are able to control the intravascular volume effectively and thus reduce the risk of overinfusion.

Clinical Experience with CAVH in Interstitial Lung Edema

In what follows, the effect of dehydration with CAVH on pulmonary function is demonstrated in intensive care patients with multiorgan failure under mechanical ventilation and some informative case reports are included.

Case 1. A 10-year-old girl developed severe pulmonary insufficiency with circulatory failure and acute renal failure after cardiac surgery. In addition to respiration with pure oxygen, continuous extracorporeal oxygenation had to be carried out (Fig. 2). By continuous fluid removal of approximately 100 ml/h with CAVH, an increase in arterial pO_2 with simultaneous reduction of oxygen transfer in the oxygenator was achieved within 20 h, so that mechanical ventilation alone was finally sufficient. The child could be taken off the respirator after several days.

Case 2. A 16-year-old girl was admitted to the hospital after suicidal poisoning with a high, lethal dose of paraquat (ca. 30 g). Paraquat is a very toxic herbicide causing acute renal failure, a typically progressive ARDS such as lung damage beginning with interstitial lung edema, developing into progressive deterioration of gas exchange, and resulting finally in severe interstitial fibrosis. The complete anuric renal failure could be compensated by CAVH for more than 3 weeks (Fig. 3). Nevertheless, the patient died in the end from irreversible pulmonary fibrosis with uncontrollable respiratory insufficiency as a result of the paraquat intoxication. But the time for survival is longer than usual with this dose of paraquat.

During the whole time of treatment, CAVH was performed with filtration volumes of approximately 10 l per day. From the 5th day on, the patient was mechanically ventilated. Later on, peritoneal dialysis was performed additionally because of the tentative (but false) diagnosis of a hemorrhagic pancreatitis. However, peritoneal dialysis had only negative effects on pulmonary function, namely, decreased lung compliance and lung volume (FRC).

During the first days of ventilation therapy and CAVH application, pulmonary function improved considerably. During the first 60 h after onset of mechanical ventilation ca. 3.5 l fluid were removed from the patient by arteriovenous hemofiltration. As a result, all examined respiratory parameters improved (Fig. 3). The inspired oxygen concentration (F_IO_2) could be lowered from 0.8 to 0.3, alveoloarterial oxygen tension gradient ($AaDO_2$) was reduced from 450 mmHg to 113 mmHg, pulmonary diffusing capacity (D_{CO}) rose from 3.6 to 6.6 ml $\cdot$ min^{-1} $\cdot$ mmHg^{-1}, lung volume (FRC) went from 1.1 to 2 l and dynamic compliance rose from 34 to 49 ml/cmH_2O.

At the 11th day after paraquat intake 1 l fluid was oversubstituted because of a balance error. This overhydration caused an increase in the interstitial pulmonary edema and worsened the physiologic respiratory parameters: The D_{CO} was reduced from 3.9 to 2.1 ml $\cdot$ min^{-1} $\cdot$ mmHg^{-1}, FRC from 1.2 to 0.8 liters, and compliance from 44 to 29 ml/cmH_2O. (It is remarkable that $AaDO_2$ rose only insignificantly.)

This deterioration could be reversed during the next few days with massive dehydration by CAVH. Nevertheless, the progressive paraquat-caused pulmonary interstitial fibrosis could not be stopped. Later on (approximately after the 17th day) respiratory function deteriorated progressively and the girl died of hypoxemia 1 month after the paraquat intake.

Encouraged by these results, the Vienna intensive care group (Benzer and coworkers) began to apply CAVH to patients with multiorgan failure. In a preliminary study [4] 32 patients with multiorgan failure and severe respiratory insufficiency were treated with CAVH. The multiorgan failure occurred as postoperative complications (after abdominal or thoracic surgery), after severe polytrauma with hemorrhagic shock, and after obstetric problems (such as eclampsia).

When adequate oxygenation could not be assured by increasing inspiratory oxygen concentrations (F_IO_2) and PEEP level, as well as changing the inspiratory/expiratory time ratio (inversed ratio ventilation), CAVH was started.

The therapeutic effect upon respiratory function is estimated, among others, by means of the $AaDO_2$-quotient (alveolar – arterial pO_2/alveolar pO_2) and by

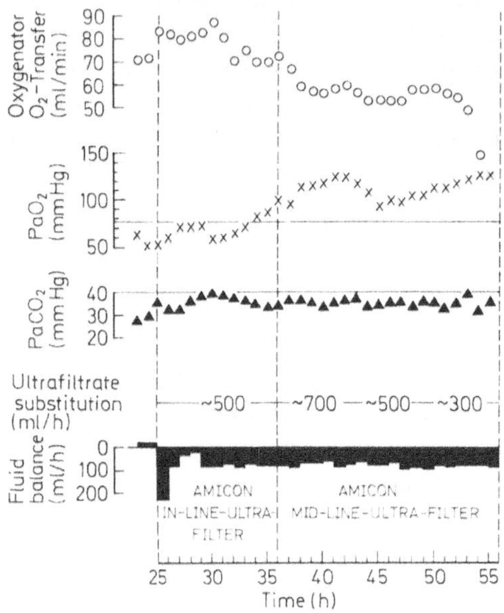

Fig. 2. Respiratory, circulatory, and renal failure after cardiac surgery in a 10-year-old girl. Intensive care therapy with mechanical ventilation ($F_IO_2=1.0$), extracorporeal oxygenation and arteriovenous hemofiltration. Registration against time (hours after operation) of the following parameters: oxygen gas flow through the oxygenator (Oxygenator O_2 transfer), arterial pO_2 (PaO_2), arterial pCO_2 ($PaCO_2$), ultrafiltrate substitution rate, and fluid balance per hour

means of a special therapy score (PIF) which is

$$PIF = PEEP\ (cmH_2O) \cdot I{:}E\ ratio \cdot F_IO_2$$

The results (mean values) are listed in Table 1.

Thus, CAVH significantly supports the oxygenating effect of mechanical ventilation. Furthermore, the elevated pulmonary vascular resistance decreases, while systemic circulation remains stable.

Fluid balance (substitution by Ringer's lactate solution) was obtained without mechanical pumping support and adapted in correspondence to the circulatory

Table 1. Effect of CAVH (mean values)

CAVH application	Before	After		
		12 h	36 h	60 h
PIF	13.2	9.7	7.4	5.5
$AaDO_2$-quotient	0.69	0.58	0.54	0.52
PaO_2	100	131	128	120 mm Hg
$PaCO_2$	38	36	38	37 mm Hg
Blood urea nitrogen	59	59	69	65 mg/dl
Serum creatinine	2.5	2.4	2.6	2.3 mg/dl

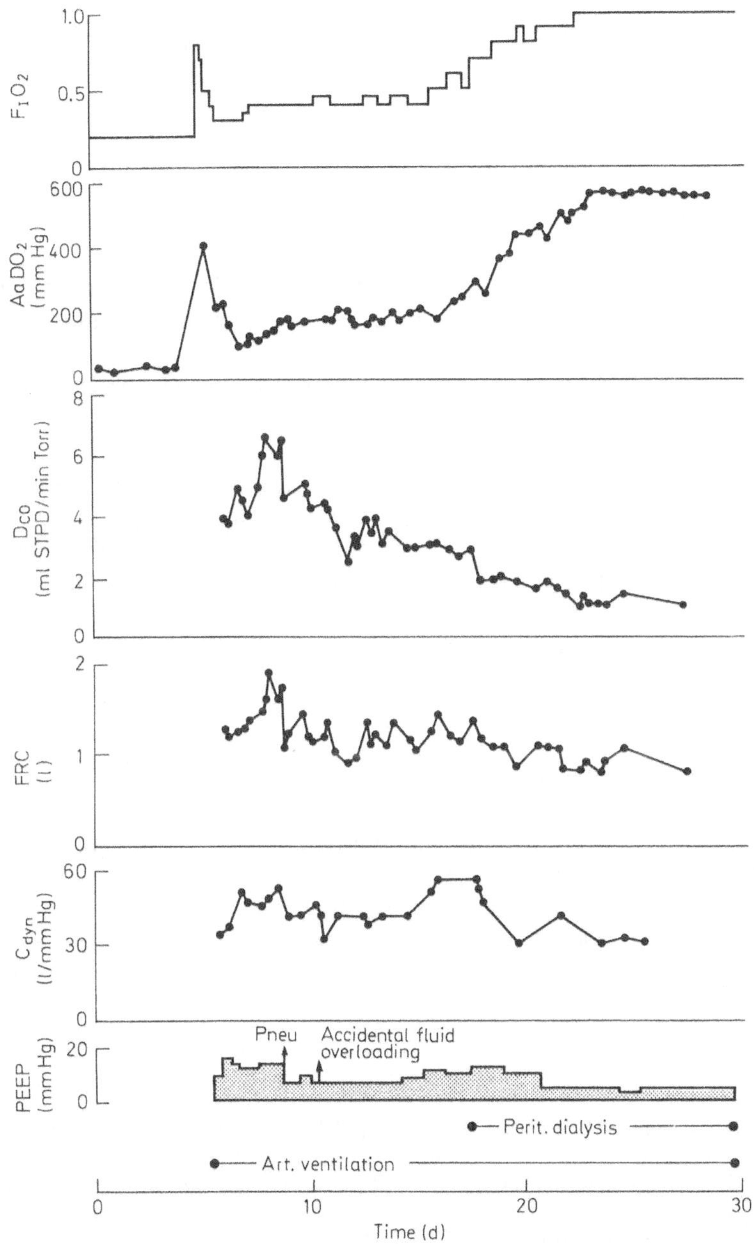

Fig. 3. Paraquat poisoning in a 16-year-old girl: inspiratory oxygen concentration (F_IO_2), alveoloarterial oxygen tension difference ($AaDO_2$), pulmonary diffusing capacity for CO (D_{CO}) with a rebreathing technique, lung volume (FRC), dynamic compliance (C_{dyn}), and positive end-expiratory pressure (PEEP) level against time (days after intoxication)

Table 2. Fluid intake and fluid balance after start of CAVH

CAVH application	0–12 h	12–36 h	36–60 h	
Fluid intake	11 500	18 700	19 100	ml/24 h
Fluid balance	− 3490	− 360	+ 320	ml/24 h

needs (Table 2). The survival rate of 47% for these patients with multiorgan failure under CAVH is better than survival rates common for combinations of respiratory and renal failure found in the literature.

The advantages of the method consist in unlimited parenteral and/or enteral nutrition, possibility for rapid correction of the fluid and electrolyte balance, low frequency of complications (no mechanical pump system).

Some disadvantages have to be pointed out: cumulative errors in the fluid balance are possible, invasive monitoring (Swan-Ganz catheter) is necessary, the method itself is invasive.

In our opinion, however, the advantages outweigh the disadvantages. Furthermore, it may be possible that toxic oligopeptides can also be eliminated by CAVH; in septic patients Hörl et al. [3] found considerable amounts of proteolytic activity in the hemofiltration fluid indicating the transfer of protease-like oligopeptides. Likewise, it is still unknown whether an elimination of low molecular proteins could provoke a depletion syndrome.

Conclusion

1. Interstitial pulmonary edema causes a severe deterioration of the pulmonary gas exchange, but with relatively late clinical manifestation.
2. The most important therapeutic steps are mechanical ventilation with PEEP and a strictly controlled fluid balance avoiding any fluid overload.
3. In this situation CAVH offers the possibility of eliminating fluid rapidly and of controlling fluid balance effectively without any handicap to parenteral or enteral nutrition. First clinical results in severe intensive care cases encourage us to pursue this new therapeutic approach.

References

1. Demling RH, Manohar M, Will JA, Belzer FO (1979) The effect of plasma osmotic pressure on the pulmonary microcirculation after hemorrhagic shock. Surgery 86:323
2. Fleming WH, Bowen JC (1972) The use of diuretics in the treatment of early wet lung syndrome. Ann Surg 175:505
3. Hörl WH, Stepinski J, Gantert C, Hörl M, Heidland A (1981) Evidence for the participation of proteases on protein catabolism during hypercatabolic renal failure. Klin Wochenschr 59:751
4. Koller WF, Benzer HM, Pauser GF (1985) CAVH in acute respiratory failure. In: Sieberth HG, Mann H (eds) Continous arteriovenous hemofiltration (CAVH). Karger, Basel
5. Lucas GE, Weaver D, Higgins RF, Ledgerwood AM, Johnson SD, Bouwman DL (1978) Effects of albumin versus non-albumin resuscitation on plasma volume and renal excretory function. J Trauma 18:564

6. Lundsgaard-Hansen P, Pappova E (1973/1974) Respiratorische Insuffizienz, kolloid-osmotischer Druck und Albumintherapie. Infusionstherapie 1:624
7. Skillman JJ, Parkikh BM, Tanenbaum BJ (1970) Pulmonary arteriovenous admixture. Improvement with albumin and diuresis. Am J Surg 119:440
8. Skillman JJ (1972) Treatment of acute respiratory distress syndrome: role of albumin and diuretics. In: Forscher BK, Lillehei RC, Stubs SS (eds) Shock in low- and high-flow states. Excerpta Medica, Amsterdam
9. Staub NC (1978) Pulmonary edema. Chest 74:559
10. Staudacher C, Di Carlo V, Chiesa R, Cristallo M (1979) Morphological alterations in shock lung. An electron microscopic study. In: Mayrhofer-Krammel O, Schlag G, Stoeckel H (eds) Akutes progressives Lungenversagen. Thieme, Stuttgart, p 8 (Intensivmedizin, Notfallmedizin, Anaesthesiologie Bd. 16)
11. Sturm JA (1985) Traumatischer Schock und die Lunge: Gefäßschädigung und Volumentherapeutika im Experiment. Springer, Berlin Heidelberg New York Tokyo
12. Tranbaugh RF, Lewis FR, Christensen JM, Elings VB (1980) Lung water changes after thermal injury. Ann Surg 192:479
13. Virgilio RW, Rice CL, Smith DE, James DR, Zarkins CK, Hobelmann CF, Peters RM (1979) Crystalloid vs colloid resuscitation: is one better? Surgery 85:129
14. Weil MH, Henning RJ, Morissette M, Michaelis S (1978) Relationship between colloid osmotic pressure and pulmonary artery wedge pressure in patients with acute cardio-respiratory failure. Am J Med 64:643

Ultrafiltration During Cardiopulmonary Bypass

D. J. Magilligan

Introduction

Crystalloid prime with hemodilution has been a great advantage to cardiac surgeons, for in addition to decreasing blood requirements it has also resulted in improved pulmonary and renal function [1]. Postoperative weight gain and an increase of up to 33% in the measured extracellular fluid space [2] are the disadvantages of dilution perfusion. In most patients this excess water is well tolerated and rapidly excreted. Certainly in renal failure patients, this excess fluid load may be detrimental. However, we are also interested in patients with severe preoperative fluid overload, in whom, even with adequate renal function, the additional water volume particularly in the lungs, may lead to organ dysfunction. We first set out to evaluate the use of ultrafiltration during cardiopulmonary bypass in a laboratory setting and have now instituted its use in a clinical setting. The following is a report of that experience.

Materials and Methods

Laboratory Evaluation

Animal Model

Mongrel dogs weighing between 25 and 30 kg were anesthetized with i.v. pentobarbital (20 mg/kg). Anesthesia was maintained with halothane (1.0%). Ventilation was carried out through a cuffed endotracheal tube with a tidal volume of 20 ml/kg at a range of 8–12/min delivered by a Bird Mark 7 Respirator (Bird, Palm Springs, CA). A polyethylene catheter was inserted into a jugular vein and advanced into the right atrium for fluid infusion. A Swan-Ganz catheter (American Edwards, Santa Ana, CA) was inserted into the pulmonary artery via a jugular vein and a lung water catheter (American Edwards, Santa Ana, CA) – a 5 French catheter with a distal opening for sampling and injection and a thermistor at its distal tip – was inserted into the femoral artery and positioned in the abdominal aorta. The Swan-Ganz and lung water catheters were connected to pressure transducers and pulmonary artery pressure (Ppa), systemic arterial pressure (Psa), and EKG were recorded continuously. Pulmonary capillary wedge pressure (Ppcw) and thermodilution cardiac outputs were determined before bypass and 30 min after bypass. Cardiac index was calculated using body surface area derived from animal body weight [3]. Hematocrit, hemoglobin, electrolytes, and colloid-oncotic pressure (COP) (Weil Oncometer, Instrument Laboratories, Lexington, MA) were obtained before bypass and 30 min after bypass. The COP-Ppcw hydrostatic pressure gradient which estimates Starling's forces was calculated pre- and postbypass.

Cardiopulmonary Bypass

A median sternotomy was performed and the animal heparinized (3 mg/kg body weight). The left femoral artery and both venae cavae were cannulated and connected to a Sarns modular heart lung machine (Sarns, Ann Arbor, MI), using a Bently Temptrol Q-200A bubble oxygenator (Bentley, Irvine, CA). The oxygenator was primed with a solution of 1500 ml Ringer's lactate, 12.5 g mannitol, 500 mg calcium gluconate, and 1500 IU heparin. The animal was placed on cardiopulmonary bypass and mechanical ventilation was turned off with the lungs partially inflated at 20 mmHg. The left heart was vented by a cannula placed into the left ventricle through the right superior pulmonary vein. Venae cavae were snared and bypass flow maintained at 100 ml/min/kg with lactated Ringer's solution added to maintain this flow. In group 1, the animals were kept at normothermia with the heart beating for 120 min and then weaned from bypass. In group 2, the animals were cooled to 28 °C and 150 ml cardioplegic solution was instilled into the aortic root immediately after cross clamping and at 20, 40, 60, and 80 min. The cardioplegic solution consisted of Isolyte-S (McGaw, Irvine, CA), to which was added 20 mEq KCl 30 mEq $NaHCO_3$, 15 gm dextrose to total 1000 ml. The resultant composition was: $K^+ = 25$ mEq/L, Na^+ 178 mEq/L, $Cl^- = 109$ mEq/L, $Mg^{++} = 2.7$ mEq/L, $NaHCO_3^- = 50$ mEq/L, pH = 7.9, osmolarity = 460 mosmol/L.

Ultrafiltration

An Amicon Diafilter-20 (Amicon, Lexington, MA) was interposed between the arterial inflow and venous return of a standard cardiopulmonary bypass circuit (Fig. 1). Ultrafiltration could be turned on or off by clamping the filter inflow without disturbing the total bypass flow. The rate of ultrafiltration was controlled by adjusting a screw clamp on the filtrate outflow of the diafilter. An attempt was

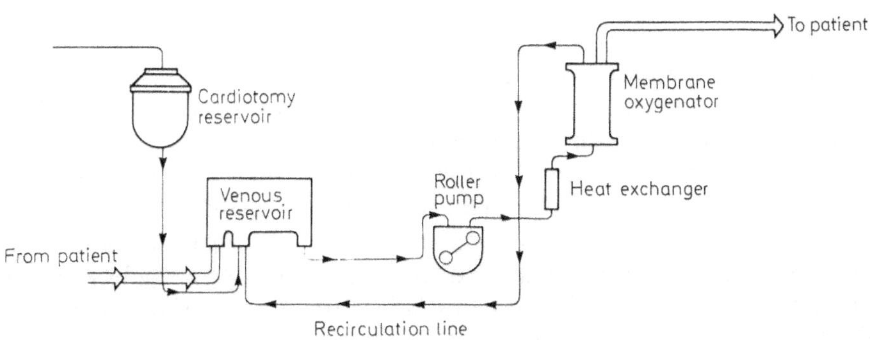

Fig. 1. The basic perfusion setup using a membrane oxygenator and separate heat exchanger

made to remove all priming fluid, all fluid added during bypass, and additional fluid was removed if bypass flows and pressures could be maintained.

Lung Water

Thermal Dye. Extravascular lung water (EVLW) was determined from the extravascular thermal volume of the lung (ETV), as measured by the double indicator dilution technique using indocyanine green dye as the intravascular indicator and the transfer of heat as the extravascular indicator. Through the right atrial catheter 10 ml iced indocyanine green dye (25 mg dye diluted to 50 ml at 5 °C) was injected. Thermal curves were sensed through the thermistor at the tip of the lung water catheter and also through this catheter blood was withdrawn and dye concentration measured by a densitometer (Waters Instrument, Rochester, MN) and both curves inscribed on a strip-chart recorder. The thermal and dye curves were analyzed on-line by a Lung Water Computer (American Edwards, Santa Ana, CA), which gave a digital recording of cardiac output, dye decay time, thermal decay time, dye mean transit time, thermal mean transit time, and extravascular lung water. The average of three readings was taken, divided by body weight, and expressed as ml/kg.

At the conclusion of seven of the experiments, gravimetric lung water was determined by the method of Pearce and associates [4] as modified by Holcroft and Trunkey [5], with a correction for lung blood water.

Clinical Experience

Patient Selection

We used ultrafiltration in 48 cardiac surgical patients; 33 of the 48 had the ultrafilter inserted at the start of bypass since they had evidence of excess body water preoperatively. Thirteen had the ultrafilter installed after the start of bypass because of any combination of the following: long pump run, excessive pump reservoir volume, and/or low hematocrit. One patient had ultrafiltration preoperatively to improve nutrition in the face of severe fluid overload. One patient had ultrafiltration postoperatively because of diuretic-resistant severe fluid overload.

Cardiopulmonary Bypass

All patients underwent cardiopulmonary bypass with moderate systemic hypothermia (28 °C), nonblood prime, and a membrane oxygenator (Sci-Med, Minneapolis, MN). Topical cooling was exployed, except in reoperations when it was technically difficult; the left heart was routinely vented; and caval tapes were not routinely employed except when a right atriotomy was performed. Crystalloid cardioplegia (modified St. Thomas solution) was routinely employed. Flows were maintained at 2.5 l/min/m^2 and lactated Ringer's solution was added as needed to maintain flow. When the hematocrit dropped below 18%, whole blood was added to the perfusate. Intake fluid volumes were a summation of i.v. crystalloid, blood, perfusate, and cardioplegia. Output volume was a summation of urine, ultrafiltrate, and blood loss.

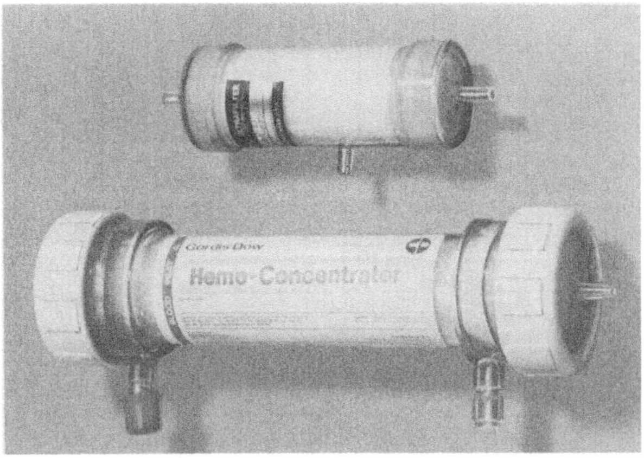

Fig. 2. Ultrafiltration can be accomplished with the use of the Diafilter (*top*) (Amicon, Lexington, MA) or the Hemoconcentrator (C. R. Bard, Santa Ana, CA)

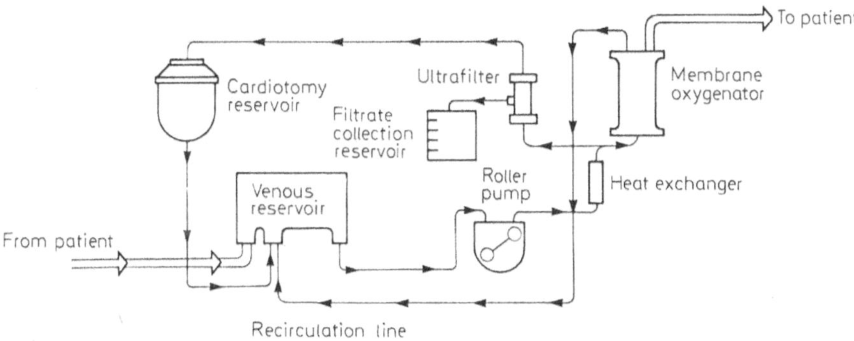

Fig. 3. When ultrafiltration is instituted at the start of bypass it is inserted in a branch of the line between the heat exchanger and the oxygenator

Ultrafiltration

A Diafilter-20 (Amicon, Lexington, MA) was used in most patients and a Hemoconcentrator (CR Bard, Santa Ana, CA) in the early experience. An attempt was made to remove all priming fluids, all fluid added during bypass, and any additional fluid as long as bypass flows and pressure could be maintained.

The Amicon device is composed of 5000 polysulfone hollow fibers with an internal diameter of 200 μ ± 10% and an active surface area of 0.25 m^2. The high permeability of the membrane allows flux of water and solutes with a mol. wt. <50000 daltons. It is compact (5 in.) and does not require suction to produce an effective transmembrane gradient (Fig. 2).

The Hemoconcentrator is composed of cellulose acetate hollow fibers with an internal diameter of 200 μ and has an active surface area of 1.8 m^2. The membrane allows a flux of water and solutes with a mol. wt. <60000 daltons and requires the addition of suction to generate transmembrane pressures (Fig. 2).

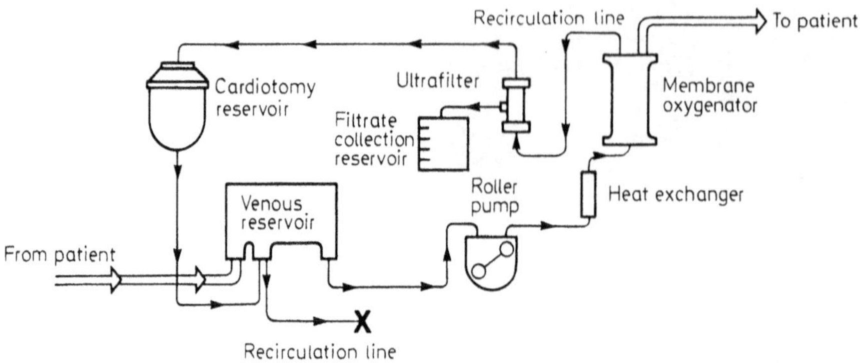

Fig. 4. When ultrafiltration is instituted during bypass, it is interposed in the recirculation line without disrupting flow to the patient

The basic cardiopulmonary bypass set up at Henry Ford Hospital is shown in Fig. 1. When ultrafiltration was set up prior to bypass it was inserted in a tubing branch immediately before the oxygenator. The blood exiting from the ultrafilter was returned to the cardiotomy reservoir (Fig. 3). When the ultrafilter was added during bypass it was simply placed in the recirculation line (Fig. 4).

Lung Water

EVLW was determined as in the animals using the Lung Water Computer (American Edwards, Santa Ana, CA). Injection was into a catheter, whose tip was positioned in the right atrium, and sampling was from a lung water catheter positioned in the distal aorta via the common femoral artery.

Statistical Methods

Comparisons between pre- and postbypass values were made using Student's *t*-test for paired data. A probability ≤ 0.05 was considered significant on the laboratory experiments.

Results

Laboratory Evaluation

All animals were successfully weaned from bypass without the need for catecholamine support. In group 1 (120 min bypass with empty beating heart), the amount of fluid added to the control animals and the ultrafiltered animals was similar. The amount of fluid removed in the control group by renal excretion was 180 ml and in the ultrafiltered animals (filtered + urine) was 2288 ml, and this was significantly different ($P < 0.01$). Although the COP, Ppcw, and COP-Ppcw gradients all changed in a direction favoring the accumulation of lung water, the pre- and postbypass differences were similar in control and ultrafiltered animals. However, the postbypass increase in EVLW was significantly less in the ultrafiltered animals (Table 1).

Both control and ultrafiltered animals in group 1 showed a marked, but similar, decrease in CI postbypass. The cardiac output enters into the equation for the

Table 1. Comparison of animals undergoing 120 min normothermic bypass with empty beating heart with and without ultrafiltration (group 1)

	Control	Ultrafiltration	Difference (P)
Number	4	4	–
Fluid in	2350 ±1090 SD ml	2750 ±500 SD	0.480
Fluid out	180 ± 232 ml	2288 ±315	0.002[a]
Δ Ppcw	↑ 1.0 ± 3.9 mmHg	↑ 2.5 ± 6.0	0.596
Δ COP	↓ 6.9 ± 2.8 mmHg	↓ 8.2 ± 1.5	0.650
Δ COP-Ppcw	↓ 11.2 ± 4.4 mmHg	↓ 10.5 ± 3.2	0.860
Δ CI	↓ 1.20 ± 0.3 l/min/m^2	↓ 1.65 + 0.8	0.310
Δ EVLW	↑ 2.83 ± 0.5 ml/kg	↑ 1.03 ± 0.2	0.007[a]

Values represent mean and SD, Δ represents mean change between pre- and postbypass values
[a] $P < 0.05$

Table 2. Comparison of animals undergoing 90 min cold cardioplegic arrest followed by 30 min of recovery with and without ultrafiltration (group 2)

	Control	Ultrafiltration	Difference (P)
Number	2	4	–
Fluid in	2775 ± 25 SD ml	3425 ± 96 SD	0.001[a]
Fluid out	110 ±120 ml	2710 ±258	0.001[a]
Δ Ppcw	↑ 4.0 ± 1.4 mmHg	↑ 1.8 ± 5.2	0.597
Δ COP	↓ 10.5 ± 0.4 mmHg	↓ 7.8 ± 2.4	0.205
Δ COP-Ppcw	↓ 14.3 ± 1.5 mmHg	↓ 10.5 ± 4.7	0.355
Δ CI	↓ 0.90 ± 0.8 l/min/m^2	↓ 0.65 ± 0.3	0.430
Δ EVLW	↑ 3.40 ± 0.4 ml/kg	↑ 0.95 ± 1.1	0.049[a]

Values represent mean and SD, Δ represents mean change between pre- and postbypass values
[a] $P < 0.05$

measurement of lung water as follows:

$$\mathrm{EVLW} = \mathrm{MTT}_{\mathrm{thermal}}\mathrm{MTT}_{\mathrm{dye}} \times \mathrm{CO}$$

where EVLW is extravascular lung water, MTT is mean transit time, and CO is cardiac output. Because the postbypass decrease in CO might have had an effect on the EVLW accuracy, a second group of animals was studied using cold, potassium cardioplegic arrest to maintain postbypass CO near normal levels and to eliminate any possible effect that a low CO might have on EVLW measurement.

In group 2 (90 min cardioplegic arrest and 30 min recovery), significantly more fluid was added to the ultrafiltered animals than to the control animals ($P < 0.01$). The amount of fluid removed in the control group was 110 ml (urine) and in the ultrafiltered group was 2710 ml, a significant difference ($P < 0.01$). Again, the COP, Ppcw, and COP-Ppcw gradients changed in a direction favoring the accumulation of lung water, but the pre- and postbypass differences were similar in control and in ultrafiltered animals. In addition, the postbypass change in CI was very small and similar in control and ultrafiltered animals (Table 2).

Table 3. Comparison of concentration of solutes in plasma and ultrafiltrate in animal experiments

	Plasma	Ultrafiltrate	Difference
Na^+ (mEq/l)	142 ±0.8	140 ±0.8	0.225
K^+ (mEq/l)	4.0±0.6	3.7±0.6	0.636
Cl^- (mEq/l)	114 ±3.3	122 ±5.4	0.051
Ca^{++} (mg/dl)	7.5±1.4	5.2±0.5	0.098
PO_4^{--} (mg/dl)	3.2±0.8	2.6±0.9	0.538
Urea nitrogen (mg/dl)	14.3±5.5	13.3±2.5	0.724
Total protein (gm/dl)	3.9±	0	0.000[a]

[a] $P < 0.05$

The concentration of solutes in plasma and ultrafiltrate is shown in Table 3. As expected, the composition of the filtrate was similar to plasma and there was no protein in the ultrafiltrate. The lack of protein in the ultrafiltrate was confirmed using a microtechnique for measuring protein (Biuret method).

Clinical Experience

1. Ultrafiltration at the start of cardiopulmonary bypass was done in 33 patients. The amount of ultrafiltrate during bypass ranged from 1000 ml to 6600 ml and averaged 2728 ml. This resulted in an average intraoperative fluid balance of −638 ml, and an average intraoperative weight gain of 1.9 kg. In eleven of these 33 patients pre- and postoperative measurements of extravascular lung water (EVLW) were made using the thermal-dye technique. The postoperative EVLW (823 ml) was significantly lower than the preoperative EVLW (1119 ml) ($P < 0.05$).

2. In 13 patients ultrafiltration was started after bypass had begun, because of a long perfusion and for excessive pump reservoir volume and/or low hematocrit (<17%). The ultrafilter was easily interposed in the recirculation line during bypass in these patients and resulted in a mean ultrafiltration volume of 1619 ml and an average fluid balance of +595 ml.

3. One patient with severe congestive heart failure (CHF), sepsis, respiratory failure, and nutritional depletion had ultrafiltration preoperatively. After ultrafiltration for 4 days, which allowed an intake of 3000 kcal/day with a nitrogen balance of +3.29/day and without weight gain, the patient underwent successful MVR and CABG.

4. One patient returned to the hospital after AVR with no improvement in CHF and resistance to maximal diuretic therapy. Ultrafiltration was instituted through an A-V dialysis shunt with a 7.4 kg weight loss in 7 days and improvement in radionucleide ejection fraction from 37% to 60%.

Discussion

Dilution perfusion, for all its advantages, will result in decreased plasma colloid-oncotic pressure and an elevated interstitial water content [6]. Since further increases in body water might be detrimental to an already fluid overloaded patient, ultrafiltration has a logical place in the cardiopulmonary bypass apparatus. However, reports of its use during bypass have been limited [7, 8].

One reason for the limited use of ultrafiltration during bypass has been the inability to accurately measure organ water content by methods that are not destructive. Although crystalloid hemodilution has been shown to result in increased water content in lungs [9], heart, kidney, and gastrointestinal tract [10], the technique to measure organ water was wet to dry weight and not clinically applicable. The thermal-dye double indicator dilution technique for measuring EVLW is simple, can be repeated, and correlates more closely with gravimetric lung water than the previously used isotope techniques [11]. Establishment of this technique in our laboratory with previous documentation of a close correlation with gravimetric lung water ($R = 0.95$) in 28 measurements over a wide range [12] allowed us to repetitively measure lung water. We showed an increase in EVLW during routine bypass in dogs and demonstrated that the increase in EVLW was significantly less when ultrafiltration was employed during bypass. The correlation between thermal-dye and gravimetric lung water was close ($R = 0.96$) in seven of the present experiments in which both were measured. This experience has been published [13].

In conclusion, our laboratory evaluation of ultrafiltration during cardiopulmonary bypass showed that large amounts of water should be safely removed with a lowering of EVLW compared with control animals. Ultrafiltration used clinically has been safe and effective in removing up to 6 l plasma water during bypass. At the present time, we recommend its use for: (a) patients requiring open cardiac surgery who have excess body water as demonstrated by clinical evaluation, radiographic examination, or elevated thermal-dye EVLW, (b) long bypass with accumulation of large reservoir volumes and/or low hematocrit, (c) improved nutritional support in the fluid overloaded patient, and (d) for improvement in cardiac function in the fluid overloaded diuretic-resistant patient.

References

1. Lilleaasen P, Stokke O (1978) Moderate and extreme hemodilution in open heart surgery: fluid balance and acid-base studies. Ann Thorac Surg 25:127–133
2. Breckenridge IM, Digerness SB, Kirklin JW (1970) Increased extracellular fluid after open intracardiac operation. Surg Gynecol Obstet 131:53–56
3. Davis LE (1963) Treatment and management of burns. Veterinary Scope 8:7–11
4. Pearce ML, Yamashita J, Beazell J (1965) Management of pulmonary edema. Circ Res 16:482–488
5. Holcroft JW, Turnkey DD (1974) Extravascular lung water following hemorrhagic shock in the baboon. Ann Surg 180:480–487
6. English TAH, Digerness S, Kirklin JW (1971) Changes in colloid osmotic pressure during and shortly after open intracardiac operation. J Thorac Cardiovasc Surg 61:338–341
7. Darup J, Bleese N, Kalmar P, Lute G, Pokar H, Polonius MJ (1979) Hemofiltration during extracorporeal circulation. Thorac Cardiovasc Surg 27:227–230
8. Romagnoli A, Hocker J, Keats A, Milan J (1976) External hemoconcentration after deliberate hemodilution. In: Abstracts from the annual meeting of the American Society of Anesthesiology. Am Society of Anesthesiology, Park Ridge, p 269

9. Demling RH, Hick RE, Edmunds LH Jr (1976) Changes in extravascular lung water during venovenous perfusion. J Thorac Cardiovasc Surg 71:291–294
10. Utley JR, Wachtel C, Cain RB, Spaw EA, Collins JC, Stephens DB (1980) Effects of hypothermia, hemodilution, and pump oxygenation on organ water content, blood flow, and oxygen delivery and renal function. Ann Thorac Surg 31:121–133
11. Holcroft JW, Hopewell P, Sheldon GF, Lipanski A, Hoeffel J, Osborn JO (1973) Thermodilution for measurement of lung water: comparison with isotope and gravimetric methods. Circulation 48 [Suppl 4]:447
12. Magilligan DJ Jr, Oyama C, Levin N (1981) Interstitial and intraalveolar pulmonary edema – reversal by ultrafiltration. Crit Care Med 9:257
13. Magilligan DJ Jr, Oyama C (1984) Ultrafiltration during cardiopulmonary bypass: Laboratory evaluation and initial clinical evaluation. Ann Thorac Surg 37:33–39

Experiences with Continuous Arteriovenous Hemofiltration in Surgical Intensive Care Patients

F. E. Isemer, M. Hölscher, H. H. Hildebrand, and R. Sievert

Introduction

After 2 years of experience with continuous arteriovenous hemofiltration (CAVH) (1979–1981) we now predict that intermittent conventional hemodialysis and hemofiltration will be used in the future only for limited indications.

During these 2 years, a total of 32 surgical patients were treated with CAVH postoperatively. The results for treating uremia are completely satisfactory. In contrast to intermittent hemodialysis and hemofiltration, CAVH offers significant advantages especially for surgical intensive care patients.

In intensive care patients variable fluid removal permits hyperalimentation already in the stage of beginning renal insufficiency. Because of extensive apparatus and personnel effort, hemodialysis and mechanical hemofiltration are used for treatment only when the patient is already uremic. The circulation system of these patients often tolerates continuous fluid removal and continuous fluid substitution better than acute fluid removal by intermittent hemodialysis or hemofiltration.

Since accurate fluid balancing is possible by CAVH, installation of a bedscale is not required. Also in our experience CAVH requires relatively little personnel effort. In addition, no special mechanical equipment or energy supply is necessary. The vascular access for this method can be installed simply and quickly. For these practical reasons we decided to utilize CAVH in the last 2 years.

Patients and Diseases

We treated a total of 32 patients with this method, 18 men and 14 women, whose underlying illnesses are compiled in Table 1.

About two-thirds of the patients were over 50 years old. The table shows the underlying illness of the patient at the time of surgery. Partly, double diagnoses are cited as, e.g., in the case of a patient with polytrauma who suffered from rupture of the liver in addition to multiple bone injuries.

Most patients suffered from gastrointestinal or pancreas, liver, and gallbladder diseases. Four patients underwent surgery because of perforation or bleeding of the stomach. Fifteen patients had intestinal surgery because of ileus or neoplasm. Necrotic inflammation of the pancreas was found in two cases. Nine patients were treated for disorders of liver or gallbladder.

Table 1. Summary of underlying illnesses in 32 patients who were treated with CAVH in the intensive care unit from 1979–1981 (April). – Age: 30 years, $n=4$; 40 years, $n=5$; 50 years, $n=23$. Sex: male, $n=18$; female, $n=14$

Underlying illness	
Esophagus carcinoma	1
Stomach (perforation, bleeding)	4
Intestinal (ileus, neoplasm)	15
Pancreas (necrotic inflammation)	2
Liver-gallbladder (cirrhosis, stones)	9
Struma	2
Systemic illness (neoplasm)	1
Injuries (polytrauma, burns)	4

In five of these cases posthepatitis or alcoholic cirrhosis of the liver existed which had caused varicose esophageal bleeding. The other four patients suffered from gallstones which required surgical therapy. Two patients were admitted to our intensive care unit because of severe polytrauma and two others because of burns. The postoperative clinical course was complicated in all patients.

Complications of Underlying Diseases

The most significant complications are summarized in Table 2. The primary complications entered are those which we considered to be the main cause for renal failure. Secondary organ failures are arranged according to frequency in this patient population. Among the primary complications, there were 18 cases of peritonitis, by far the most prevalant basic illness, in 14 cases it was diffuse and in 4 cases as a result of abdominal abscesses. Causes for peritonitis were perforation of gastrointestinal tract or intestinal seam insufficiency. One patient of this group survived his diffuse bilious peritonitis and has completely recovered from his

Table 2. Main postoperative complications which led to renal failure, among other things, and necessitated CAVH

Primary complications		Secondary organ failure	
	n		*n*
Peritonitis (diffuse)	14 (1[a])	Renal	31
(abscessing)	4	Pulmonary	21
Bleeding >1.5 l	10	Cardiac-circulatory	21
Secondary ileus	1	Cerebral	7
Manifested cardiac insufficiency	2	Hepatic	6
Renal failure	1[a]	Diabetes mellitus	2
		Panmyelopathy	4

[a] Surviving patients

acute renal failure. Ten patients were bleeding during the course of their illness, usually considerably more than 1.5 l. Especially patients with varicose esophageal bleeding or patients with bleeding gastric or duodenal ulcers belong to this group.

Two of the older patients developed cardiac insufficiency which could not be controlled with drugs. Despite large doses of dopamine or other vasopressors over an extended period of time, sufficient filtration pressure for hemofiltration could not be achieved and hemofiltration was discontinued.

After ileus surgery in a woman with an ovarian neoplasm, acute renal failure developed, but this patient survived.

In all the remaining cases the renal failure was not a primary complication of the underlying illness but belonged to the broader groups of "secondary organ failures." A total of 21 patients suffered from considerable pulmonary insufficiency. The criterion for pulmonary failure was volume-controlled ventilation with more than 50% oxygen. In 21 patients cardiac-circulatory insufficiency existed. This group of patients needed more than 12 γ dopamine/kg body weight per min. Seven patients were comatose because of electroencephalographically confirmed, severe cerebral damage. In six patients we observed severe liver failure, where, besides hyperbilirubinemia and hepatic enzyme imbalance, also synthesis of albumin and clotting factors were interrupted. Two patients developed severe insulin-dependent diabetes mellitus which was not observed prior to surgery. In four patients panmyelophathy became apparent during the course of illness.

It becomes evident from the summary of most significant complications that renal failure did not occur as a primary complication in this patient population but was caused by the secondary complications. As a rule all patients exhibited "multiple organ failure" in the course of CAVH with an average of three secondary organ failures besides the underlying illness and the primary complication. One exception was the female patient with a primary renal failure after ileus surgery.

Indications for Use of CAVH and Outcome

In all patients the indication for CAVH was oliguria. Our patient population with "multiple organ failure" required hyperalimentation as well as specific drug therapy. This by itself caused volume problems in renal failure, requiring early, high continuous fluid removal.

Specific indications for CAVH were: Moderate overhydration in 17 patients who had peripheral edema and pulmonary congestion; only one patient was severely overhydrated, thus 6 l fluid had to be removed within 24 h.

Electrolyte imbalance, particularly hyperkalemia with values exceeding 5.5 meq/l as a result of renal failure, was the indication for CAVH in 16 patients. It has to be pointed out that the hyperkalemia of these patients could be well controlled with a large filtrate turnover of 20 l/day.

In six patients hypernatremia with values above 160 meq/l was the main indication. Hypernatremia was observed in 20% of the cases. It was often partly iatrogenic due to the high sodium content of medications. Probably because CAVH

Table 3. Indications for hemofiltration in the surgical observation unit 1979–1981 (April)

Oliguria	$n=32$
Overhydration	
Moderate	17
Severe	1
Electrolyte imbalance	
K^+	16
Na^+	6
Urea-N	
<100 mg/dl	8
>100 mg/dl	24
Creatinine	
<6 mg/dl	16
>6 mg/dl	16

Table 4. Length of treatment and successes with CAVH

Days	PRF	Elimination of		
		HV	EI	UR
	(*n*)	(*n*)	(*n*)	(*n*)
< 3 ($n=8$)	8			
<14 ($n=22$)	20	30[a]	30	30
>14 ($n=2$)	1			

[a] Two patients with primary cardiac insufficiency could not be treated successfully

PRF, persistent renal failure; HV, hypervolemia; EI, electrolyte imbalance; UR, uremia

is now started early, lately we have hardly seen hypernatremia in acute renal failure.

Blood urea nitrogen (BUN) was below 100 mg/dl in eight patients, and in 24 patients over 100 mg/dl. Creatinine was below 6 mg/dl in 16 patients, and in the other 16 patients over 6 mg/dl. These values reflect the catabolic metabolism of our severely ill patient population. Therefore, in these patients a high fluid turnover was necessary to compensate uremia.

Filtrate output achieved was 600–800 ml/h or 15–20 l/day. With this exchange volume even severe imbalances of the potassium metabolism could be controlled. The length of time a hemofilter could be used for a particular patient varied considerably, but usually lasted up to 5 days.

Table 4 shows the length of treatment and the results achieved with CAVH. Eight patients were treated up to 3 days; renal failure persisted in all of them. Twenty-two patients were treated up to 14 days; in 20 of them the renal failure persisted and in two, renal function recovered. Two patients were treated over 14 days; in one of them renal function was restored.

CAVH made hyperalimentation and adequate drug therapy possible for all patients. The consequences of acute renal failure such as electrolyte imbalance as well as uremia could be well controlled. In three patients renal function recovered by CAVH, two patients survived. Two patients with manifested cardiac insufficiency could not be treated adequately since not enough pressure for filtration could be achieved.

Conclusions

We have treated a patient population with "multiple organ failure" who had significant complications and several secondary organ failures besides the severe basic illness. On the average, we observed two other organ failures in addition to the renal failure and the underlying illness. Therefore the prognosis of these patients was uncertain. The effectiveness of CAVH therapy, thus, cannot be measured by the survival rate of the patients but only by the criteria for control of renal insufficiency.

Survival of the patients was only possible when the causative chain of complications could be effectively interrupted. This was the case in a 59-year-old patient whose lung and kidney failures could not be eliminated until the bilious peritonitis was sanitized surgically first.

When CAVH has to be considered for intensive care in conjunction with ventilation, pace markers, etc., in our opinion, it offers considerable advantages over intermittent hemodialysis and hemofiltration.

Potentials and Pitfalls of Continuous Arteriovenous Hemofiltration

Intensive Care Potentials of Continuous Arteriovenous Hemofiltration

P. Kramer and G. Biege

Arteriovenous hemofiltration offers a number of possibilities in intensive care and monitoring [4], which can sometimes be decisive for the use of the method (Fig. 1).

Arterial Blood Pressure

Since there is a catheter in the femoral artery, continuous arterial pressure measurements can be made. Thereby the arterial blood line has to be occluded behind the pressure line connection for the short time of pressure recording. The correlation with cuff pressure or pressure measured in the radial artery is for clinical practice good enough to use the access to the femoral artery (Fig. 2). Although

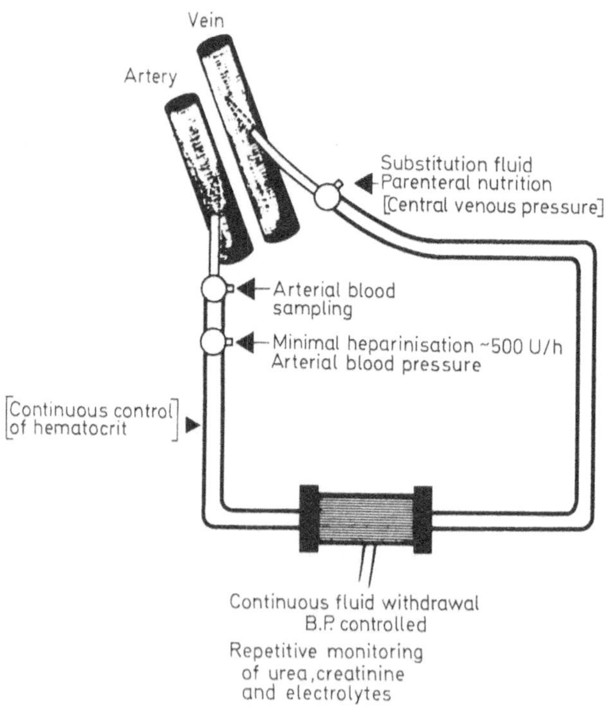

Fig. 1. Schematic illustration of the various intensive care potentials of the extracorporeal CAVH circuit

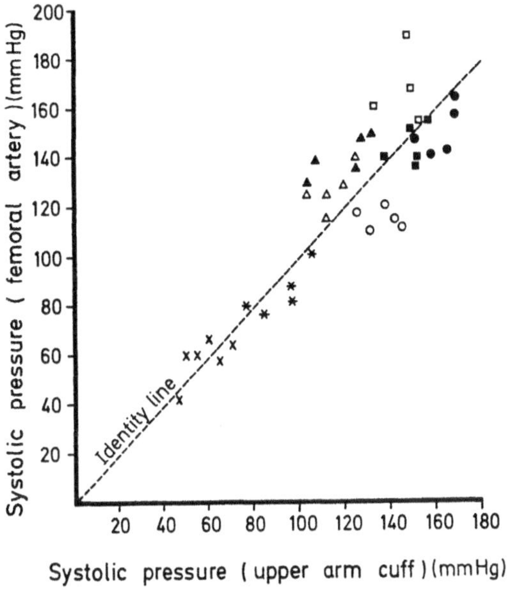

Fig. 2. Comparison between systolic pressure measured in the femoral artery and with an upper arm cuff

the shunting of blood is only small, the increase of central arterial pressure after occlusion is measurable; in adults a transient increase of 5 mmHg was observed. This may be different in small children, in whom the proportion of the shunting is higher; an increase of central arterial pressure by 20 mmHg is not unusual.

Central Venous Pressure

The venous catheter permits measurement of central venous pressure when extracorporeal circulation is interrupted temporarily, but it must be stressed that the venous pressure measured in the femoral vein is 5–8 cm H_2O higher than in the vena cava. If this difference is taken into account the femoral vein pressure is a useful parameter for intensive supervision.

Arterial Blood Sampling

The cannula in the femoral artery may be used for repeated arterial blood sampling for blood gas analysis provided that this is carried out under strictly sterile conditions.

Pressure-Dependent Fluid Removal

As the filtration rate depends on the hydrostatic pressure, blood-pressure dependent fluid removal can be taken advantage of. If the ultrafiltrate-collecting container is attached to the patient's bed frame at the proper height, fluid is withdrawn only when the blood pressure exceeds a preselected limit.

Ultrafiltrate Analysis

Since the composition of the ultrafiltrate is very similar to the glomerular filtrate, the concentration of a number of substances and electrolytes such as urea, creatinine, uric acid, glucose, sodium, potassium, chloride, and phosphate [6], can also be measured in the ultrafiltrate instead of in the blood.

Cooling

A very important capability of CAVH is cooling. The arterial and the venous tubings are placed in ice water and the effect on body temperature is seen within an hour: even high body temperature is easily controlled and may be titrated to any wanted level. The cooling has no effect on the filtration rate. On the contrary lowering body temperature usually results in circulatory stabilization [5] with an improvement of filtration rate. Cooling is very important for the prevention of cerebral edema [2].

Blood Volume

As shown by the group in Aachen [7], continuous measurement of the hematocrit or of blood volume can also be made in the arterial line. This may eventually become an important parameter for adapting the ultrafiltration rate to the refilling rate.

Obligatory Heparinisation

The dose of heparin necessary for arteriovenous hemofiltration (<10 IU/kg/h) corresponds approximately with the dose which would be given to any intensive care patient for prophylaxis of thrombosis. Since the continuous heparin supply can never be interrupted during CAVH without prior additional administration of heparin, to prevent thrombosing of the hemofilter, optimal prophylaxis against thrombosis is also provided for the large blood vessel catheters.

Hyperosmolar Parenterals

All parenterals including 40% glucose solution can be introduced through the venous cannula under optimal conditions, since dilution with substitution fluid and fully heparinized blood first occurs extracorporeally, then entering a large-caliber vein at high flow rate. The osmolality of a 40% glucose solution is reduced from 1500 to 350 mosmol/l. The possibility of optimal parenteral feeding of patients with complicated acute renal failure from the first day on is a significant advance toward the improvement of the prognosis [1].

Diagnostic Hemoperfusion

Arteriovenous hemofiltration permits "diagnostic hemoperfusions" with minimal effort. In this method, arteriovenous blood bypasses the hemofilter flowing through a small charcoal cartrigde for 10–30 min. The cartrigde adsorbs microorganisms for bacteriological diagnosis. According to our preliminary results, this seems to be an important advance in combatting sepsis, since it is possible to accumulate microorganisms on the charcoal which are not detected with conventional blood cultures [3, 6].

References

1. Abel RM, Beck CH, Abbott WM, Ryan JA, Barnett GO, Fischer JE (1973) Improved survival from acute renal failure after treatment with intravenous essential L-amino acids and glucose. Results of a prospective double-blind study. N Engl J Med 288:695
2. Botarell EH, Lougheed WM, Scott JW, Vandewater SL (1956) Hypothermia and interruption of carotid, or carotid and vertebral circulation in the surgical management of intracranial aneurisms. J Neurosurg 13:1–42
3. Keller F, Feldmann K, Abshagen U, Hennemann H, Barz R (1981) Diagnostic hemoperfusion for rapid detection of bacteremia. Klin Wochenschr 59:425
4. Kramer P, Böhler J, Kehr A, Gröne HJ, Schrader J, Matthaei D, Scheler F (1982) Intensive care potential of continuous arteriovenous hemofiltration. Trans Am Soc Artif Intern Organs 18:28–31
5. Maggiore Q, Pizzarelli F, Zoccali C, Siscia S, Nicolo F, Parlongo S (1981) Effect of extracorporeal blood cooling on dialytic arterial hypotension. Proc Eur Dial Transplant Assoc 18:597–601
6. Matthaei D, Kramer P, Grieben K, Schrader J, Ansorg R, Scheler F (1985) Advantages of CAVH in the management of acute renal failure. Nephrology (to be published)
7. Stiller S, Mann H (1980) Continuous monitoring of blood volume during hemodialysis. Proc Eur Dial Transplant Assoc 7:167

Differential Indications for the Use of Continuous Arteriovenous Hemofiltration

P. Kramer

Choice of Mode of Treatment

The number of publications and case reports on continuous arteriovenous hemofiltration (CAVH) has increased exponentially [1, 6–8] as a result of various reasons all related to clinical practice, including:

1. Overhydration resistant to diuretics is a common problem in all intensive care units and the resulting restriction of fluid administration or the time-consuming discussion about the indication of a hemodialysis is an unpleasant experience of most physicians and surgeons.
2. CAVH is a simple procedure, which may be started by any physician or surgeon who has experience with the Seldinger technique for insertion of femoral catheters.
3. The pumpless ultrafiltration driven by cardiac contraction force is not expected to work and thus impresses most withnesses of visible "urine output" of the artificial glomerulus more than do other innovations.
4. The new kidney replacement therapy has made it possible to treat patients in the specialist's intensive care unit (hopefully with the nephrologist as a consultant). Thus, various specialists such as general and thoracic surgeons, anesthesiologists and cardiologists eventually collected more practical experience with this method than did nephrologists.

It is a matter of discussion whether this development has improved the prognosis of patients with acute renal failure (ARF) and whether CAVH may be a useful renal replacement therapy in all cases of ARF. Therefore, it must be made absolutely clear that the author who first described this technique in 1977 [2] objects to the use of CAVH in simple uncomplicated ARF: Patients who are able to get up, who have no serious circulatory or pulmonary complication, who have to be hospitalized only because of ARF, should best be treated by venovenous single-needle hemodialysis with volume-controlled ultrafiltration.

In Table 1 the choice of mode of treatment is displayed for different patients in different clinical situations as practised in Göttingen. Intermittent hemodialysis is the treatment of choice in adults with uncomplicated ARF, in massive hyperkalemia, and in intoxications. Intermittent venovenous pump-driven hemofiltration is the treatment of choice in elderly patients with serious cerebrovascular or coronary sclerosis but otherwise uncomplicated ARF. Continuous peritoneal dialysis is the treatment of choice in patients with ARF due to acute hemorrhagic

Table 1. Choice of mode of treatment as it is practised in Göttingen University Hospital 1984

	HD	HF	CAVH	CPD	IPD
Children (< 12 years) Uncomplicated renal failure	(+)	(+)		+	+
Adults (13–65 years) Uncomplicated renal failure	+	+			
Elderly patients (> 65 years) Uncomplicated renal failure		+			
Serious vascular sclerosis (coronary-, cerebro-)		+	(+)	+	(+)
No vascular access				+	+
Acute renal failure "multiple organ failure" (circulatory and pulmonary failure)		(+)	+	(+)	
Acute renal failure due to acute pancreatitis				+	
Acute renal failure with massive hyperkalemia (e.g., hemolysis)	+	(+)			
Intoxication and acute renal failure	+	(+)			

HD, hemodialysis, venovenous
HF, hemofiltration, venovenous
CAVH, continuous arteriovenous hemofiltration
CPD, continuous peritoneal dialysis
IPD, intermittent peritoneal dialysis

pancreatitis, in patients without vascular access, and in small children. (In children > 10 kg CAVH has been used recently if cardiopulmonary problems were predominant.)

During the past 15 years, the proportion of patients with uncomplicated ARF has fallen in some areas to below 10%. Most anuric patients today present multiple organ failure, whereby renal failure is the final complication. And particularly in these patients the intermittent hemodialysis or hemofiltration displays its unphysiologic (sometimes lethal) effects.

In chronic renal failure the side effects of the unphysiologic intermittent treatment have to be balanced against the patient's freedom from the machine. In critically ill patients, however, one should follow as closely as possible the functions of the natural kidney, which are 24-h per day correction of water, electrolyte, and acid-base disorders, as well as for elimination of waste products.

In the past, before 1977, we have treated these patients with continuous peritoneal dialysis taking into account the risk of peritonitis, the loss of proteins, and the difficulty to control fluid balance. Besides that diaphragmatic breathing excursions were limited by intraperitoneal fluid so that an already critical respiratory situation generally became worse.

Therefore, CAVH was immediately accepted as the better continuous kidney replacement therapy by anesthesiologists, general surgeons, and cardiologists. Figure 1 gives an idea of the frequency of CAVH use and of the different basic illnesses complicated by ARF treated early in 1982 in four different intensive care units of the University Hospital in Göttingen. Frequency and indications have not changed very much since that time.

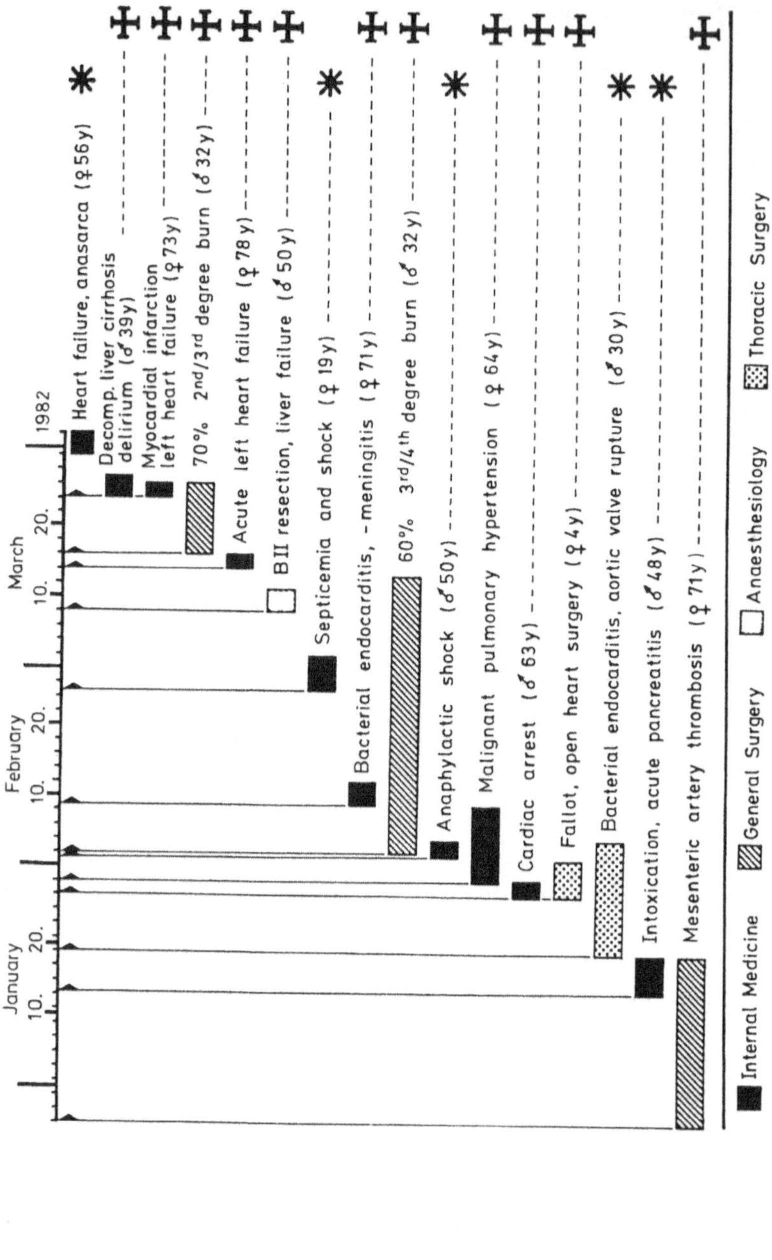

Fig. 1. Frequency of use and indication for CAVH in early 1982 at four different intensive care units of the Unviersity Hospital in Göttingen

Table 2. Advantages and disadvantages of CAVH in comparison with intermittent mechanical hemofiltration

Advantages	Disadvantages
Gentle circulatory effect	Low efficiency
Higher effective fluid withdrawal possible	Not applicable with femoral cannulation in serious atherosclerosis
Metabolic steady state	Only for the bedridden patient
No risk of air embolism	
No filter rupture	
No power connection or consumption	
No specially trained personnel	
No investment costs	

Indication for the use of CAVH is determined, on the one hand, by the potentials [3–5] and risks of this new procedure in comparison with conventional hemodialysis, pump-driven hemofiltration, or continuous peritoneal dialysis, and, on the other hand, by necessary measures which must be taken, particularly with complicated acute renal failure; these may sometimes be decisive for the application.

The engagement is worthwhile, particularly in cases of ARF, because the kidneys recover completely in most patients. Arguments for the use of arteriovenous hemofiltration are rarely unequivocal. Of course, if there is no machine available – unfortunately true in health care for 70% of the world population – and if peritoneal dialysis cannot be carried out due to diaphragmatic defect, paralytic ileus, extensive peritoneal adhesions, or blockage of the peritoneal catheter with fibrin clots, there will be no other choice in the future than to make use of this new procedure.

Fortunately, in the Western part of the world we have still the opportunity in most cases to use machines for the treatment of ARF. To that extent, the new method must compete with conventional procedures, particularly with pump-driven hemofiltration, which has proven itself especially in the treatment of ARF in the intensive care area, due to controlled withdrawal of fluid and independence from water supply. In comparison with intermittent mechanical hemofiltration, CAVH has advantages and disadvantages, which are displayed in Table 2.

Because of continuous withdrawal of fluid, the procedure is close to physiologic conditions and has only few negative effects on the circulation. For this reason, more effective fluid withdrawal is possible than with intermittent mechanical hemofiltration [6]. The metabolism is in a steady state and electrolytes may be maintained constant, which is of importance for controlled parenteral nutrition based on daily nitrogen balance.

Since no roller pumps are used, air embolism is practically precluded. Positive pressure prevails in the extracorporeal system. Filter ruptures practically never occur, as a result of low perfusion pressures. If there is a defect in the hemofilter, this is discovered immediately after beginning extracorporeal blood circulation.

The procedure requires no power connection and to that extent is suitable for catastrophes. Simple execution avoids the need for specially trained personnel.

The fact that no investment costs are necessary is of great importance, particularly in planning for treatment of ARF, because machines obtained specifically for the treatment of ARF are often not fully utilized.

The main disadvantage of the procedure is its low efficiency, i.e., it is effective only with long-term use. This must be taken into consideration, particularly in cases of poisoning and massive hyperkalemia.

The described technique of using the cannulated femoral artery and vein as circulatory access can be used in cases of high-grade atherosclerosis only in the sense of an "ultima ratio," when it is not desired to make use of a Scribner shunt. In addition, this procedure has so far been used with femoral catheters in bedridden patients only. The catheters now available are so flexible that the patients can bend their legs and may be moved, as necessary, in bed. There should be no mobilization of the patients, as would be possible with conventional hemodialysis, hemofiltration, or intermittent peritoneal dialysis.

According to the experience of four different intensive care units, with a total of more than 250 patients, the following indications for the application of CAVH are suggested:

1. *General indications:* overhydration resistant to diuretics; no hypercaloric nutrition possible; hyperkalemia; azotemia
2. *Specific indications:* lung diffusion disturbances and circulatory failure; natriurectic-resistant hypernatremia; cerebral edema; controlled parenteral nutrition; anuric kidney protection
3. *Questionable indications:* poisoning; massive hyperkalemia (such as in hemolysis)

General indications, in which CAVH may be used as an alternative to conventional methods, include:
1. Overhydration resistant to diuretics, when it is not possible to obtain sufficient urine output even with high doses of furosemide and the infusion volume, particularly the parenteral nutrition, has to be restricted
2. "Normal" hyperkalemia, in the course of azotemia, but CAVH treatment should be started early and a plasma water exchange rate of approximately 10 l/day should be achieved.

There are some specific indications in which CAVH is superior to the conventional intermittent procedure. This applies especially to disturbances of lung diffusion coupled with circulatory failure or severe circulatory instability, so that adequate intermittent fluid withdrawal is not possible. Natriuretic-resistant hypernatremia (for example, after resuscitation) is another specific indication. In such cases it is important to normalize high plasma sodium levels gently but continuously over a period of 2 days by substituting plasma water with sodium-free solutions. Cerebral edema may be treated with continuous dehydration using CAVH and a high normal sodium concentration in the substitution fluid. The continuous fluid deprivation is essential and cannot be achieved with intermittent treatment.

Daily nitrogen balance and energy balance requires a steady state of metabolism and nutrition. Thus, controlled parenteral nutrition in catabolic renal failure cannot be achieved with intermittent renal replacement therapy.

For the recovery of kidney function it is essential to maintain constantly high normal plasma sodium concentration (150 meq/l), positive base excess (+5 meq/l), and hydration as much as possible with respect to lung and heart function.

Exogenous poisoning is a questionable indication for the use of CAVH. In this case, hemodialysis should be used for poisoning with low molecular weight substances, or hemoperfusion and pump-driven hemofiltration for poisoning with highly protein bound and high molecular weight substances. In no case should massive hyperkalemia, as occurring with hemolysis or with extensive tissue destruction, be treated by CAVH alone: in that case, hemodialysis must be used as soon as possible.

References

1. Kaplan AA, Longecker RE, Folkert VW (1983) Suction-assisted continuous arterio-venous hemofiltration. Trans Am Soc Artif Intern Organs 29:408–412
2. Kramer P, Wigger W, Rieger J, Matthaei D, Scheler F (1977) Arteriovenous hemofiltration: a new and simple method for treatment of over-hydrated patients resistent to diuretics. Klin Wochenschr 55:1121–1122
3. Kramer P, Kaufhold G, Gröne HJ, Wigger W, Rieger J, Matthaei D, Stokke T, Burchardi H, Scheler F (1980) Management of anuric intensive-care patients with arterivenous hemofiltration. Int J Artif Organs 3:225–230
4. Kramer P, Schrader J, Bohnsack W, Grieben G, Gröne HJ, Scheler F (1981) Continuous arteriovenous haemofiltration. A new kidney replacement therapy. Proc Eur Dial Transplant Assoc 18:743–749
5. Kramer P, Böhler J, Kehr A, Gröne HJ, Schrader J, Matthaei D, Scheler F (1982) Intensive care potential of continuous arteriovenous hemofiltration. Trans Am Soc Artif Intern Organs 18:28–31
6. Lauer A, Saccaggi A, Ronco C, Belledonne M, Glabman S, Bosch JP (1983) Continuous arteriovenous hemofiltration in critically ill patients. Clinical use and operational characteristics. Ann Intern Med 99:455–460
7. Lysaght JM, Schmidt B, Gurland HJ (1984) Filtration rates and pressure driving force in AV filtration: an experimental study. Blood Purification (in press)
8. Synhaivsky A, Kurtz SB, Wochos DN, Schniepp J, Johnson WJ (1983) Acute renal failure treated by slow continuous ultrafiltration. Mayo Clin Proc 58:729–733⟨1⟩

Limitations and Pitfalls of Continuous Arteriovenous Hemofiltration

P. Kramer

Limitation: Blood Pressure

The driving force of arteriovenous hemofiltration is the blood pressure gradient between artery and vein. For this reason, a decompensated cardiac or circulatory failure places a limit on the use of this procedure. Adequate fluid withdrawal can only be obtained with systolic blood pressures higher than 60 mmHg, with a hematocrit below 40%, and rather low colloid-osmotic pressure. With a systolic blood pressure of 70 mmHg, filtration rates of 2–4 ml/min are observed. In our expierence, a low filtration rate of 180 ml/h is sufficient for the improvement of heart failure with low cardiac output (CO) in oligoanuric patients. In patients with cardiogenic shock, frequent thrombosis of the hemofilter may occur, but the overall elimination of fluid may be sufficient to improve the patient's condition. Not infrequently, "prerenal kidney failure" exists in these patients and the excretion function of the kidney starts again, when cardiac output has slightly improved.

Although arteriovenous hemofiltration is superior to the natural kidney with respect to the elimination of water in case of low blood pressure [4, 5], it is only justified in cardiogenic shock, when venovenous pump-driven hemofiltration or conventional hemodialysis are not available.

In view of the low extracorporeal blood flow (2%–5% of CO), an additional volume load for the heart by continuous arteriovenous hemofiltration (CAVH) can be precluded. If CAVH is used in small children, however, blood pressure reduction due to blood shunting may be significant. Continuous peritoneal dialysis may be preferable if the blood line occlusion of the extracorporeal circuit causes the central arterial blood pressure to increase more than 10 mmHg.

Limitation: Fluid Turnover

A low filtration rate below 6 ml/min does not suffice for compensation of uremia. Figure 1 shows the steady-state plasma creatinine as a function of the ultrafiltrate substitution rate. The values were obtained from patients in whom we were able to maintain a constant ultrafiltration and substitution rate for at least 48 h. According to the figure the inverse relationship between plasma creatinine and substitution rate is very similar to that between plasma creatinine and glomerular filtration rate. Exchange volumes greater than 6 ml/min or 8.6 l/day are necessary

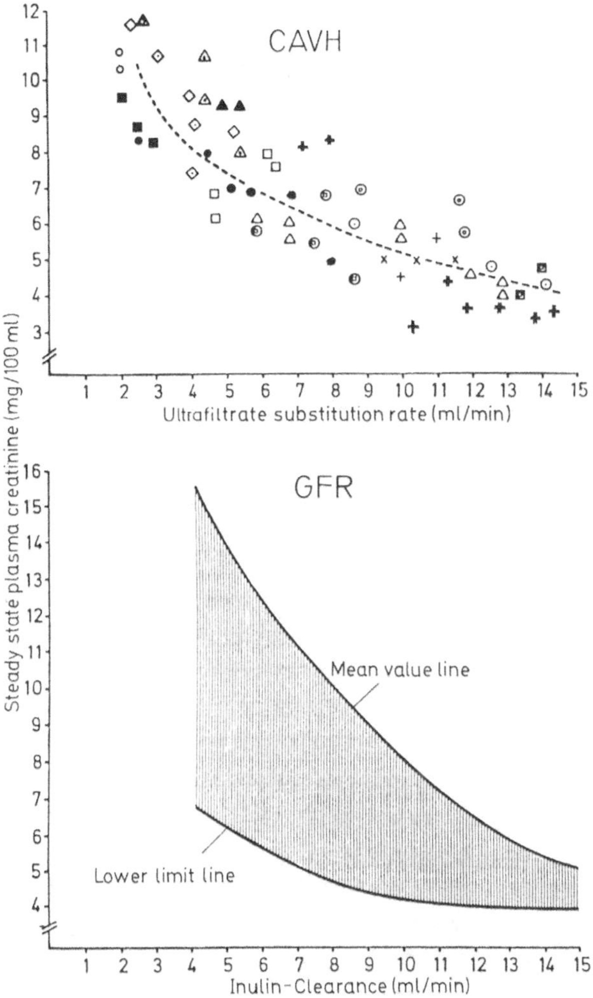

Fig. 1. Steady-state plasma creatinine in relation to ultrafiltrate substitution rate and glomerular filtration rate

to obtain adequate compensation of uremia and for prevention of hyperkalemia. Isotonic ultrafiltration only without substitution of potassium-free fluid results inevitably in hyperkalemia. In some patients with catabolic acute renal failure (ARF), a higher fluid turnover is required in order to achieve blood urea nitrogen (BUN) levels below 120 mg/dl. In these cases occasionally hemodialysis may be required. On the other hand, in our experience optimal parenteral nutrition may cause an impressive fall of the BUN level.

In patients with low-normal colloid-osmotic pressure and hematocrit values below 40%, exchange volumes between 10 and 20 l can be achieved with a systolic pressure of 100 mmHg. Even severe catabolic renal failures can be treated exclusively with CAVH.

A particularly impressive clinical course is shown in Fig. 2, where the subject is a 30-year-old patient with 60% third-fourth degree burns, whose anuric renal

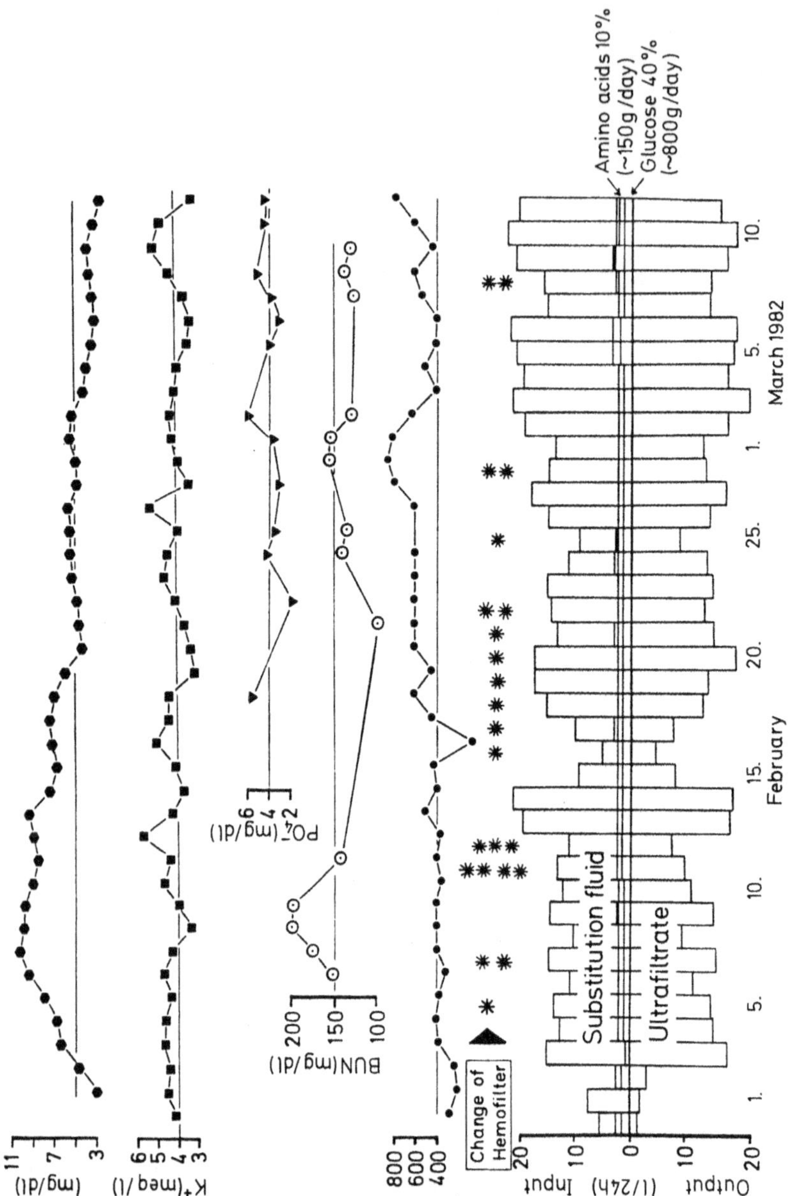

Fig. 2. Clinical course of a 30-year-old patient with 60% burns treated exclusively by CAVH

failure was treated for 6 weeks exclusively with CAVH. Systolic blood pressures were approximately 100 mmHg during the entire treatment. With total parenteral nutrition, it was possible to achieve anabolism. BUN fell below 150 mg/dl, although the amino acid supply was 150 g/day. Potassium and phosphate had to be substituted [5], indicating cellular build-up or anabolism. During the first week plasma, creatinine, and BUN rose as a result of insufficient fluid turnover. During this period intermittent hemodialysis could have been used to improve azotemia. Therefore, in a hospital with frequent use of CAVH easy access and skilled performance of all conventional kidney replacement methods must be available.

Limitation: Hematocrit

Inadequate filtration rates were observed when hematocrit was above 45%. High hematocrit values were observed particulary in cor pulmonale and other pulmonary affections with secondary polyglobulia. In these cases it is recommended to carry out predilution: The substitution solution is infused into the arterial three-way valve instead of the venous three-way valve. This way, filtration rates are generally much higher and the hemofilters remain open longer. But it is not simple to perform predilution CAVH. Fluid dosing must be very accurate and in most cases suction is needed to obtain a negative fluid balance. Venovenous hemodialysis is certainly the better kidney replacement therapy in these cases, unless intermittent treatment is not tolerated.

Pitfall: Fluid Balance

Because of the high fluid turnover, small systematic errors in dosing of substitution fluid or measuring of ultrafiltrate may amount to several liters false positive or negative fluid balance within a few days. This has been a painful experience with manual fluid balancing and it was the main stimulus for developing flow balances. But besides the improvement of devices for measuring fluids, the clinical viewpoint is of utmost importance. Knowing this pitfall, the clinician should always make up his mind about the patient's water metabolism before reading the input/output protocol. A thorough investigation of cutaneous turgor, the search for pitting edema or ascites, the auscultation of the lungs, the estimation of sweat secretion and saliva flow, as well as the measurement of body temperature, pulse rate, central venous pressure, arterial pressure, and finally the analysis of blood gases should be considered for a firm decision concerning whether the patient needs more or less fluid.

"Don't trust the written fluid balance."

Pitfall: Blood Loss Due to Tubing Disconnection

A disconnection of the extracorporeal blood-conducting tubing system is immediately followed by blood loss up to 250 ml/min. Unfortunately, there have been to our knowledge three cases, in whom lethal blood loss occurred after disconnection of the CAVH system. In these cases more than one of the following causes were responsible for this avoidable complication:

1. Patient restless and insufficiently supervised
2. Inappropriate femoral indwelling catheter
3. Femoral CAVH catheter not sutured to the skin
4. Catheter, tubing, and hemofilter connections without Luer lock

With regard to (1), all cases were restless and insufficiently supervised. Hemofilter and tubing were covered by a blanket. Usually the nurse left the patient alone for just a few minutes. In one case, however, disconnection with lethal blood loss occurred during rounds, with doctors and nurses standing beside the patient's bed being absorbed in discussion about laboratory data. Therefore, the following measures should be taken: (a) preferably use intermittent hemodialysis in restless patients; (b) never leave a restless patient on CAVH alone; (c) always leave hemofilter, blood conducting tubings, and vascular access uncovered and visible from all points of the room; (d) in restless patients the arterial blood line should be connected to a pressure monitor with lower alarm limits.

With regard to (2), in one case lethal blood loss occurred from a broken catheter, in another a disconnection occurred between silicone and teflon components. Minor but continuous bleeding with a wrong catheter may occur along a kink if it is located in the vascular wall. Therefore, the following measures should be taken: (a) use only catheters specially made for CAVH, which have to last for weeks; (b) make sure that a new catheter made for CAVH has safe connections between silicone and teflon parts.

With regard to (3), in one case the venous catheter was not sutured to the skin and pulled out by the unattended patient. The lethal blood loss did not occur from the femoral vein but from the femoral artery, the blood flowing through the CAVH system out of the venous catheter. Therefore, the following measures should be taken: (a) always suture the femoral catheters safely to the skin; (b) check the sutures every day; (c) tape the arterial and venous tubing to the thigh for protection of the sutures against pulling.

With regard to (4), use of catheters and tubings without screw connections for CAVH is obsolete. This is also true for all infusion or monitor tubings connected to the extracorporeal blood circuit. Serious blood loss was observed after disconnection between hemofilter and tubing.

Very efficient measures to be taken are: (a) refuse tubings without screw connections such as the Luer lock; (b) refuse screw connections which are difficult to handle; (c) use only CAVH systems, which have a safe connection between hemofilter and tubing.

Pitfall: Dehydration

The continuous slow water withdrawal by means of CAVH allows a serious dehydration without hypotension. Skin folds put up at the front head or thigh may stand up for an hour or so as an obvious sign of extensive dehydration. In most cases negative fluid balance improved gas exchange of the lungs. Apparently this measurable therapeutic effect is so impressive, that many clinicians forget about the main disadvantage of dehydration: Delayed recovery of kidney function. If patients receive parenteral nutrition solutions without sodium, they may even be-

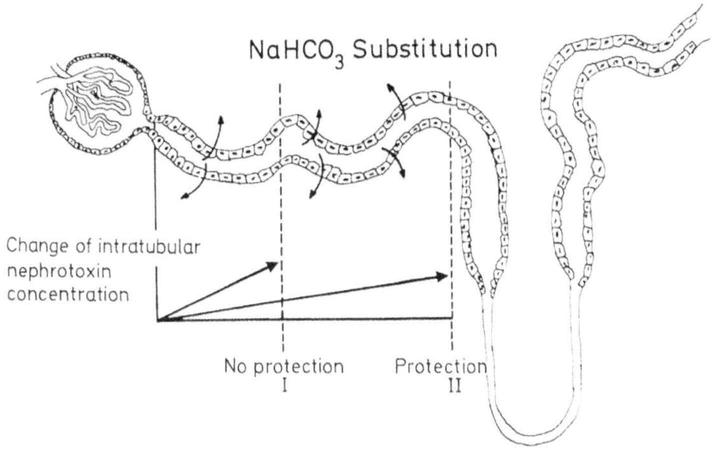

Fig. 3. Schematic illustration of the theoretical relationship between sodium bicarbonate loading and protection of the proximal tubules in anuric kidneys

come hyponatremic. It is a matter of discussion whether the combination of serious dehydration and hyponatremia in CAVH patients was the reason for prolonged anuria.

Acute organic renal failure is an unfavorable sign with respect to prognosis in patients with multiple organ failure, and recovery of kidney function is considered a good prognostic sign. Thereby the kidney does not only play a passive indicator role. Endocrine and peptide degradation function and other not yet known functions are, besides the excretion function, of utmost importance for the survival of patients. This is a reasonable assumption, which provides the basis for a new intensive care program called *proximal tubule protection*. The clinical experience that sodium and bicarbonate may protect against impending ARF is extrapolated for protection of the anuric kidney [3]. It is well known that during ARF glomerular filtration continues at a low level [1, 2, 6–8], whereby the filtrate is reabsorbed more or less totally along the proximal tubule.

In patients with multiorgan failure who developed acute tubular necrosis, the nephrotoxins continue to enter the tubular fluid via glomerular filtration. Depending on the rate at which the filtrate is reabsorbed, the continuing toxic effect on the tubular cells may be quite different, whether the fluid is totally reabsorbed in the first part of the proximal tubule or as a result of delayed reabsorption later along the tubule. In any case, the exposure of the single tubular cell to nephrotoxins should be less with reduced proximal tubule reabsorption and this may affect the glomerular filtration [9]. Figure 3 illustrates this theoretical relationship.

Under the assumption that this mechanism is valid, hydration, high plasma sodium and bicarbonate levels should delay reabsorption along the proximal tubule [7]. Hydration may disturb cardiac and pulmonary function, but maintaining a plasma sodium of 150 meq/l and a base excess of +5 meq/l does not. This program so far is very deliberate and has only very preliminary clinical support, but it may be only performed by means of CAVH. By infusion of either NaCl or $NaHCO_3$ concentrate during ongoing CAVH with regular substitution fluid the concentration of sodium and bicarbonate may be maintained at any preselected level. This is by no means possible with intermittent treatment. Also the level of hydration may be better controlled with continuous fluid removal and sodium substitution.

In summary: CAVH may be used for protection of the anuric kidney, but it may also be a very efficient method for continuous proximal tubule damaging with maintenance of anuria.

Pitfall: Inadequate Diagnostic Measures

The simplicity of CAVH and a possible lack of cooperation with the nephrologist may result in inadequate diagnostic measures in patients with complicated ARF. It is absolutely necessary to search "aggressively" for the cause of ARF before CAVH is started. The patient must be seen by a nephrologist and the whole spectrum of nephrological and urological diagnostic measures must be used to identify the cause of renal failure. Avoidable complications related to the unreflected use of CAVH were seen in patients with anuria due to dissecting aortic aneurism or traumatic retroperitoneal bleeding. Therapeutic measures were delayed for days in patients with postrenal failure who were "put on CAVH" because it is so simple.

Diagnostic and therapeutic measures concerning the natural kidney are certainly more important for the overall prognosis of the patient than is the early use of CAVH. In some cases it may be necessary to use a conventional kidney replacement therapy instead of CAVH. This decision needs the specialist. CAVH may improve the prognosis of patients with complicated ARF, provided the nephrologist is brought in as a consultant.

References

1. Catell WR, McIntosh CS, Moseley IFA (1973) Excretion urography in acute renal failure. Br Med J II:575
2. Fry IK, Catell WR (1971) Radiology in the diagnosis of renal failure. Br Med Bull 27:148
3. Kopp KF (1978) Success of sodiumbicarbonate induced metabolic alcalosis in the reversal and prevention of acute oliguric renal failure. XIVth Int Congr Intern Medicine, Rome, 1978
4. Kramer P, Kaufhold G, Gröne HJ, Wigger W, Rieger J, Matthaei D, Stokke T, Burchardi H, Scheler F (1980) Management of anuric intensive-care patients with arteriovenous hemofiltration. Int J Artif Organs 3:225–230
5. Kramer P, Schrader J, Bohnsack W, Grieben G, Gröne HJ, Scheler F (1981) Continuous arteriovenous haemofiltration. A new kidney replacement therapy. Proc Eur Dial Transplant Assoc 18:743–749
6. Myers BD, Chui F, Hilberman M, Michaels A (1979) Transtubular leakage of glomerular filtrate in human acute renal failure. Am J Physiol 6:F319
7. Pitts RF (1972) Physiologie der Niere und der Körperflüssigkeiten. Schattauer, Stuttgart
8. Reubi FC, Vorburger C, Tuckmann J (1973) Renal distribution volumes of indocyanine green (^{51}Cr) EDTA and ^{24}Na in man during acute renal failure. J Clin Invest 52:223
9. Schnermann J (1975) Regulation of single nephron filtration rate by feedback – facts and theories. Clin Nephrol 3:75

Chronic Renal Failure

Slow Continuous Ultrafiltration – Supplemental Therapy to Intermittent Hemodialysis

E. P. Paganini

Introduction

Increasingly sophisticated medical technology in the past 10 years has brought greater diagnostic accuracy with less patient invasion and morbidity, but these procedures are extraordinarily complex and costly. The development, therefore, of a relatively simple procedure that offers patient stability while allowing aggressive medical intervention is an important advance.

Acute renal dysfunction, whether medical or surgical, poses major therapeutic challenges. The application of dialytic techniques in the mid-1950s was rewarded with marked improvement in morbidity and mortality [12, 20]. At that time, attempts at "continuous hemodialysis" met with promising results [18] but the equipment was cumbersome and the extracorporeal volume needed was large. Intermittent forms of hemodialysis grew in popularity and the basic designs changed. A greater understanding of the underlying pathophysiology of both acute and chronic renal failure ensued, and intermittent hemodialysis became the main support for control of fluid and electrolyte balance, as well as uremia.

Fluid control, however, remained a problem in oliguric acute renal failure (ARF). The use of larger volumes of fluid for hyperalimentation or as a vehicle for pressor agents or antibiotics necessitated daily dialytic support. Although intermittent isolated ultrafiltration was used, a substantial number of patients could not be supported in this manner because of hemodynamic instability. Continuous ultrafiltration techniques were initially developed for these patients.

Definitions

Many extracorporeal techniques are employed to treat renal failure, some for uremic control, others for fluid balance. As the literature grows, it is of utmost importance to establish baseline definitions of these techniques to allow accurate comparisons of similar procedures (Table 1).

The primary goal of slow continuous ultrafiltration (SCUF) is either removal or balance of fluid. The rate of filtration (*CF*) is regulated by the desired fluid intake plus projected weight loss. An ultrafiltration rate of 5 ml/min is the usual range; replacement is generally not postdilutional but achieved by either hyperalimentation or fluid/drug administration via other access sites. Continuous arterio-

Table 1. Working definitions of various extracorporeal techniques applied in fluid and uremic control

Hemodialysis	A diffusion-based mode of blood cleaning wherein ultrafiltration is limited to the removal of excessive body water. The aim is uremic control as well as fluid and electrolyte balance. It can be intermittent (HD) or continuous (CAVHD)
Hemofiltration	A convective mode of blood cleaning wherein large fluid exchanges account for virtually all solute removal. The aim is uremic control as well as fluid and electrolyte balance. It can be intermittent (HF) or continuous (CAVH)
Ultrafiltration	The removal of plasma water as well as small molecular weight substances (electrolytes, urea) in an attempt at fluid balance. It can be intermittent (IUF) or continuous (SCUF)

venous hemofiltration (CAVH), on the other hand, is continuous postdilutional hemofiltration. The *QF* here dictates replacement volume. The goal is not only fluid balance but also azotemic control. Exchange rates are generally 8 ml/min. Enhanced *QF* applying negative pressure to the hemofilter has been advocated as a technique for increasing longevity of the individual cartridge [5]. This should be approached with caution since exceeding the optimal filtration fraction of the device and promoting significant postcartridge blood inspissation may adversely affect both flow characteristics and cellular integrity. There may, however, be a place for this augmentation if predilutional CAVH is performed. In continuous arteriovenous hemodialysis (CAVHD), [4] a pumpless circuit is used in series with a dialyzer and furnished with a continuous dialysate flow for the diffusive control of uremia. It is said to have a much better solute removal capacity than CAVH.

Design of Circuitry

Access

All continuous techniques are intimately tied to an adequately functioning access site. If blood flow is poor because of arterial inadequacy or venous obstruction, the characteristics of the circuitry will change which might limit the ultrafiltration rate. Lower *QF* would therefore allow only for SCUF, not being able to handle the volumes necessary for CAVH. As *QB* falls, circuitry clotting is enhanced.

Access can be either percutaneous [9] or via surgically constructed portals such as arteriovenous shunts [14] or fistulae [10]. The arterial access site is perhaps the most crucial since this is where the driving force for movement of blood as well as the development of transmembrane pressures will originate. We have favored the use of a lower arm Scribner shunt over percutaneous femoral arterial and venous cannulations for several reasons. Mobility is not hampered by access via an A-V shunt; the patient can be moved from bed and seated, or walked without concern for damage to either cannulae or vessels. Care should be taken, however, in placement of the A-V shunt [11]. Distal circulation must be maintained to avoid ischemic injury, and appropriate testing (Allen test) should be employed. The choice of access site also depends upon venous condition. Placement of a shunt in a vein subjected to multiple intravenous catheterizations should be avoided, since venous stenosis/occlusion will lead to poor blood flow through the shunt and, ultimately, failure of the procedure.

Surgical expertise is a necessity. Although viewed as "minor" surgery, continuous renal replacement therapy cannot be accomplished without proper shunt. Time is needed to choose the vessels, dilate them when necessary, avoid vessel damage or torsion, and stabilize the implants. By simply following established surgical procedures and giving attention to small details, the A-V shunt can offer a powerful, useful access site for continuous as well as intermittent replacement support.

No major complications have been reported with long-term indwelling arterial and venous catheters during CAVH, but the patients generally have been much younger than those we are seeing. With an elderly population, it would seem reasonable to avoid blind entry into a possibly atherosclerotic artery which may dislodge plaques with consequent distal emboli. Also catheters made in the United States are not optimal for use with percutaneous arterial puncture. Their smaller bore size and tapered design do not allow optimal transmission of arterial pressure to the arterial line and consequently QB as well as QF are dampened. With appropriate catheter and patient selection, however, percutaneous cannulation allows quick access to the blood supply without a major scheduling problem.

Both access procedures may result in three complications: infection, thrombosis, and bleeding. Infection at the site of entry is not an infrequent occurrence and results in a cutaneous cellulitis rather than a deep-seated local infection, it is easily treated with adequate skin preparation prior to entry and continued local aseptic technique and antiseptic maneuvers during therapy. We have not encountered any systemic infections related to access in the more than 80 patients treated with SCUF or CAVH. We have also established A-V shunts for support in patients with sepsis and found no local infection or seeding of the access site as long as appropriate antibiotic therapy had been used for treatment of the original sepsis.

Thrombosis of the arterial and/or venous lines of the access site has several causes. Systemic blood pressure will dictate blood flow through the A-V shunt, so that with low pressures and consequent poor flows, the incidence of clotting rises. We have used an A-V shunt for SCUF even at mean arterial pressures of 50–55 mmHg. Below this value, however, blood flow is so compromised that thrombosis formation is inevitable. Technical factors such as deformed tubing, improperly placed catheter tips, and damaged or poorly chosen blood vessels will lead to poor blood flow and subsequent clotting.

Early recognition of thrombosis and reversal of the underlying abnormality is crucial for salvage of the access site. We have found that pinching the arterial area of the shunt and clearing a small area distal to the pinch by "milking" the shunt produces a clear area. When the pinch is released, blood will flow briskly into the clear area, thus attesting to the potency of the shunt. If, however, blood flow is retrograde or absent, then early arterial insufficiency or total thrombosis should be suspected. This allows for earlier detection of thrombosis than waiting for the separation of plasma from red cells, and is performed on a regular basis by the bedside nurse.

Local bleeding is another problem rarely encountered with A-V shunt placement since there is direct visualization of the arterial and venous catheters. However, with the use of heparin or systemic anticoagulation either secondary to medications or disease, continued oozing may occur. This is treated by applying local pressure to the area and correcting the underlying cause of the bleeding.

Traumatic damage to the shunt is accompanied by bleeding. Admittedly rare, this complication is totally avoidable by immobilizing the system. Care should be taken that stress is not placed on either arm of the shunt, which leads to local necrosis of the vessel wall with subsequent lysis of the supporting tissue. This will also be accompanied by profuse bleeding. Control of bleeding and establishment of another site of entry should be undertaken immediately. So far, we have not had such an incident.

Blood and Ultrafiltration Tubing and Control

The arterial venous tubing for SCUF is designed to offer a short arterial and variable length venous line. Made of polyvinyl chloride (Fig. 1), this shorter form of tubing will avoid dissipation of pressure to overcome the resistances found in the larger varieties. The tubing can also be used with CAVH but its principal use has been with SCUF.

Ultrafiltration should be controlled to avoid overzealous fluid removal and the development of intravascular depletion with vascular collapse. Control is achieved with the use of a screw clamp on the ultrafiltrate line [14], or by attaching the ultrafiltrate line to an i.v.-infusion pump and "dialing in" the desired amount of fluid to be removed for that hour (Fig. 2). The advantages and disadvantages of both methods are listed in Table 2. Although the infusion pump is much more precise and does not require frequent readjustments of the screw clamp, it does not permit early detection of a drop in ultrafiltration rate, a crucial element in the early diagnosis of ultrafilter clotting or access thrombosis.

When hemodialysis is offered as a method of azotemic control, the circuitry is quite simple. We leave the arterial arm of the shunt attached to the SCUF circuitry and merely attach the arterial hemodialysis blood line directly to the venous SCUF line while the venous dialysis line is connected to the venous area of the shunt. In this manner, SCUF continues in series while hemodialysis proceeds. We have not encountered any problems with clotting of the hemodialysis line or

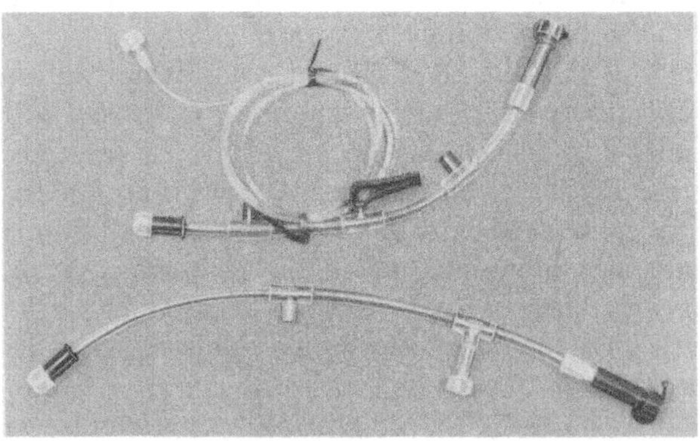

Fig. 1. Arterial and venous tubing used for SCUF and CAVH

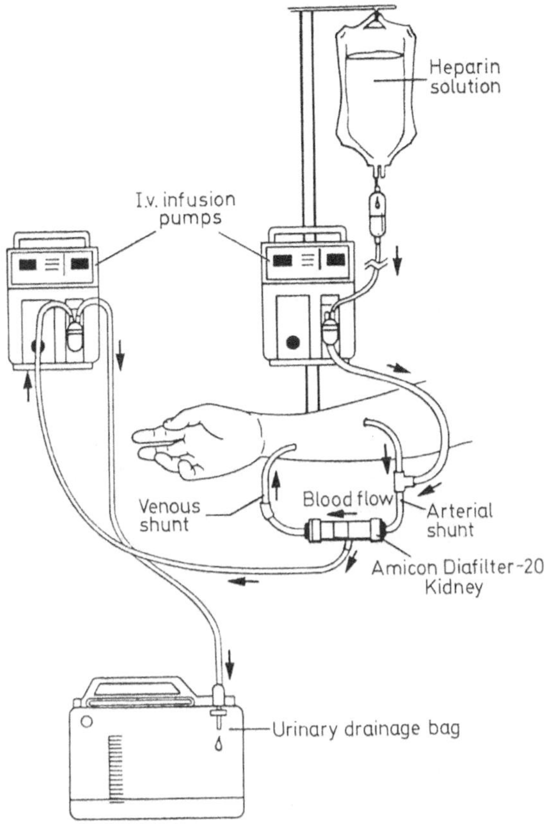

Fig. 2. Design of SCUF circuitry using i.v.-infusion pumps for control of ultrafiltration rate

Table 2. Advantages and disadvantages of various ultrafiltration control techniques for SCUF

	Ease of operation	Accuracy of rate	Ease in evaluating early UF change	Create negative pressure on membrane
I.v.-infusion pump controlled	+	+	±	+
Screw-clamp controlled	−	±	+	−

ultrafilter damage, and have been able to reestablish the SCUF circuit at the end of hemodialysis.

Clinical Applications of Slow Continuous Ultrafiltration

Supplemental Therapy to Intermittent Hemodialysis

Fluid balance has been one of the primary goals in the therapy of ARF. This end point is facilitated in patients with nonoliguric failure (500 cc/24 h) but often patients with oliguria or anuria are receiving large volumes of fluid in the form of pressor agents, antibiotics, or hyperalimentation. This volume imbalance leads to fluid excess states or suboptimal delivery of therapy as, e.g., inadequate caloric delivery secondary to imposed fluid restriction.

Until recently, fluid removal was accomplished by various forms of dialytic intervention including daily hemodialysis, isolated ultrafiltration, or peritoneal dialysis [21]. Hemodynamic instability, rapid volume shifts, or patient intolerance often made effective fluid balance difficult if not impossible to attain [6, 22].

The separation of ultrafiltration from diffusive dialysis technique (isolated ultrafiltration) allowed for greater vascular stability in the chronic dialysis population [7, 19]. Bergström et al. [1] noted that removal of significant volumes of fluid was not accompanied by hypotensive episodes in patients unable to tolerate an equal volume loss during standard hemodialysis. This superior stability is thought to be secondary to the active participation of the venous system in the maintenance of both preload and central cardiopulmonary volumes despite reduction of total peripheral resistance and total body water [2, 13]. When this same technique was applied to hemodialysis patients with incipient congestive heart failure, increased cardiac output with lowered afterload and maintenance of the cardiopulmonary volume was again obtained [13].

Standard isolated ultrafiltration techniques, however, require specialized material. The equipment is available in centers which provide hemodialysis, but nurses must be trained to operate it. Also, while the actual hourly rate of fluid removal can be adjusted, the technique is an intermittent form of therapy, and hence elicits a variable hemodynamic response. Avoiding the paradoxical drop of intravascular volume in the face of increasing cardiac output would eliminate further renal insult and perhaps allow for accelerated return of normal renal function.

Although ultrafiltration was used for oliguric patients with ARF, a method for continuous fluid removal was also sought when hemodynamic instability prevented standard dialytic intervention, or when a way of reducing daily intermittent replacement therapy was needed [8, 14, 16]. Since therapy was indeed continuous, the rate of removal per unit of time could be lowered so that the removal of fluid from the intravascular space would not exceed the refilling rate. This therefore provided hemodynamic stability and allowed for daily fluid losses to exceed intake.

Using SCUF as a continuous form of ultrafiltration and relying on standard diffusive techniques for solute control, we have managed to reduce the need for hemodialysis intervention much the same way as reported by Dodd et al. [3]. This approach has permitted the infusion of adequate hyperalimentation with resultant positive amino acid balance, despite the oliguria and hemodynamic instability found in this patient population [15]. Patients who have been unable to be supported by diffusive dialysis, were subjected to CAVH for azotemic control. However, the majority of oliguric patients receiving continuous therapy underwent SCUF [17].

References

1. Bergström J, Asaba H, Furst P, Oules R (1976) Dialysis ultrafiltration and blood pressure. Proc Eur Dial Transplant Assoc 13:293

2. Chen WT, Chaignon M, Omvik P, Tarazi RC, Bravo EL, Nakamoto S (1978) Hemodynamic studies in chronic hemodialysis patients with hemofiltration/ultrafiltration. Trans Am Soc Artif Intern Organs 24:682–686
3. Dodd NJ, Turney JH, Parsons V, Weston MJ (1982) Continuous haemofiltration maintains fluid balance and reduces haemodialysis requirement in acute renal failure. Proc Eur Dial Transplant Assoc 19:329–333
4. Geronemus R, Schneider N (1984) Continuous arteriovenous hemodialysis (CAVHD): a new modality for treatment of acute renal failure. Trans Am Soc Artif Intern Organs 13:42 (Abstract)
5. Kaplan AA, Longnecker RE, Folkert VW (1984) Continuous arteriovenous hemofiltration. A report of six months' experience. Ann Intern Med 100:358–367
6. Keshaviah P, Shapiro FL (1982) A critical examination of dialysis-induced hypotension. Am J Kidney Dis 2:290–301
7. Khanna R, Popowniak KL, Magnusson MO, Nakamoto S (1973) Control of ascites in patients on chronic hemodialysis by modified ultrafiltration using a Dow Hollow Fiber Capillary Kidney (DHFCK). Trans Am Soc Artif Intern Organs 2:31 (Abstract)
8. Kramer P, Wigger W, Rieger J, Matthaei D, Scheler F (1977) Arteriovenous hemofiltration: a new and simple method for treatment of overhydrated patients resistant to diuretics. Klin Wochenschr 55:1121–1122
9. Kramer P, Böhler J, Kehr A, Gröne HJ, Schrader J, Matthaei D, Scheler F (1982) Intensive care potential of continuous arteriovenous hemofiltration. Trans Am Soc Artif Intern Organs 28:28–32
10. Lauer A, Saccaggi A, Ronco C, BelleDonne M, Glabman S, Bosch JP (1983) Continuous arteriovenous hemofiltration in the critically ill patient. Clinical use and operational characteristics. Ann Intern Med 99:455–460
11. Light JA (1975) A review of vascular access management. Dialysis and Transplant 4:20
12. Merrill JP (1952) Medical progress. The artificial kidney. N Engl J Med 246:17–27
13. Paganini EP, Fouad F, Tarazi RC, Bravo EL, Nakamoto S (1979) Hemodynamics of isolated ultrafiltration in chronic hemodialysis patients. Trans Am Soc Artif Intern Organs 25:422–425
14. Paganini EP, Nakamoto S (1980) Continuous slow ultrafiltration in oliguric acute renal failure. Trans Am Soc Artif Intern Organs 26:201–204
15. Paganini EP, Flaque J, Whitman G, Nakamoto S (1982) Amino acid balance in patients with oliguric acute renal failure undergoing slow continuous ultrafiltration. Trans Am Soc Artif Intern Organ 28:615–620
16. Paganini EP, Flaque J, Whitman G, O'Hara P, Nakamoto S (1983) Slow continuous ultrafiltration in oliguric acute renal failure. Blood Purification 1:53 (abstract)
17. Paganini EP, O'Hara P, Nakamoto S (1984) Slow continuous ultrafiltration in hemodialysis resistant oligurie acute renal failure patients. Trans Am Soc Artif Intern Organs 30:173–178
18. Scribner BH, Caner JE, Buri R, Quinton W (1960) The technique of continuous hemodialysis. Trans Am Soc Artif Intern Organs 6:88–103
19. Silverstein ME, Ford CA, Lysaght MJ, Henderson LW (1974) Treatment of severe fluid overload by ultrafiltration. N Engl J Med 291:747–751
20. Smith LH Jr, Post RS, Teschan PE et al. (1955) Post 1 = 1 traumatic renal insufficiency in military casualties; management, use of artificial kidney, prognosis. Am J Med 18:187–198
21. Teschan PE, Ahmad S, Hull AR, Nolph KD, Shapiro FI (1980) Daily dialysis – applications and problems. Trans Am Soc Artif Intern Organs 26:600–602
22. Van Stone JC, Bauer J, Carey J (1982) The effect of dialysate sodium concentration on body fluid compartment volume, plasma renin activity and plasma aldosterone concentration in chronic hemodialysis patients. Am J Kidney Dis 2:58–64

Continuous Pump-Driven Hemofiltration in Renal Failure

K. Bischoff and M. Doehn

For a long time imbalances of fluid metabolism in patients with impaired renal function could only be treated with intermittent conventional dialysis. While this method suffices for ambulatory chronic renal failure patients, those with acute renal failure (ARF) present various problems in the intensive care unit. Clinically, overhydration is usally the main concern. Setups for conventional dialysis, however, are often not at hand.

For the treatment of overhydration Silverstein et al. [13] introduced supplementary ultrafiltration in 1974 for chronic dialysis patients. 1977 Kramer et al. [7] reported their experience with arteriovenous hemofiltration. With straight arteriovenous ultrafiltration the filtration rate between 200 and 600 ml/h was rather low for emergency cases. Therefore, we inaugurated the pump-driven continuous ultrafiltration by which filtration rates of 500–1000 ml/h can be achieved without difficulty. Also, the filtration rate does not depend on the blood pressure.

We made this method available for wide clinical use in the intensive care unit. An emergency apparatus was developed, with the aid of a manufacturer, which can handle the special requirements of an intensive care unit.

Pump-driven ultrafiltration was mainly used for two indications:

1. Overhydration, including the necessary fluid removal for parenteral hyperalimentation and infusion of drugs
2. Compensation of uremia

The following summarizes our experiences with pump-driven venovenous hemofiltration.

Patients and Method

Twenty patients with ARF from the surgical intensive care unit were treated with continuous venovenous hemofiltration. The underlying illnesses of the patients are displayed in Table 1. Six patients suffered from a shock after polytrauma and

Table 1. Underlying illness of patients with acute renal failure who were treated with continuous venovenous hemofiltration ($n=20$)

Polytrauma	6 (30%)
Gram negative sepsis after second operation	12 (60%)
Esophageal varicose bleeding	2 (10%)

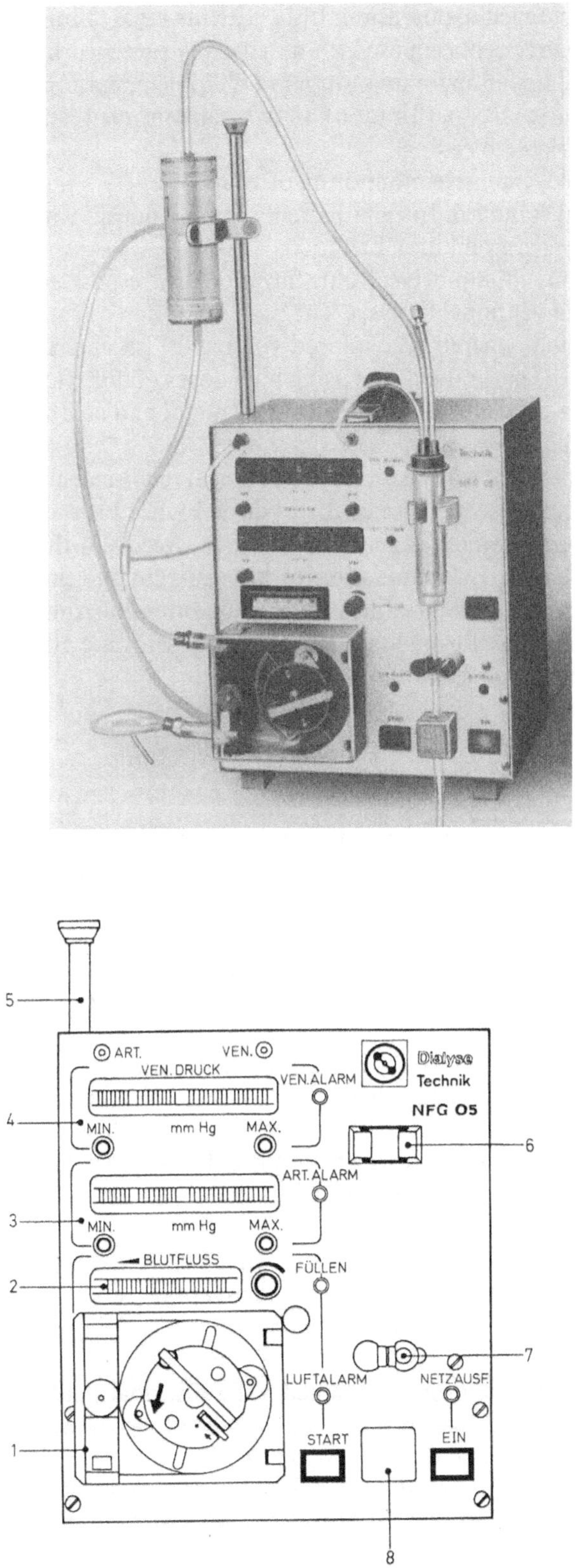

Fig. 1. Diagram and picture of the emergency apparatus (Dialyse-Technik, Karlsruhe) developed for continuous venovenous hemofiltration. *1* Blood pump, *2* Blood flow indicator, *3* Arterial pressure monitor, *4* Venous pressure monitor, *5* Filter holder, *6* Bubble trap holder, *7* Air trap, *8* Clamp

developed ARF as a result of prolonged hypotension. In 12 patients renal failure seized on account of a gram-negative septicemia which was usually preceded by second operations after extensive upper abdominal surgery (Whipple operation, excision of necrotic pancreas, gastric ulcer perforation). In two patients renal failure occurred after esophageal varicose bleeding.

All patients had to be ventilated. Intensive monitoring of vital parameters was performed according to the usual standard. In eight patients cardiac output was determined additionally with the thermodilution method.

The indication for continuous pump-driven ultrafiltration corresponded mostly with the indication for conventional dialysis. The patients suffered from ARF and increasing fluid retention, whereby the infused volume for parenteral nutrition was not eliminated via the natural kidneys using high doses of diuretics and dopamine. Besides that, urea concentration rose above 80 mg/dl and creatinine concentration above 4 mg/dl.

The length of ultrafiltration treatment was adapted to the clinical requirements and, in one case, was almost continuously performed for 14 days. Figure 1 shows the simple apparatus with a diagram which was used in all cases. Access to the vascular system was usually achieved by cannulation of a large central vein, mostly the jugular or subclavian vein. For ultrafiltration, the diafilter-20 (Amicon) was used. For prophylaxis against thrombosis, 500 IU/h heparin were administered into the blood line before using the diafilter.

Results

At a filtration rate of 15 ml/min, 20–24 l plasma water could be substituted per day. Since the patients were usually overhydrated, up to 6 l ultrafiltrate were taken off during the first 24 h. Ultrafiltrate was later substituted with Ringer's solution together with 100–500 mEq bicarbonate per day. On the average 25 mEq of sodium bicarbonate were added per liter substitution solution. Dosage was determined according to blood gas analysis which was evaluated several times per day in ventilated patients.

As a result of the initial dehydration, in most cases the respiratory situation improved. Depending on the initial condition, oxygen content of the respiration air could be lowered down to 20% during the course of the first day. With this volume removal, also central venous pressure decreased from the initial 15–20 cm to 5–7 cm H_2O. The mean arterial pressure remained constant between 60–80 mmHg in normotensive and hypotensive patients.

In patients, hypertensive due to hypervolemia, pressure could be reduced to normal. Patients with hypertension, however, were more the exception. Cardiac output remained constant with volume removal and was between 3 and 6 l per min.

Plasma electrolyte concentrations could be maintained within normal limits with continuous ultrafiltrate substitution when individual substitution requirements according to the basic illness were taken into account.

Blood urea nitrogen (BUN) and plasma creatinine could be lowered and maintained constant with permanent ultrafiltration substitution rate, whereby the daily ultrafiltration volume was chosen so that BUN was kept between 60 and 80 and plasma creatinine between 3 and 5 mg/dl.

Sometimes, with a high filtration rate, the loss of body heat, through the ultrafiltrate and tubing was too high and therefore infusion solutions were warmed up with a blood heater. On the other hand, we used this effect to lower the elevated temperature in septic patients.

In summary, it can be said that renal function disorders could be compensated successfully with our method for up to 14 days despite difficult circulatory situations. This length of time was usually sufficient since renal function either improved or the patient died from cardiocirculatory failure as a result of "multiple organ failure." Of the patients we observed, approximately 40% survived and 60% died.

Discussion

The good tolerance of pre- and postdialytic ultrafiltration could be confirmed in several experiments [2, 5, 6]. The reason for this, according to Vlaho et al. [14], is small loss of catecholamines, while Shinaberger [12] believes it to be the isotonic fluid removal with constant plasma osmolality. Certainly constant and slow fluid removal by prolonged ultrafiltration methods plays a part in the extraordinarily low circulatory stress [9]. The clinical use of ultrafiltration alternatively or parallel to hemodialysis was published by various authors [8, 11, 13].

It was introduced in 1977 by Kramer et al. [7] in the form of arteriovenous hemofiltration as a separate method. Also in 1977, Pogglitsch et al. [10] and later in 1981 Brandt et al. [3] reported about the treatment of edemas in patients with cardiac insufficiency with straight ultrafiltration via a pump using the "single needle" method.

It was called hemofiltration which has been given a different definition in the meantime [4]. Henderson et al. [4] reported in 1980 about changes in hemodynamic parameters of congestive cardiac insufficiency caused by ultrafiltration. The pressure in the right atrium decreased and the mean arterial pressure remained constant, as in our patient population. Cardiac output improved in these patients probably because the stroke volume was optimized through the Frank-Starling mechanism.

In 1978 Asaba et al. [1] reported about temporary, 3–4 h ultrafiltration for the treatment of overhydration in patients with cardiac insufficiency, cirrhosis of the liver and nephrotic syndrome.

Paganini and Nakamoto described in 1980 [9] continuous slow ultrafiltration in six patients as a supplementary measure to chronic intermittent hemodialysis.

The procedure we introduced serves first of all for straight fluid removal and is therefore ultrafiltration by definition. In its continuation, after volume overload is removed, it serves predominantly for fluid balancing as well as for the elimination of uremic substances and then has to be termed continuous hemofiltration.

In the way of effort, pump-driven ultrafiltration is a simple procedure that can be performed in every intensive care unit. Its use as continuous hemofiltration requires only few additional measures and controls. We believe therefore, that this form of dehydration and detoxification of patients with renal insufficiency in intensive care units constitutes an important alternative to conventional intermittent hemodialysis and hemofiltration which usually require a dialysis unit in the neighborhood. Our procedure can be performed successfully in any hospital, independent of a special department, exclusively with the resources of an intensive care unit. For one, this eliminates the necessity of transporting vitally endangered patients to other centers, and secondly provides the possibility to treat nontransportable patients in intensive care units without dialysis equipment.

References

1. Asaba H, Bergström J, Fürst P, Shaldon S, Wiklund S (1978) Treatment of diuretic-resistant fluid retention with ultrafiltration. Acta Med Scand 204:145
2. Bergström J, Asaba H, Fürst P, Oules R (1976) Dialysis, ultrafiltration, and blood pressure. Proc Eur Dial Transplant Assoc 13:293
3. Brandt D, Pogglitsch H, Harpf H, Holzer H, Klein W (1981) Die Ultrafiltration in der Therapie der schweren kongestiven Herzinsuffizienz. Herz 13:30
4. Henderson LW, Colton C, Leber H, Quellhorst E (1980) Hemofiltration. Trans Am Soc Artif Intern Organs 26:788
5. Ing TS, Vilbar RM, Shin KD, Viol GW, Bansal VK, Geis WP, Hano JE (1978) Predialytic isolated ultrafiltration. Dialysis Transplant 7:557
6. Ing TS, Chen WH, Daugirdas JT, Kwaan HC, Hano JE (1980) Isolated ultrafiltration and new techniques of ultrafiltration during dialysis. Kidney Int 18:77
7. Kramer P, Wigger W, Rieger J, Matthaei D, Scheler F (1977) Arterio-venous hämofiltration: a new and simple method for treatment of over-hydrated patients resistant to diuretics. Klin Wochenschr 55:1121
8. Ono T, Taniguchi Y, Katoaka H, Ishitobi T, Kunitomo T, Kikuchi T (1980) Designing therapeutic modes in nondialytic ultrafiltration. Trans Am Soc Artif Intern Organs 26:205
9. Paganini EP, Nakatomo S (1980) Continuous slow ultrafiltration in oliguric acute renal failure. Trans Am Soc Artif Intern Organs 26:201
10. Pogglitsch H, Waller J, Giessauf W, Holzer H, Katschnigg H (1977) Die Behandlung therapiefraktärer Ödeme mittels Hämofiltration. Intensivmed Prax 14 [Suppl II]:104
11. Shaldon S, Beau MC, Deschodt G, Lysaght MJ, Ramperez P, Mion C (1980) Continuous ambulatory hemofiltration. Trans Am Soc Artif Intern Organs 26:210
12. Shinaberger JH (1977) Dialysis. In: Gonick HC (ed) Current nephrology, vol 1. Pinecliff Medical, Pacific Palisades, p 311
13. Silverstein ME, Ford CA, Lysaght MJ, Henderson LW (1974) Treatment of severe fluid overload by ultrafiltration. N Engl J Med 291:747
14. Vlaho M, Glöckner W, Mies R, Sieberth HG (1980) Einsatz der Hämofiltration beim Nierenversagen. Med Welt 31:1308

Diagnostic Hemoperfusion During Continuous Arteriovenous Hemofiltration in Patients with Septicemic Acute Renal Failure

D. Matthaei, R. Ansorg, and P. Kramer

Often acute renal failure (ARF) is induced or maintained by septicemia and the kidneys do not recover as long as the surgical or internistic measures to remove the source of infection are not successful. The detection of bacteria in arterial blood cultures is often extremely difficult for the clinican [4]. Otherwise, specific antibiotic therapy of the bacteremia is an essential therapeutic measure for the course of illness.

Here, a method for germ extraction through diagnostic hemoperfusion developed by Keller et al. [3] seems to be a decisive advance, judging from the first results of the group from Würzburg [2, 3]. Similar to charcoal hemoperfusion in intoxications, it is possible to bind the germs to charcoal particles by using small charcoal filters for hemoperfusion in bacteremia. The earlier-mentioned authors describe a perfusion of the charcoal cartridge with a blood-flow rate of about 100 ml/min in the extracorporeal shunt. For this procedure the Seldinger technique was utilized (femoral artery) and the blood was returned into a vein. In some patients without arterial access, pump-driven venovenous perfusion was necessary. Besides this the authors mentioned a one-time heparinization of an initial dose of 5000 IU heparin.

There is no explanation yet why the germs accumulate on the activated charcoal. For diagnostic hemoperfusion a high blood-flow rate (100 ml/min) is re-

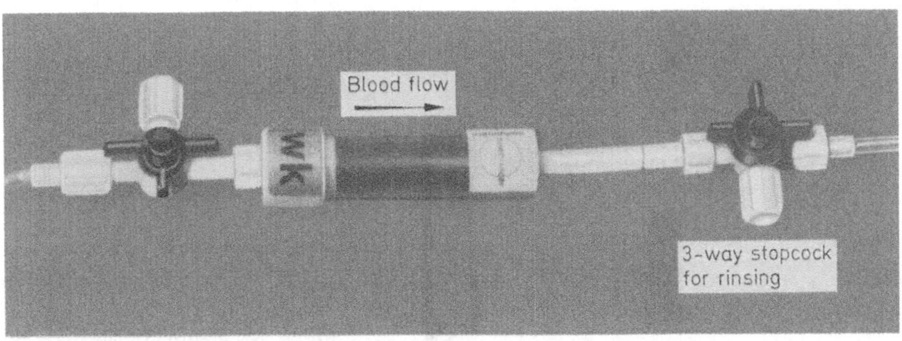

Fig. 1. Newly developed cartridge for diagnostic hemoperfusion with prefabricated connections and sterile three way stopcocks. (Boehringer, Mannheim, with permission)

quired, according to the initiators, which according to our experience can be achieved utilizing the arteriovenous shunt during CAVH.

For this reason it seems that diagnostic hemoperfusion can be performed easily especially in patients on continuous arteriovenous hemofiltration if bacteremia is suspected in the clinical course.

In our hospital, diagnostic hemoperfusion was performed so far in four patients who were treated with CAVH over a prolonged period of time. A small charcoal hemoperfusion cartridge was developed especially for this diagnostic clinical experiment. The new charcoal cartridge, shown in Fig. 1, will be available shortly.

Preparation of the Setup

After perfusion with saline, the cartridge is placed into the arteriovenous shunt using two new three-way stopcocks at each end of the cartridge for connection with the arterial and venous blood lines. To date, these new three-way stopcocks still have to be adapted to the system. For further clinical use, three-way stopcocks that fit onto the system correctly should be supplied which will make handling of the filters much easier (Fig. 2). By hemoperfusion through large lumenal CAVH catheters, blood-flow rates of 100–150 ml/min were observed in our patients. During 20 min perfusion, a total of approximately 3 l blood came into contact with the charcoal.

At present, no experiments are known that explain the relationship between germ yield and length of perfusion. Therefore, the mentioned time seems to be sufficient especially with regard to interruption of continous arteriovenous hemofiltration during the time of diagnostic hemoperfusion. The hemofilter should be filled with heparinized saline during the interruption if diagnostic perfusion is applied longer than 30 min or if the patient was on a low dose of heparin (<400 IU/h) because of high bleeding risk. The heparin dose required to keep the small charcoal cartridge unclotted is approximately 500 IU/h, which is infused into the arterial blood line of the system.

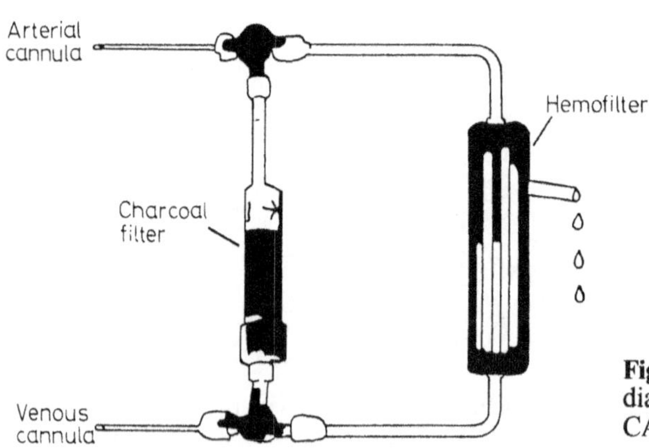

Fig. 2. Schematic illustration of diagnostic hemoperfusion in the CAVH system

First Clinical Results

In two clinical cases a germ yield was achieved that was not possible with previously and simultaneously drawn blood cultures. In two other perfusion cartridges used by us no germs were detected. But conventional blood cultures also showed no growth in these cases.

In one of the two successful diagnostic hemoperfusions the Candida test was positive which did not show up in conventional cultures. In the second case a mixed septicemia with three kinds of germs was found – only one kind was found in the conventional culture. This colonization was confirmed post mortem in the liquor of the ventricle.

Our first clinical results with diagnostic hemoperfusion seem to support the positive reports of Keller et al. The use of this method in patients with continuous arteriovenous hemofiltration should be considered in the future when bacteremia is suspected but no positive results are obtained with conventional cultures. The described method has to be evaluated first in more extensive clinical testing before any definitive statements can be made. Besides that, particular practical problems with the method have to be resolved and theoretical questions about colonization on the charcoal have to be answered.

Still, advocating use of this method seems to be justified already at this point in patients with acute renal failure and suspected bacteremia, since their general bad condition can only be improved through direct germ detection and specific antibiotic therapy.

If the germs are not identified bacteremia generally contributes to the exacerbation of the underlying illness of these patients and specifically maintains the renal failure. The experience with hemoperfusion in poisonings rules out any negative consequences for the patient with the method described here [1].

References

1. Hennemann H, Richter IE, Brunswig D, Röckel A, Kult J, Sattenlöhner W, Heidland A (1977) Hämoperfusion – Pro und Kontra. Klin Wochenschr 55:533
2. Keller F (1981) Die Hämoperfusion als neues diagnostisches Verfahren zur Erkennung von Septikämien. Habilitationsschrift, Würzburg
3. Keller F, Feldmann K, Abshagen U, Hennemann H, Barz R (1981) Diagnostic haemoperfusion for rapid detection of bacteremia. Klin Wochenschr 59:425
4. Milligan SL, Luft FC, McMurray StD, Kleit StA (1978) Intra-abdominal infection and acute renal failure. Arch Surg 113:467

Intestinal Substitution in Arteriovenous Hemofiltration – An Experimental Study on Inexpensive Long-Term Application of Continuous Arteriovenous Hemofiltration

M. Trautmann, H. J. Gröne, E. Heuer, and P. Kramer

Introduction

Arteriovenous hemofiltration was first used in 1977 for the dehydration of diuretic-resistant patients [1]. For treatment of renal insufficiency by arteriovenous hemofiltration, the plasma water withdrawn from the patient has to be replaced by a potassium-free Ringer's lactate solution. This solution is ordinarily fed into the venous line of the blood-carrying tubing system through a three-way valve, and is therefore administered to the patient intravenously [2]. We considered the possibility of supplying the substitution solution intestinally. Through reabsorption of the solution, the intestine takes over the role of the renal tubule system, supplementing the hemofilter which only performs the function of the renal glomeruli.

With intestinal administration of the substitution solution, its sterility does not have to be considered. From this, we anticipated reduction of treatment costs and basic simplification, since the patient would be able to prepare the substitution solution in the kitchen from tap water and electrolyte powder of appropiate composition. We also hoped to pave the way to a still hypothetical detoxification of the hemofiltrate, followed by intestinal return to the patient. We expected that elimination of the necessity for sterility would also simplify the possibility of such a detoxification.

Methods and Results

Intestinal Administration of Human Hemofiltrate in Normal Animals

The first question to be answered was whether the intestine is able to absorb hemofiltrate or subsitution solution in relevant amounts, without discomfort, diarrhea, or regurgitation. To answer this question, human hemofiltrate was fed into the small intestine of dogs through an implanted catheter.

The following procedure proved successful for the implantation of the intestinal catheter: After exposure of the stomach, a silicone tube was inserted into the interior of the stomach through a small incision on the front of the stomach. It was pushed forward by palpating through the pylorus to a distance of approximately 15 cm into the duodenum. The free, external end of the catheter was

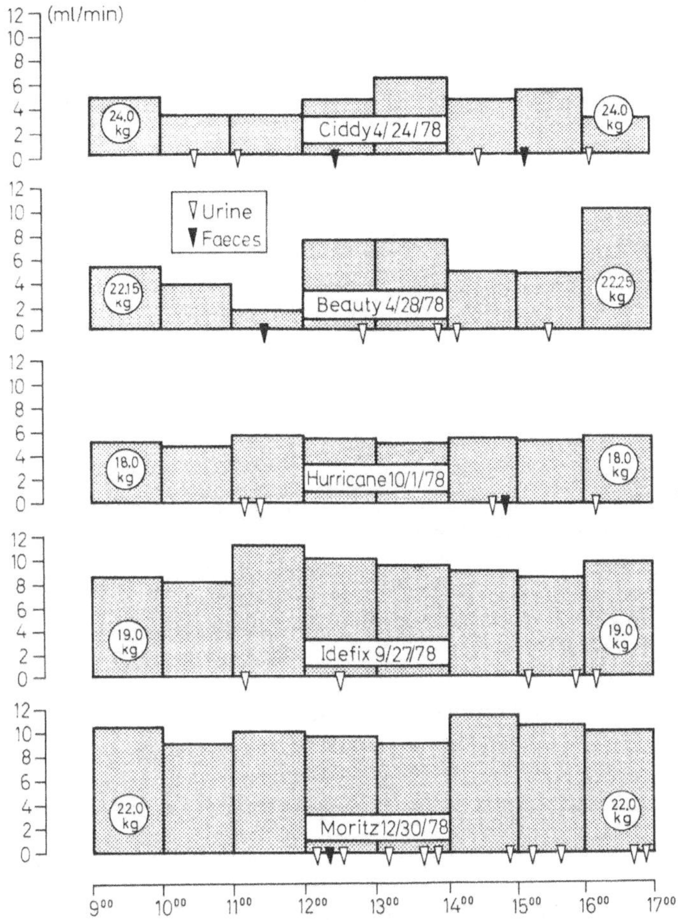

Fig. 1. Test protocol: intestinal administration rate of human hemofiltrate; bowel movement, micturition, and body weight before and after administration of hemofiltrate

passed between two ribs from the peritoneal cavity through a subcutaneous tunnel to the neck region, where it came through the skin using a specially developed skin button.

Human hemofiltrate was infused into the duodenum of five dogs through the first successfully implanted catheters. Figure 1 shows the results of this study, in which the dogs received between 5 and 10 ml/min for 8 h. None of the dogs showed signs of discomfort, diarrhea, or regurgitation. All five dogs had solid stools and distinctly increased diuresis. The body weight of all animals remained constant.

We concluded from this that complete intestinal reabsorption of the administered fluid takes place.

The study results were the prerequisite for treating uremic dogs with arteriovenous hemofiltration and intestinal filtrate substitution.

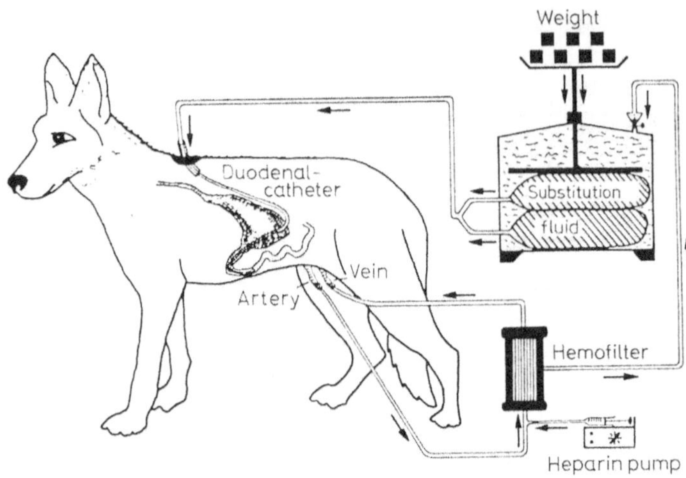

Fig. 2. Experimental arrangement: arteriovenous hemofiltration with intestinal ultrafiltrate substitution using a weight driven substitution box

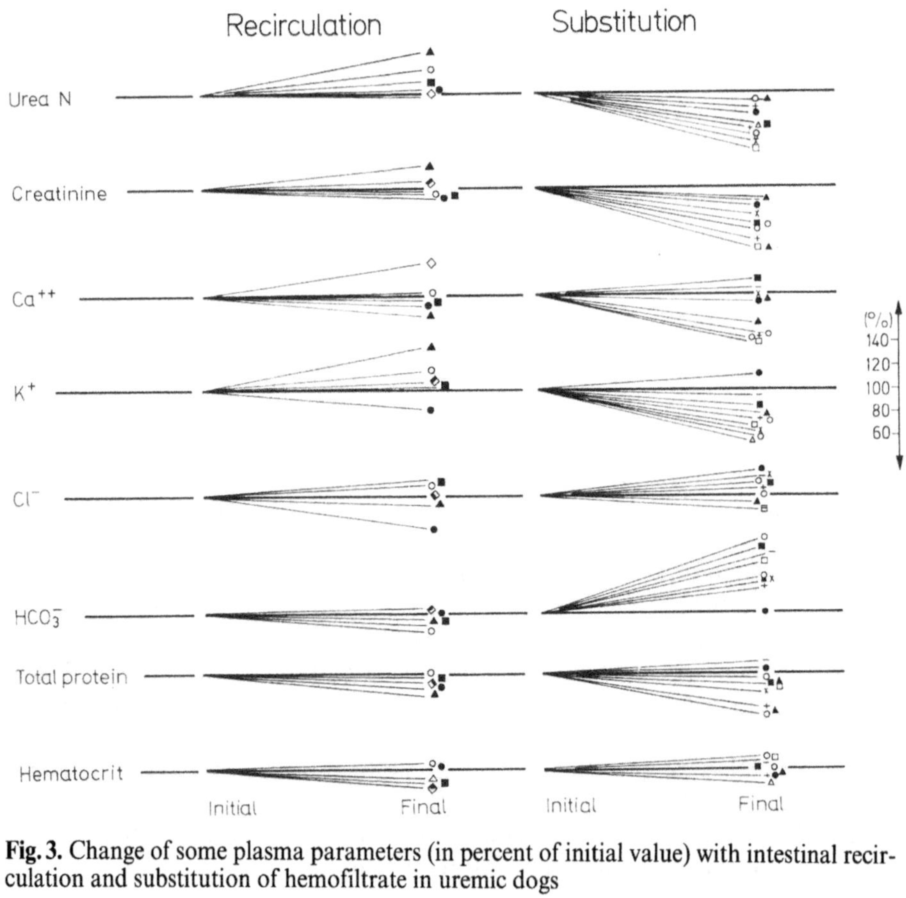

Fig. 3. Change of some plasma parameters (in percent of initial value) with intestinal recirculation and substitution of hemofiltrate in uremic dogs

Intestinal Recirculation and Substitution of Autologous Hemofiltrate in Uremic Dogs

Uremia was produced by arterial embolization of the renal arteries with glass microspheres [3]. With this method, the embolization material is injected directly into the renal artery with contrasting agent, using an angiography catheter. Adequate embolization of the kidneys was assumed when there was arterial stasis with photosensor monitoring, and the contrasting agent image of the vessel tree did not change any longer. With this intervention, the serum creatinine level of the animals reached values between 12 and 15 mg/dl after a few days.

In an acute test which lasted approximately 20 h, the arteria and vena femoralis were then cannulated with large-bore indwelling catheters and an ultrafilter (D-20, Amicon) was connected. Heparin was introduced continuously into the arterial line of the tubing system through an infusion pump. Depending on the arteriovenous blood pressure gradient, filtration rates of 5–10 ml/min were obtained (for experimental system, see Fig. 2).

First, autologous hemofiltrate was recirculated through the intestinal catheter in a control group of five uremic dogs. Since this did not change the azotemia, we followed it with a second test in which 10 dogs received a potassium-free Ringer's lactate solution instead of the ultrafiltrate. The fluid balancing was controlled by a simple, weight-driven substitution apparatus [4, 5]. Figure 3 shows the changes in percent of the initial value of some plasma parameters occurring under the two different experimental protocols. Neither the substitution nor the recirculation of the filtrate into the intestine led to a hemoconcentration, as demonstrated by hematocrit and total serum protein.

Table 1. Changes of some plasma parameters under arteriovenous hemofiltration with intestinal filtrate substitution in the uremic dog with the highest exchange rate

	Initial	Final
Hct (vol %)	20.0	20.0
Total protein (g/100 ml)	4.6	4.0
Urea-N (mg/100 ml)	162.0	80.0
Creatinine (mg/100 ml)	14.6	6.9
K^+ (mmol/l)	4.7	3.2
Po_4^{---} (mg/100 ml)	10.8	7.7
Ca^{++} (mg/100 ml)	13.5	7.9
Na^+ (mmol/l)	151.0	121.0
Cl^- (mmol/l)	100.0	86.0
HCO_3^- (mmol/l)	18.0	26.5
BE (meq/l)	− 8.2	+ 4.8
pH	7.20	7.49
Cholesterol (mg/100 ml)	195.0	145.0
Triglycerides (mg/100 ml)	50.0	36.0

► Duration of hemofiltration, 18 h ◄
► Total fluid exchange, 13.5 l ◄

Serum concentrations of urea-N and creatinine in the control group with filtrate recirculation showed a distinct increase, which indicates nonselective reabsorption of these substances through the intestine. The increase is explained by the increase of the uremia.

In the main group with intestinal substitution of the filtrate, on the other hand, a distinct decrease of these parameters was observed. The degree of correction of the azotemia here depended upon the ultrafiltrate exchange rate, the initial values, and finally on whether the uremia had reached "steady-state" conditions before beginning the test. The effect of intestinal ultrafiltrate substitution is shown in Table 1, using the dog with the highest exchange rate. Total fluid exchange of 13.5 l led to complete and even excessive correction of the acidosis within 18 h, and to decrease of the urea and creatinine concentrations of more than 50%. The serum levels of potassium and phosphate were also distinctly lowered.

Conclusions

The results permit the following conclusions:

1. The intestine of dogs is able to reabsorb hemofiltrate or substitution solution in an amount up to 10 ml/min.
2. Since electrolytes and low molecular weight (uremic-derived) substances contained in the hemofiltrate are also absorbed intestinally, recirculation of the filtrate is not suitable for therapy of azotemia.
3. Intestinal substitution of the ultrafiltrate with nonsterile, potassium-free Ringer's lactate solution, on the other hand, leads to the correction of acidosis and azotemia and can, in principle, therefore be considered as a therapeutic possibility for patients.

Possible Clinical Applications

In particular, we see the following possible future applications for intestinal ultrafiltrate substitution:

1. With conventional hemofiltration, partial oral substitution could be undertaken with any beverage by adding NaCl and sodium bicarbonate capsules. Thus, sterile substitution solution could be avoided and the posthemofiltration thirst [6, 7] could be reduced. However, there is a danger that liquid may remain in the stomach, which could very rapidly lead to circulatory collapse. Use would therefore have to be limited initially to a few, specially chosen patients.
2. Arteriovenous hemofiltration with intestinal substitution through a duodenal catheter could be used for treatment of acute renal failure if there is no ileus. Such a procedure would be conceivable in exceptional situations in which either there is not enough equipment because too many patients require treatment, or enough sterile substitution fluid is not available.
3. Due to low filtration rate, arteriovenous hemofiltration offers the possibility of intestinal substitution trough an implanted catheter even with terminal re-

nal insufficiency. By using nonsterile substitution fluid, the costs for treatment of chronic renal failure could be substantially lowered. An external, long-term functioning arteriovenous shunt would be a prerequisite, which is not yet available at this time.

References

1. Kramer P, Wigger W, Rieger J, Matthaei D, Scheler F (1977) Arterio-venous hemofiltration: A new and simple method for treatment of overhydrated patients resistant to diuretics. Klin Wochenschr 55:1121
2. Kramer P, Tiffin MC (1981) Arterio-venöse Hämofiltration. Video, University of Göttingen
3. Wolf KJ (1978) Therapeutische Embolisation von Organarterien. Tierexperimentelle Untersuchungen, erste klinische Erfahrungen, Einführung eines neuen Embolisationsmaterials. Fortschr Geb Röntgenstr 128:414
4. Kramer P, Seegers A, De Vivie R, Matthaei D, Trautmann M, Scheler F (1978) Therapeutische Möglichkeiten der Hämofiltration. Verh Dtsch Ges Inn Med 84:1226
5. Kramer P, Seegers A, De Vivie R, Matthaei D, Trautmann M, Scheler F (1979) Therapeutic potential of hemofiltration. Clin Nephrology 11:145
6. Wigger W, Girndt J (1977) Zwischenfälle bei der Hämofiltration im Vergleich mit der Hämodialyse. In: Hämofiltration, edited by Scheler F and Henning HV, Dustri-Verlag, München-Deisenhofen: 17
7. Kramer P, Wigger W, Matthaei D, Langescheid C, Rieger J, Fuchs C, Rumpf KW, Scheler F (1978) Clinical experience with continuously monitored fluid balance in automatic hemofiltration. Artificial Organs 2:145

Cerebral Edema: Treatment by Continuous Arteriovenous Hemofiltration – A Case Report

B. Demierre, P. Kramer, and O. Spoerri

Introduction

Based on numerous studies on the cause of cerebral edema, [3, 18] different therapeutic approaches have been proposed. Reviving the idea of Hippocrates, Cushing recommended subtemporal decompressive operation [6]. Quincke suggested [23] the repeated lumbar puncture and when contraindicated Cushing advocated [7] cisternostomy. Weed and McKibben [27] first demonstrated in cats that the brain bulk could be decreased by infusing hypertonic saline.

In 1956 the intravenous use of urea became a conventional treatment in neurosurgery [12]. This was later followed by intravenous mannitol [28] and intravenous or oral glycerol [26]. Furosemide [10], corticosteroids [14, 21], hypothermia [5], hyperventilation [17], and barbiturates [25] are still today commonly used treatments in many neurological and neurosurgical units.

Most of these therapeutic measures are either not very efficient or may have undesired side effects.

Based on the positive results with fluid restriction [11, 15], CAVH was used with success in a case with traumatic cerebral edema and renal failure.

Case Report

A 22-year-old man was admitted to hospital after a traffic accident. He presented hypovolemic shock, multiple fractures, and pneumothorax. The patient was somnolent after transient unconsciousness. After correction of hypovolemia the patient's orientation improved. Neurological examination revealed only anterograde and retrograde amnesia; neurological status was normal. Within 24 h after admission the patient developed renal failure. Three days after the accident he became rapidly disoriented and somnolent. He was then transferred to our hospital for exclusion of intracranial bleeding. The laboratory data before transfer revealed hypokalemia, thrombocytopenia and elevated plasma creatinine. The fluid balance was positive (1740 ml/24 h) and the central venous pressure elevated (14 cm H_2O).

At neurological examination in our hospital the patient was somnolent (grade 10 according to Glasgow scale), he reacted to the calling of his name and to pain

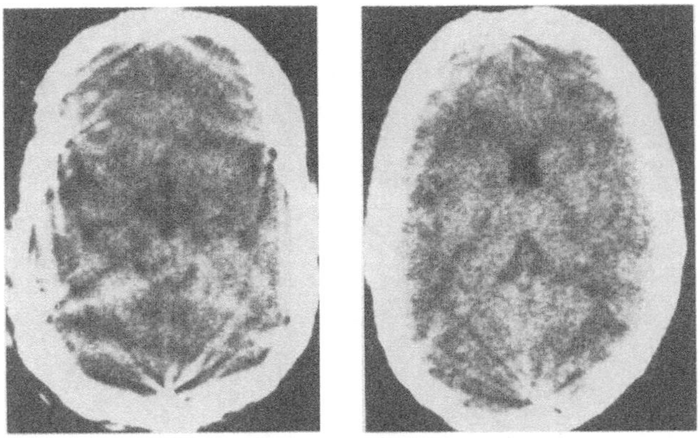

Fig. 1. Noncontrast CT scan 3 days after accident. The brain edema is visualized by partial effacement of basal cisterns and small ventricles

with coordinate flection. Lung auscultation and chest X-ray confirmed the diagnosis of pneumothorax and pulmonary edema.

The CT scan showed no incidence of intracranial bleeding, but partial narrowing of basal cisternae, ventricular system, and cortical sulci indicating cerebral edema (Fig. 1).

Therefore, the intracranial pressure (ICP) was measured with an epidural transducer (Ladd system). Initially the pressure was clearly elevated ranging between 28 and 32 mmHg in spite of 80 mg dexamethasone given 1 h before insertion.

Because of renal failure, continuous arteriovenous hemofiltration (CAVH) was started. The clinical and biochemical data and the fluid balance (input/output) are displayed in Table 1. ICP decreased to normal values (8–12 mmHg) during the first hour of hemofiltration with a negative fluid balance of 445 ml and remained normal during the 10 following hours.

After this period the patient had a negative fluid balance of 5429 ml resulting in hemoconcentration indicated by the increase of the hemoglobin concentration from 9.7 to 13.1 g/dl. The systemic arterial pressure and pulse rate remained rather stable without using catecholamines. The central venous pressure, however, decreased from +16 to −0.5 cm H_2O.

The general clinical condition of the patient improved with respect to cooperation in spite of sedatives and the stress of CPAP respiration. Unfortunately, the ICP could not be traced on paper and the transducer had to be removed later because of technical problems. But the second CT scan 1 week later showed the disappearance of cerebral edema signs (Fig. 2).

Although the neurological status of the patient improved, the kidney function did not recover as a result of septicemia. Thus, the patient was on CAVH for 6 weeks and died finally from a bleeding complication.

Cerebral edema is defined as bulk increase of the brain as a result of elevated water content [9]. According to Klatzo [13] two types of cerebral edema may be distinguished: vasogenic and cytotoxic.

Table 1. Clinical and biochemical data with fluid balance

Time (h)	−1	CAVH ↓ 0	1	2	3	4	5	6	7	8	9
SAP (mmHg)	140/90	130/75	140/80	140/85	120/75	130/75	140/90	130/85	130/80	140/90	120/75
PR (per min)		56	57	59	80	60	58	65	60	70	60
CVP (cmH_2O)	+16	+6.5	+5	+4.5	+2.5	+2.5	+0.5	±0	−0.5		+0.5
ICP (mmHg)	28–30	28–32	8–12	14	15	13					11
Hemoglobin (g/dl)	9.7	10.1	11.7				12.2			13.1	
Sodium (meq/l)	142	134	136				135			140	
Potassium (meq/l)	5.1	5.7	5.4				5.6			5.5	
Creatinin (mg/dl)	11.2										8.3
pH		7.402	7.379				7.369			7.369	
Infusion (ml)			395	495	96	96	96	96	96	496	471
Total infusion (ml)			–	890	986	1082	1178	1274	12370	1866	2337
Withdrawal (ml)			745	860	920	880	850	740	750	770	850
Total withdrawal (ml)			–	1605	2525	3405	4255	4995	5745	6415	7265
Urine (ml)			–	38	36	38	30	20	10	8	26
Total urine (ml)			95	133	169	207	237	257	267	275	301
Gastric tube (ml)			–	–	200	200	200	200	200	200	200
Total withdrawal (ml)			840	1738	2894	3812	4692	5452	6212	6890	7766
Balance (ml)			−445	− 848	−1908	−2730	−3514	−4178	−4842	−5024	−**5429**

SAP, systemic arterial pressure; PR, pulse rate; CVP, central venous pressure; ICP, intracranial pressure

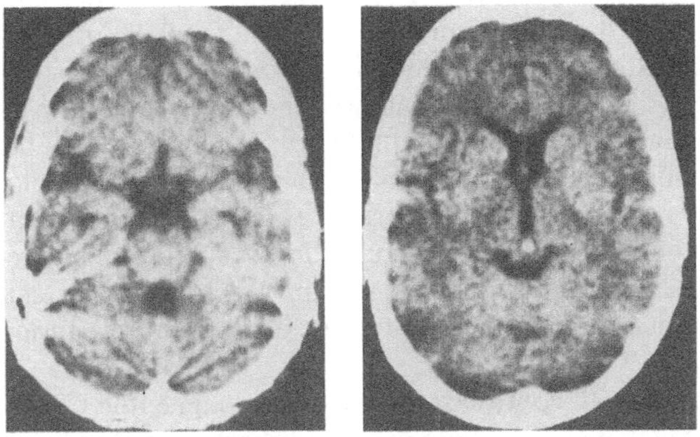

Fig. 2. Noncontrast CT scan 1 week after CAVH. The brain edema has disappeared

Vasogenic edema is characterized by increased capillary permeability. Edema is the result of extracellular fluid and plasma protein accumulation principally localized in the white matter. It is observed in tumors, infarction, hemorrhage, encephalopathy, purulent meningitis, and trauma.

Cytotoxic edema is characterized by increase of cellular volume in the white and gray matter, whereby the cells contain more water and sodium. The extracellular volume is decreased and the capillary permeability for large molecules is normal. It is observed in hypoxia, hypoosmolality as in water intoxication, and also in purulent meningitis [9, 13, 19, 20].

A third type of cerebral edema, called interstitial, is mainly found in hydrocephalus and is not a matter of this contribution [9].

The therapeutic effect of corticosteroids is obvious in vasogenic edema, particularly in tumors but not in cytotoxic edema [9, 20]. Osmotic therapy, however, reduced cerebral edema in both types.

In the case presented, edema most likely was a combination of these two types. Because of renal failure one was reluctant to use barbiturates for lowering ICP.

According to several studies [2, 24, 28] the dehydration by means of mannitol causes metabolic acidosis due to interruption of cell metabolism and renal failure. In addition, accumulation of mannitol in the cerebrospinal fluid may cause a rebound effect with reversed fluid shifting. The osmotherapy in the case presented was contraindicated because of renal insufficiency.

Dehydration by means of fluid restriction in cerebral edema remains controversial. Some neurosurgeons continue to use dehydration in acute cases, in order to obtain serum hyperosmolality [11, 15]; this, however, is not without danger, particularly in polytraumatized patients. The intravascular volume must be maintained for sufficient cerebral blood supply, whereby the cerebral blood flow depends more on cardiac output than on systemic arterial pressure [8]. In order to maintain sufficient intravascular volume and iso- or hyperosmolality, continuous arteriovenous hemofiltration was used.

This simple kidney replacement therapy is certainly superior to conventional hemodialysis particularly with respect to cerebral edema. Although it has been demonstrated that hemodialysis can reduce ICP [1, 4], the rapid fluid and solute removal can provoke not only "disequilibrium syndrome" as a result of serum hypoosmolality [22] but also reduced cerebral blood perfusion. These negative effects may be prevented by using CAVH, which allows continuous isoosmotic ultrafiltration. Slow continuous isoosmotic fluid withdrawal takes into account the factors influencing the refilling rate. The fluid shift from extra- to intravascular space depends mainly on the colloid-osmotic pressure, which is increased by effective withdrawal of isotonic fluid. The reduction of intravascular volume remains small, if ultrafiltration does not exceed the refilling rate to a great extent. By this means cardiac output, systemic blood pressure, and cerebral perfusion should be maintained.

In addition to dehydration with controlled intravascular volume, the CAVH allows the maintenance of high plasma sodium by using a substitution fluid with high sodium concentration [16]. This has the advantage of additional cellular dehydration and kidney protection in a state of dehydration.

In the patient reported, isotonic fluid removal was effective to normalize ICP and the cerebral blood perfusion pressure was certainly improved. The rapid decrease of ICP in this case is the result of a more homogenous dehydration than would have been obtained by hyperosmotic agents and hemodialysis.

In order to confirm this observation further investigations are presently being conducted in patients with cerebral edema of different origin.

References

1. Bada HS, Chua C, Salmon JH, Hajjar W (1979) Changes in intracranial pressure during exchange transfusion. J Pediatr 94:129–132
2. Becker DP, Vries JK (1972) The alleviation of increased intracranial pressure. In: Brock M, Dietz H (eds) Intracranial pressure. Springer, Berlin Heidelberg New York, pp 309–315
3. Bell BA (1983) A history of the study of cerebral edema. Neurosurgery 13:724–728
4. Berman W, Pizzi F, Schut L, Raphaely R, Holtzapple P (1975) The effects of exchange transfusion on intracranial pressure in patients with Reye syndrome. J Pediatr 87:887–891
5. Botterell EH, Lougheed WM, Scott JW, Vandewater SL (1956) Hypothermia, and interruption of carotid, or carotid and vertebral circulation, in the surgical management of intracranial aneurysms. J Neurosurg 13:1–42
6. Cushing H (1908) Subtemporal decompressive operations for the intracranial complications associated with bursting fractures of the skull. Ann Surg 47:641–644
7. Cushing H (1909) Some principles of cerebral surgery. JAMA 52:184–192
8. Davis DH, Sundt TM (1980) Relationship of cerebral blood flow to cardiac output, mean arterial pressure, blood volume, and alpha and beta blockade in cats. J Neurosurg 52:745–754
9. Fishman RA (1975) Brain edema. N Engl J Med 293:706–711
10. Galle B, Staudacher M (1968) Einfluß entwässernder Medikamente auf den Liquordruck beim Schädelhirntrauma. Med Klin 63:16–20
11. Hao-Hui L (1980) Dehydration therapy and hypotension in post-resuscitation cerebral edema, and application of intra-ocular pressure measurement – a review of resuscitation work, part I. Resuscitation 8:195–209
12. Javid M, Settlage P (1956) Effect of urea on cerebrospinal fluid pressure in human subjects. Preliminary report. JAMA 160:943–949
13. Klatzo I (1967) Neuropathological aspects of brain edema. J Neuropathol Exp Neurol 26:1–14

14. Kofman S, Garvin JS, Nagamani D (1957) Treatment of cerebral metastases from breast carcinoma with prednisolone. JAMA 163:1473–1476
15. Kramer G (1972) Probleme der Entwässerungstherapie bei schweren Schädel-Hirntraumen. Hefte Unfallheilkd 111:242–244
16. Kramer P, Böhler J, Kehr A, Gröne HJ, Schrader J, Matthaei D, Scheler F (1982) Intensive care potential of continuous arteriovenous hemofiltration. Trans Am Soc Artif Intern Organs 18:28–31
17. Lundberg N, Kjällquist A, Bien C (1959) Reduction of increased intracranial pressure by hyperventilation. A therapeutic aid in neurosurgical surgery. Acta Psychiat Scand [Suppl] 34:139
18. Lundberg N, Kjällquist A, Kullberg G, Pontén U, Sundbärg G (1974) Non-operative management of intracranial hypertension. In: Krayenbühl H (ed) Advances and technical standards in neurosurgery. Springer, Wien New York, pp 3–59
19. Meinig G, Reulen HJ, Magawly C (1973) Regional cerebral blood flow and cerebral perfusion pressure in global brain edema induced by water intoxication. Acta Neurochir (Wien) 29:1–13
20. O'Brien MD (1979) Ischemic cerebral edema: a review. Stroke 10:623–628
21. Prados M, Strowger B, Feindel W (1945) Studies on cerebral edema. Arch Neurol Psychiat 54:290–300
22. Prill A (1969) Die neurologische Symptomatologie der Niereninsuffizienz. Springer, Berlin Heidelberg New York
23. Quincke H (1905) Die diagnostische und therapeutische Bedeutung der Lumbalpunktion. Klin Vortr Dtsch Med Wochenschr 31:1825–1829
24. Rosomoff HL (1962) Distribution of intracranial contents after hypertonic urea. J Neurosurg 19:859–864
25. Shapiro HM, Galindo A, Wyte SR, Harris AB (1973) Rapid intraoperative reduction of intracranial pressure with thiopentone. Br J Anaesth 45:1057–1061
26. Virno M, Chiavarelli S, Cantore GP (1961) Azione der glicerolo sull'edema cerebrale del coniglio dopo craniectomia. Gazz Int Med Chir 66:3509–3515
27. Weed LH, McKibben PS (1919) Pressure changes in cerebrospinal fluid following intravenous injection of solutions of various concentrations. Am J Physiol 48:512–530
28. Wise BL, Chater N (1962) The value of hypertonic mannitol solution in decreasing brain mass and lowering cerebrospinal fluid pressure. J Neurosurg 19:1038–1043

Subject Index

GPSR Compliance

The European Union's (EU) General Product Safety Regulation (GPSR) is a set of rules that requires consumer products to be safe and our obligations to ensure this.

If you have any concerns about our products, you can contact us on ProductSafety@springernature.com

In case Publisher is established outside the EU, the EU authorized representative is:

Springer Nature Customer Service Center GmbH
Europaplatz 3
69115 Heidelberg, Germany

Batch number: 10704763

Printed by Printforce, the Netherlands